ON FREUD'S "THE QUESTION OF LAY ANALYSIS"

The questions of what psychoanalysis is, and does, and who can and should practice it, remains key within the modern profession. Has the invaluable material packed into Freud's *The Question of Lay Analysis* (1926) been underestimated by contemporary psychoanalysis? This book explores how the issues raised in this paper can continue to impact contemporary Freudian theory and practice. The chapters examine why the arguably litigious nature of the paper might be contributing to its neglect and underestimation.

The editors of this book put forth a hypothesis: is there an underlying, still unrecognized, but heartrending factor underlying the century-old quarrel between "lay analysts" and what might be described as medically or psychiatrically trained analysts? They then brought together a selection of major contemporary psychoanalytic thinkers from around the world to attempt to bridge the seemingly unbridgeable gap between medical and non-medical analysis, using *The Question of Lay Analysis* as a central pivot. The work of the key figure, in social and historic terms, on this issue, Theodor Reik, is also duly honored.

On Freud's "The Question of Lay Analysis" will be of great interest to all psychoanalysts and psychoanalytic psychotherapists.

Paulo Cesar Sandler, MD, MSci, is a training analyst at Sociedade Brasileira de Psicanalise de São Paulo; and a psychiatrist at the Institute of Medicine of Rehabilitation of the Hospital das Clinicas, Faculdade de Medicina, Universidade de São Paulo, Brazil. He is Honorary Associate of Academia Lancisiana, Rome; former Director of the Mental Health Center at Faculdade de Saude Publica da Universidade de São Paulo; former Editor of *Revista Brasileira de Psicanalise* and former Director of the Publishing Department of SBPSP.

Gley Pacheco Costa, MD, is a founding member and training analyst of the Brazilian Psychoanalytic Society of Porto Alegre, Brazil, and Professor of Psychiatry and Psychotherapy at Mário Martins University Foundation, Porto Alegre, Rio Grande do Sul.

THE INTERNATIONAL PSYCHOANALYTICAL ASSOCIATION CONTEMPORARY FREUD TURNING POINTS AND CRITICAL ISSUES SERIES

Series Editor: Gabriela Legoretta (Montreal)

IPA Publications Committee

Titles in this series

On Freud's "Group Psychology and the Analysis of the Ego"
Edited by Ethel Spector Person

On Freud's "Mourning and Melancholia"
Edited by Leticia Glocer Fiorini, Thierry Bokanowski, and Sergio Lewkowicz

On Freud's "The Future of an Illusion"
Edited by Mary Kay O'Neil and Salman Akhtar

On Freud's "Splitting of the Ego in the Process of Defence"
Edited by Thierry Bokanowski and Sergio Lewkowicz

On Freud's "Femininity"
Edited by Leticia Glocer Fiorini and Graciela Abelin-Sas

On Freud's "Constructions in Analysis"
Edited by Thierry Bokanowski and Sergio Lewkowicz

On Freud's "Beyond the Pleasure Principle"
Edited by Salman Akhtar and Mary Kay O'Neil

On Freud's "Negation"
Edited by Mary Kay O'Neil and Salman Akhtar

On Freud's "On Beginning the Treatment"
Edited by Christian Seulin and Gennaro Saragnano

On Freud's "On Narcissism: An Introduction"
Edited by Joseph Sandler, Ethel Spector Person, and Peter Fonagy

On Freud's "Inhibitions, Symptoms and Anxiety"
Edited by Samuel Arbiser and Jorge Schneider

On Freud's "Observations on Transference-Love"
Edited by Ethel Spector Person, Aiban Hagelin, and Peter Fonagy

On Freud's "Creative Writers and Day-Dreaming"
Edited by Ethel Spector Person, Peter Fonagy, and Sérvulo Augusto Figueira

On Freud's "A Child Is Being Beaten"
Edited by Ethel Spector Person

On Freud's "Analysis Terminable and Interminable"
Edited by Joseph Sandler

On Freud's "The Unconscious"
Edited by Salman Akhtar and Mary Kay O'Neil

On Freud's "Screen Memories"
Edited by Gail S. Reed and Howard B. Levine

On Freud's "Formulations on the Two Principles of Mental Functioning"
Edited by Lawrence J. Brown

ON FREUD'S "THE QUESTION OF LAY ANALYSIS"

Edited by

Paulo Cesar Sandler and Gley Pacheco Costa

CONTEMPORARY FREUD
Turning Points and Critical Issues

Routledge
Taylor & Francis Group
LONDON AND NEW YORK

First published 2019
by Routledge
2 Park Square, Milton Park, Abingdon, Oxon OX14 4RN

and by Routledge
52 Vanderbilt Avenue, New York, NY 10017

Routledge is an imprint of the Taylor & Francis Group, an informa business

British Library Cataloguing-in-Publication Data
A catalogue record for this book is available from the British Library

Library of Congress Cataloging-in-Publication Data
Names: Sandler, P. C. (Paulo Cesar), editor. | Costa, Gley Pacheco, 1944– editor.
Title: On Freud's the question of lay analysis : contemporary Freudian turning points and critical issues / edited by Paulo Cesar Sandler and Gley Pacheco Costa.
Description: Abingdon, Oxon ; New York, NY : Routledge, 2019. | Series: The International Psychoanalytical Association Contemporary Freud Turning Points and Critical Issues series | Includes bibliographical references and index.
Identifiers: LCCN 2018048150 (print) | LCCN 2018050417 (ebook) | ISBN 9780429021091 (Master) | ISBN 9780429667640 (Pdf) | ISBN 9780429662201 (MobiPocket) | ISBN 9780429664922 (ePub3) | ISBN 9780367075088 (hardback : alk. paper) | ISBN 9781782206293 (pbk. : alk. paper)
Subjects: LCSH: Freud, Sigmund, 1856–1939. | Psychoanalysis.
Classification: LCC BF109.F74 (ebook) | LCC BF109.F74 O52 2019 (print) | DDC 150.19/52—dc23
LC record available at https://lccn.loc.gov/2018048150

ISBN: 978-0-367-07508-8 (hbk)
ISBN: 978-1-78220-629-3 (pbk)
ISBN: 978-0-429-02109-1 (ebk)

Typeset in Palatino
by Apex CoVantage, LLC

CONTENTS

SERIES EDITOR'S FOREWORD
Gabriela Legorreta vii

NOTES ON CONTRIBUTORS x

Introduction
Paulo Cesar Sandler and Gley Pacheco Costa 1

1 The question of lay analysis: then and now
Ron Spielman 6

2 Wayward analysis
Ester Hadassa Sandler 24

3 Who I think the layman is to Freud: comments on Sigmund Freud's "The Question of Lay Analysis"
Jose Luiz Freda Petrucci 37

4 Some notes about alike applications of psychoanalysis
Irina Panteleeva 46

5 Theodor Reik: the analyst of silence and surprise
Avedis Panajian 70

6 From word to deed: why psychoanalysis needs laypersons?
Bernd Nissen 96

7 The analyst and his odyssey: like Ulysses, we must not forget the return journey . . .
Monica Horovitz 122

8 The problem of pluralism in psychoanalysis
Charles Hanly 135

9 On "The question of lay analysis" by Sigmund Freud
Abel Fainstein 168

10 Psychoanalysis is lay in its essence
Cláudia Aparecida Carneiro 192

11 From the obvious to the unbridgeable
Avner Bergstein 215

12 Enduring questions: who is the lay today? Are today's judges impartial persons?
Paulo Cesar Sandler and Gley Pacheco Costa 237

INDEX 290

SERIES EDITOR'S FOREWORD

This significant series, "Contemporary Freud Turning Points and Critical Issues" was founded in 1991 by Robert Wallerstein and subsequently edited by Joseph Sandler, Ethel Spector Person, Peter Fonagy, Leticia Glocer Fiorini and, most recently, Gennaro Saragnano. Its important contributions have been of interest to psychoanalysts in many different parts of the world, and it has succeeded in creating a stimulating forum for the exchange of ideas. It is therefore my great honor, as the new Chair of the Publications Committee of the International Psychoanalytic Association to continue the tradition of this most successful series.

The objective of this series is to approach Freud's work both from a historical and a contemporary point of view. On the one hand, this means highlighting the fundamental contributions of his work that constitute the axes of psychoanalytic theory and practice. At the same time, it implies learning about and spreading the ideas of present psychoanalysts about Freud's *oeuvre*, both where they coincide and where they differ. The work presented in this series comes from psychoanalysts from different geographical regions that represent, in addition, different theoretical stances.

In this series, one sees that Freud's papers remain the subject of both deep discussion and elaboration. The extension of his work is a testimony to the richness of his legacy, with its originality, creativity and, at times, provocative thinking. His work has become a breeding ground from which new ideas and developments have arisen.

Psychoanalytic thinking has developed while preserving many of the core elements of its original formulations. This has led to a theoretical, technical and clinical pluralism that has to be acknowledged and thought through. It is therefore necessary to avoid a comfortable and uncritical acceptance of concepts in order to consider systems of increasing complexity that consider both the convergences and divergences of the categories at play.

The significance of Freud's paper "The Question of Lay Analysis" (1926) is highlighted by James Strachey's editor's note in the original publication: "Freud presented in the following pages what was perhaps his most successful non-technical account of the theory and practice of psycho-analysis, written in his liveliest and lightest style" (1926, p. 181). It is indeed remarkable to witness Freud's elucidations on the highest theoretical and clinical problems using exceptional scientific thoroughness without suppressing open questions and problems.

Without a doubt, the questions addressed by Freud 92 years ago in "The Question of Lay Analysis" continue to have great importance and pertinence today. For one thing, his dialogue with an "impartial person" should encourage psychoanalysts to engage in a much-needed dialogue with other disciplines. A dialogue should highlight and communicate the specificity of the theory and practice of psychoanalysis and convey, in this manner, that psychoanalysis aims at understanding the psychic truth and reality of the individual in their complex dynamic and structure. Moreover, by examining the important question of the personal and professional qualities needed to practice psychoanalysis, this paper addresses issues related to the complex subject of psychoanalytic training worldwide today.

The Publications Committee is pleased to publish *On Freud's "The Question of Lay Analysis,"* which constitutes the 19th volume of the "Contemporary Freud Turning Points and Critical Issues" series. Paulo Cesar Sandler and Gley Pacheco Costa have skillfully edited this new volume. They have asked ten distinguished colleagues from different regions to discuss and place Freud's ideas in the light of contemporary psychoanalytic thinking. The result is this important book, which will surely encounter the favor of every psychoanalytic student as well as individuals interested in Freud's work, its evolution and the complexity of mental life. I want to thank wholeheartedly the editors and contributors of this new volume that continues the tradition of the successful IPA book series.

Gabriela Legorreta
Series Editor
Chair, IPA Publications Committee

CONTRIBUTORS

Avner Bergstein, MA, FIPA, is a training and supervising psychoanalyst and faculty member of the Israel Psychoanalytic Society. He works in private practice with adults, adolescents and children and has worked for some years at a kindergarten for children with autism. He has authored numerous papers and book chapters elaborating on the clinical implications of the writings of Bion and Meltzer, and his papers are translated into several languages, including German, French, Italian, Spanish and Portuguese. He is the author of the book *Bion and Meltzer's Expeditions into Unmapped Mental Life: Beyond the Spectrum in Psychoanalysis*. He conducts reading seminars internationally focusing on the writings of these two authors.

Cláudia Aparecida Carneiro, MA in Clinical Psychology and Culture – University of Brasília (UnB), is a member of the Society of Psychoanalysis of Brasília (SPBsb); assistant teacher of the Institute of Psychoanalysis Virginia Leone Bicudo; psychologist and journalist. She is Director of Publications and Dissemination of the Brazilian Federation of Psychoanalysis (Febrapsi) and Editor of the "Free Association" Journal of the SPBsb; and has published papers on psychoanalytic clinic, subjective processes and sexuality, and also book chapters on writing in psychoanalysis. She works in private practice with adults and adolescents in Brasília.

Abel Fainstein, School of Medicine University of Buenos Aires. Master in Psychoanalysis. Psychiatrist. He is a full member and past president of the Argentine Psychoanalytical Association and the Latin American Psychoanalytical Federation. He is also a full member and Latin American representative of the International Psychoanalytical Association (IPA) and a professor at the APA Institute Ángel Garma.

Charles Hanly is a psychoanalyst in private practice, a training analyst at the Toronto Institute of Psychoanalysis and a Professor Emeritus (philosophy) at the University of Toronto. Hanly is the author of four books, and more than one hundred clinical, theoretical and applied papers in journals and books. Since 1985, Hanly has been active in the International Psychoanalytical Association (IPA), chairing a committee to admit previously excluded groups to join the IPA and then chairing the International New Groups Committee. He served two terms as president, from 2009 to 2013.

Monica Horovitz, MD, PhD in comparative literature, MA in Latin American literature, DESS in clinical psychology, is a full member of the Paris Psychoanalytical Society (SPP) and of the Italian Psychoanalytic Society (SPI). She is chair of "Bion in Marrakech", has been published in many texts, and works in private practice with adults and adolescents in Paris.

Bernd Nissen, Dr. phil., Psychoanalyst (DPV/IPA) in Berlin, training analyst. He is the editor of several books and co-editor of the "Jahrbuch der Psychoanalyse". He has publications in several languages on pathological organizations, autistoid dynamics, hypochondria, perversion and theory of science.

Avedis Panajian, PhD ABPP-Clinical, is one of the founders of the Psychoanalytic Center of California and the Newport Psychoanalytic Institute. He is a training and supervising psychoanalyst at the Psychoanalytic Center of California. Dr. Panajian is a Diplomate in Clinical Psychology of the American Board of Professional Psychology. He was a former board member of the American Board of Professional Psychology and a former examiner of candidates for Diplomate in Clinical Psychology. Dr. Panajian was a former examiner for the California Board of Psychology. He has received the Distinguished Educator Award from the California State Psychological Association. Dr. Panajian is a Core Faculty at the Pacifica Graduate Institute in Santa Barbara, California. He has been teaching over the past 40 years and has been teaching the works of Wilfred Bion at the Psychoanalytic Center of California for the past 25 years. He has published several clinical chapters in psychoanalytic books. Dr. Panajian is in private practice in Beverly Hills, California.

Irina Panteleeva is a member of the Russian Psychoanalytic Society and has served as a secretary of the International Department of the Russian Psychoanalytic Society. She has written several papers on projective identification, guilt and narcissism, which were published in the *Russian Psychoanalytic Bulletin* and the *Journal of Practical Psychologist* (in Russian). Her recent interests are the points of convergence of Wittgenstein's ideas and psychoanalysis, as well as application of psychoanalysis in education.

Jose Luiz Freda Petrucci, MD, training analyst, Sociedade Brasileira de Psicanálise do Rio de Janeiro; founder, Sociedade Brasileira de Psicanálise de Porto Alegre; Member of the Education Committee, FEPA; author of papers and chapters in psychoanalytical periodicals and books in Brazil.

Ester Hadassa Sandler, MD, is a training and child analyst at the Sociedade Brasileira de Psicanalise de São Paulo. She has served in many administrations of SBPSP and its Institute, and as editor of *Jornal de Psicanálise*. She has authored many papers about child analysis, pioneering the application of Bion's expansions of the contributions of Freud and Klein; she translated and co-translated the work of many authors, such as Bion, Money-Kyrle, Parthenope Bion-Talamo and Thomas Ogden.

Ron Spielman was a training and supervising analyst of the Australian Psychoanalytic Society prior to his retirement from clinical practice in 2015. He trained with the Sydney Branch of the Australian Society and qualified in 1984. Some of his (unpublished) papers give an indication of the range of his psychoanalytic interests:

"Malignant Progression", "The Mirror in Psychoanalysis", "Psychoanalysis and Attachment Theory – Partners or Rivals?", "From Basic Instincts to Higher Values", "A 100 Year Commemoration of Freud's Paper 'The Unconscious'" and "A Train of Thought Crossing a Stream of Consciousness".

Introduction

Paulo Cesar Sandler and Gley Pacheco Costa

From the editors

Who's the lay today?

> *If intolerance of frustration is not so great as to activate the mechanisms of evasion and yet is too great to bear dominance of the reality principle, the personality develops omnipotence as a substitute for the mating of the pre-conception, or conception, with the negative realization. This involves the assumption of omniscience as a substitute for learning from experience by aid of thoughts and thinking. There is therefore no psychic activity to discriminate between true and false. Omniscience substitutes for the discrimination between true and false a dictatorial affirmation that one thing is morally right and the other wrong. The assumption of omniscience that denies reality ensures that the morality thus engendered is a function of psychosis. . . . There is thus potentially a conflict between assertion of truth and assertion of moral ascendancy. The extremism of the one infects the other.*
>
> – (*Bion, 1961, p. 114*)

Are judges impartial persons?

The editors of this book, impressed by a cloudy, 100-year-old pseudo-controversy erected through a continuing misunderstanding that befell and still plagues the members of the "psycho-analytic movement" (Freud, 1914), had an idea. Namely, to publish the following book about a two-pronged matter: on the one hand, "the question of lay analysis", already the object of highly acclaimed comments, made by prestigious former presidents of the IPA and many other authors, and on the other hand, the paper from Freud with the same title, published in 1924. Would it be fit to be inserted in the highly read series "Contemporary Freud Turning Points and Critical Issues", printed under the auspices of the Publications Committee of the International Psychoanalytical Association and Karnac Books, London? Dr. Gennaro Saragnano, then directing this committee, heartily accepted the idea.

Has the invaluable material packed in *The Question of Lay Analysis* been underestimated by the current members of the psychoanalytical movement? If the answer to this question is yes – and the editors of this book suppose it is – it opens space for a new question: is the litigious content of the article a factor in the present underestimation?

This book

Worthy colleagues encompassing all generations of living analysts around the world were willing to share their thoughts about this question – alphabetically, from Argentina, Australia, Brazil, Canada, France, Germany, Israel, United States. One of them, Charles Hanly, the first non-medically trained person to attain the highest function in our movement, uniquely honors our initiative.

Without having any kind of previous contact about the theme, two among our collaborators – Ester Hadassa Sandler and Ron Spielman – had a similar idea: to make a dreamy, free-associative real letter to the discoverer of our discipline. Also dreamy is the imagined Homeric journey described by Monica Horovitz.

A kind of enlightenment about a hypothesized "layness" ethos of psychoanalysis is brought by Cláudia Aparecida Carneiro and Irina Panteleeva, who display the view of a younger generation analysts. Abel Fainstein, Avner Bergstein, Bernd Nissen and Jose Luiz Freda Petrucci bridge the seemingly unbridgeable and at the same time disentangle what seemed to be obviously bridgeable, to use Bergstein's happy naming.

Avedis Panajian makes a just and utterly due reminder about one of the most able analysts ever to appear, the pioneer Theodor Reik, who was a man deeply interested in psychoanalysis proper; who never contributed to the sad "political" partisanship, expressed by the so-called dissidences that have plagued our movement since its inception. In an effort to achieve a good enough participative representation, we invited other analysts from other main countries in which psychoanalysis thrives. All promised to send their ideas but failed to; no psychoanalytically minded editor would question their reasons.

If it is true, as Santayana (1905) observed, that "progress, far from consisting in change, depends on retentiveness. When change is absolute there remains no being to improve and no direction is set for possible improvement: and when experience is not retained, as among savages, infancy is perpetual. Those who cannot remember the past are condemned to repeat it" and if it is also true, as Marx believed, that historic facts appear twice, first as tragedy, then as farce, the editors of this book felt the need to stress, under a historically oriented non-conclusive text, of this book, the offshoots of the enduring affair of lay analysts as they can be seen in their current state (for example, Hale, 2000). Is it a "pseudo-controversy"? The editors of this book suppose it is.

In consequence, this book does not include any kind of partisan chapters; but it does include studies devoted to a psychoanalytic appreciation of the issue, with no prejudice about the previous formation of the colleagues who wrote them. Scientific appreciation, encompassing the use of the critical method, or criticism, that can be regarded as one among the origins of psychoanalysis (Kant, 1761; Sandler, 2000, 2001) differs from adopting judgmental values – the nest of warring parties.

> Patients show* that the resolution of a problem appears to present less difficulty if it can be regarded as belonging to a moral domain; causation, responsibility and therefore a controlling force (as opposed to helplessness) provide a framework within which omnipotence reigns. In certain circumstances, to be considered later, the scene is thus set for conflict (reflected in controversies such as those on Science and Religion). This situation is portrayed in the Eden and Babel myths. The significance for the individual lies in its part in obstructing the PS ⇔ D interaction. [Bion, 1965, pp. 64–65]

> [* Bion's Footnote: And not only patients. The group is dominated by morality – I include of course the negative sense that shows as rebellion against morality – and this contributed to the atmosphere of hostility to individual thought on which Freud remarked.]. . . . Much psycho-analytic "controversy" is not controversy at all. If listened to for any prolonged period, say a year, but preferably two or three, a pattern begins to emerge. . . . Controversy is the growing point from which development springs . . . but it must be a genuine confrontation and not an impotent beating of the air by opponents whose differences of view never meet. What follows is a contribution to bringing different psychoanalytic views together in agreement or disagreement. Hearing psycho-analytic controversy I have felt that the same configuration was being described and that the apparent differences were more often accidental than intrinsic; different points of view are believed to be significant of membership of a group, not of a scientific experience. Yet everyone knows that what is important is not the supposed use of a particular theory but whether the theory has been understood properly and whether the application has been sound. It may be objected that to establish this would involve consideration of every individual analyst and of the circumstances of every individual interpretation. Even so, many difficulties could be obviated by more precise definition of the point of view (vertex).
>
> (Bion, 1969, p. 303, 1970, p. 55; Sandler, 2005, p. 178)

The editors of this book put forth a hypothesis: Is there an underlying, still unrecognized, but heartrending factor underlying this century-year-old quarrel between "lay analysts" and . . . how one can qualify the other "party", one century later?

In Freud's time, this other party, delusional or not, was called medically or psychiatrically trained analysts. In looking for this underlying fact, we took into account the inversion of the groups that promoted a lawsuit, when comparing Theodor Reik's case in Austria and the IPA's case in the United States, half a century later. Being both socially instigated states, as if it was an economical quarrel between competing guilds, we considered the paradoxical pair: the interchanging functions of quantity and quality.

The eventual reader can read the chapters in any order he or she prefers. Our choice, to put them under the author's surname, in alphabetical order, seemed to us to be the most impartial possible, based in probability. To stress the probability method, we inverted – also alphabetically – this order. In the end run, and for pure coincidence, it allowed to emerge a content-related order of chapters.

The editors would like to express gratitude to the invaluable help given by Ron Spielman, who corrected the Introduction as well as Chapter 12, both in their form and content; and to all the contributors to this book, who tried to address this question. Special thanks are due to the eventual readers, whom, with most probability, and in the greatest quantity, we hardly will know personally. To them, this book is dedicated.

References

Bion, W.R. (1961). A Theory of Thinking. In: *Second Thoughts*. London: Heinemann Medical Books, 1967.

Bion, W.R. (1965). *Transformations*. London: Heinemann Medical Books.

Bion, W.R. (1969). Undated. In: Francesca Bion (Ed.), *Cogitations*. London: Karnac, 1992.

Bion, W.R. (1970). *Attention and Interpretation*. London: Tavistock Publications.

Freud, S. (1914). On the History of the Psychoanalytical Movement. *SE*, XIII.

Hale, N.G. (2000). Review of Lay Analysis: Life Inside the Controversy, by R.S. Wallerstein. *Psychoanalytic Psychology*, 17: 414–419.

Kant, I. (1761). Critique of Pure Reason. English version, by Thomas Kingsmill Abott. In: *The Great Books of the Western World*. New York: The Encyclopedia Britannica, 1994.

Marx. (1852). The 18th Brumaire of Louis Napoleon. www.marxists.org/archive/marx/works/1852/18th-brumaire/

Sandler, P.C. (2000). *As Origens da Psicanálise na obra de Kant*. Rio de Janeiro: Imago editora.

Sandler, P.C. (2001). Le Projet Scientifique de Freud en Danger un Siécle Plus Tard? *Revue Française de Psychanalyse*, Número hors-série, 181–202.

Sandler, P.C. (2005). *The Language of Bion: A Dictionary of Concepts*. London: Karnac.

Santayana, G. (1905). Flux and Constancy in Human Nature. In: *The Life of Reason*, 5 Volumes; Chapter XII of volume I, *Reason in Common Sense*. New York: Charles Scribner and Sons. Retrieved in https://archive.org/details/lifeofreasonorph01sant/page/4#donate_dropdown

1

The question of lay analysis

Then and now

Ron Spielman

My Dear Sigmund,

I have been asked to write something about your 1926 paper "The Question of Lay Analysis".

I am now retired after just over 30 years practicing as a "medical" psychoanalyst, having been a psychiatrist for some 12 years before qualifying to join your International Psychoanalytic Association in 1984. I trained with the Australian Psychoanalytic Society, which I will make relevant later.

I will not be the first to acknowledge that every time I pick up something you have written, I (like so many others!) find not only something "new", but something "awesome" in that you had some concept of issues with which we now – in 2019! – are so familiar. But you were a pioneer in so many details of issues involved in psychoanalytic practice.

My awe in this instance begins with the subheading to your title: "Conversations with an Impartial Person".

I know you have often written your papers with a sceptical reader – almost an adversary – in mind. But I read "impartial person" in this instance with a sense of your irony (do you intend this?) as I imagine you have more than made the case that such an impartial person, according to your own key concepts, cannot exist. No one can know their unconscious biases well enough to be "truly" impartial about anything! Yet, you invoke the idea of impartiality as a prelude to addressing what you clearly see as a vexed and complex issue.

You say in your very first paragraph (p. 183), "This question has its limitations in both time and place" and, indeed, it does. Perhaps more than even you knew when writing this paper in *your time* and at *your place*.

You address immediately the question of the place of psychoanalysis in the broader culture as opposed to its restriction to (or even rejection from!) medical practice.

You cannot have anticipated the irony (in present times) of your sentence:

> it (the question) does not arise in all countries with equal significance. In Germany and America it would be no more than an academic discussion; for in those countries every patient can have himself treated how and by whom he (nowadays, we have to add "or she") chooses, and anyone who chooses can as a "quack", handle patients provided only that he (or "she"! So many of your present day colleagues are now women!!) undertakes the responsibility of his actions.

We can forgive you the use of the term "quack" because we know (in house) what you mean by it (and you say so toward the end of your paper), but please don't use it too often in public as it is not "politically correct" these days to do so.

The irony suggested above is that "in America" – and perhaps "only in America" – there was a protracted period where "lay analysts" (as you write, "non-doctors") were *excluded* from becoming members of the American Psychoanalytic Association – which institution was the "Component Society" (I don't know if you are familiar with this term) in the United States of America which had "the franchise" accorded by the IPA to have responsibility for training future psychoanalysts. The APA has had many "institutes" under its umbrella – but held exclusively the right to train *only* medical persons (most often psychiatrists) in psychoanalysis.

I am happy to let you know that under the courageous leadership of one of your most admirable followers, Dr. Robert Wallerstein (himself an American) while president of the IPA from 1985 to 1989, carefully negotiated a major court case in the USA, brought against the IPA by psychologists in America, the fortunate outcome of which was to include "non-medical" mental health professionals in the trainings offered by APA institutes. In 1998, Wallerstein actually wrote a long book about his experience called *Lay Analysis – Life Inside the Experience*.

Now . . . Germany! The country which once burned your books is among the very few countries whose national health systems currently support psychoanalytic treatments with substantial public funding. (Australia is another!) Now that's an irony! If only the relevant reasons hadn't made it so.

Now, you define the "territory" of your important question (of "lay analysis"), as ever, so admirably and logically at the end of your introduction:

> Neurotics are patients, laymen are non-doctors (regrettable term!), psychoanalysis is a procedure for curing or improving nervous disorders, and all such treatments are reserved to doctors. It follows (*ergo!*) that laymen are not permitted to practice analysis on neurotics, and are punishable if they nevertheless do so. (I take the liberty of including in the brackets *my* need to add to your point.)

Not so simple in 2019!

This may well have been the "rationale" for the American Psychoanalytic Association excluding "laymen" – albeit the ones challenging their exclusion from IPA training were highly qualified professionals (psychologists and social workers).

But, as you will not necessarily know, because you published your paper in 1926, just 10 years before you tragically, for your stage of life, and urgently (because of the Nazi domination of Europe) had to hurriedly leave Vienna and migrate to London in 1936, for your own safety, that London was to become one of the most important and creative centres of psychoanalytic thought and practice – not least due to a considerable number of so-called lay analysts.

Leading among these "lay analysts" in London was your very own daughter Anna! She became such an influential contributor to our field, among so many others, for many decades after your death in 1939.

This is only to say, that again, ironically, what you were so concerned about leading up to publishing your paper on "the question of lay analysis" from Vienna in 1926 hardly was an issue at all in Britain where psychoanalysis took root in London and has flourished admirably ever since.

This is not to say that the issues you addressed in the body of your paper are now what we might nowadays term a "non-issue". They remain of significance – but only in the context, as you so presciently alluded, "to do with time and place".

I have already made the point (I hope) that "the question" is not a universal one: in at least one country (America) it *was* a major issue (but no more) and in most others in Europe and Latin America *and* – you will be surprised to learn – in India, in Israel and now in many Asian countries (Japan, Korea and China, particularly) it is not an issue at all!

Nevertheless, your "conversation with an impartial person" still retains relevance as to the "standing of psychoanalysis" in the firmament of human knowledge, alongside its acceptance, or rejection, as a method of treatment of mental disorders.

You, yourself – now famously – defined psychoanalysis in a "tri-partite" manner: as a theory of mental functioning, as a body of concepts and as a method of investigating (a "tool" you called it) and treating disorders of the mind.

I can safely let you know that psychoanalysis *has* claimed an important place in the realm of human knowledge and thought. So much of what you pioneered is taken for granted in intelligent company and so much has become part of our understanding of human behaviour on the broadest cultural level – let alone in understanding mental disorders of all kinds. A famous British poet, W.H. Auden, in a eulogy following your death wrote that you "are no longer a person, but a whole climate of opinion". What a tribute to you! You have permeated Western culture with your ideas.

The concepts derived from your work and added to by so many important contributors since you lived and worked in Vienna are our business as clinicians, and we all depend on them in our day-to-day work.

But, the realm of psychoanalysis' efficacy and relevance to treatment of mental disorder continues to be such a fraught issue – even though we continue to derive benefit for our fellow humans by deriving insights into issues of mental function through psychoanalytic investigation of the minds of those who seek us out.

Indeed, the important issue of what are the indications for psychoanalysis and its efficacy in treating what will come to be referred to as the "widening scope" (I'll tell you more about this later), has occupied considerable research efforts by many colleagues – most notably, I would consider, Peter Fonagy and his colleagues working at University College London.

In 2005, the IPA published Fonagy's "An Open Door Review of Outcome Studies in Psychoanalysis". This comprehensive review study grew out of Fonagy's and some colleagues', earlier (2002) review "What Works for Whom? A Critical Review of Psychotherapy Research".

These studies rescued our field from being criticised for "single case" anecdotal reports (of which *your* early case studies are such exemplars) and located us among those prepared to undertake rigorously controlled outcome studies.

In writing just now "the minds of those who seek us out", I was aware of how easy it would have been for me to write "our patients" – or in more modern and comprehensive terms, "our clients". But this is in fact the point of your paper: that people should be free to *seek out* suitably qualified psychoanalytically trained practitioners – *subject to the laws of the land* – which you argued may need changing.

In your **Section I**, you argue that your impartial person can never be in a position to *experience* what it is to partake in a psychoanalytic process. Were he or she to "undergo" psychoanalysis themselves, they would cease to be "impartial" – they would either become "an *advocate for*" psychoanalysis or "an *antagonist to*" psychoanalysis as a result of either successfully resolving relevant issues (in the case of the "advocate") – or having been resistant to the process and retaining unresolved hostility to the "authority figures" (in the case of the "antagonist/critic" – but I would say that, wouldn't I?).

Now, in your **Section II**, you engage in active dialogue *with* your "impartial person" – almost *as if* he were in a psychoanalytic relationship *with* you!

And here the resistances of your hypothetical impartial person become manifest: you are forced, once more, as you have done so often, into defending and advocating for psychoanalysis. You and I (and myriad colleagues) know what you are asserting is *true* – but not so accessible to anyone who has not had *an authentic experience* of the psychoanalytic process.

At the end of this Section II (p. 199) you write "How then could I expect to convince you, the Impartial Person, of the correctness of our theories, when I can only put before you an abbreviated and therefore unintelligible account of them, without confirming them from your own experiences?"

We, your modern colleagues, sense – and share – your despair!

But, I have to remind you of your own warning (in your papers on technique) against what you, yourself, called "therapeutic zeal". Your "zeal" in advocating *for* psychoanalysis is much appreciated by us all . . . but you and we, in our more sober moments, understand its futility – and, indeed, in analysis, its undesirability.

As Wilfred Bion, of whom you may have heard something at your "Wednesday Group in Heaven", was renowned for disavowing any investment at all in what we nowadays think of as "positive outcomes" of analysis – let alone therapeutic zeal itself – in his encounters with his patients.

In **Section III**, you endeavour to offer your imaginary person a "crash course" in psychoanalytic theory (let us from now on call him "IP" – because it occurs to me that nowadays in modern psychiatric and psychological treatment clinics the "IP" is a term for the "identified patient" in a family dynamic. Your "IP" shares many qualities of many modern "IPs": carrying and expressing the unrecognised – *yet denied* – pain of others!).

In your **Section IV**, you delve into the very realms which are so disconcerting to our many critics: sex!

It is this "sex" which "allows" people to challenge "what has sex got to do with disorders requiring medical treatment – if that is what you Psychoanalysts claim – and then claim that such treatments can be undertaken by non-medical persons. Are you all mad?"

Your IP even challenges you to explore ethics, conscience and ideals. What do these have to do with treatable disorders? You do rise admirably to this challenge.

Amazingly – but perhaps not so – in **Section V**, your IP expresses interest in *becoming* an analyst. How often this happens in "real life"! Our analysands (now there's a better term) so often wish to *become* psychoanalysts, don't they? Some of yours did!

The problem – as we modern analysts now understand it (on the basis of decades more actual experience than you could possibly have had) and certainly on the basis of the aggregated experience of generations of psychoanalysts in the more than 100 years since you began this all, that the *desire* to become an analyst is a complex phenomenon – particularly among those who *seek* psychoanalytic training.

Our own "candidates" are mostly "suspect" as to their unconscious motivations for even wanting to train (why on earth would anyone want to join our "impossible profession"? – yet another echo of an IP?). These conscious and unconscious "motivations" are *legitimately* the subject of exploration during any so-called training analysis. But what if they arise in the course of an "ordinary" psychoanalysis? Aren't they then even more "suspect" and likely to constitute a resistance to some or other unconscious set of issues?

Well, we nowadays would think so. But many of your analysands became psychoanalysts quite readily – and, oftentimes, quite productively. Did your acceptance of this "phenomenon" reflect your own desire for the propagation of psychoanalysis to the extent you may not have adequately analysed the relevant resistances which may have been involved in your – at your time – relatively short analyses? (Just asking.)

Nevertheless, having offered your IP a crash course in theory in the previous section, you now offer a crash course in technique!

Modern candidates will feel envy that you make it so succinct and relatively easy. But – again – you, and we all, know it isn't possible to acquire the relevant knowledge and skills without the arduous and lengthy participation in a formal psychoanalytic training, involving personal analysis together with supervision and seminars. We now call this the Eitingon Model, after your colleague and friend whom you mention on p. 228. But, under the pressures of time and money in modern times (in the early 2000s), this Eitingon Model is being modified in some societies which make up your IPA. We will have to await the consequences of all this.

Mentioning "time and money pressures" leads directly into your **Section VI**.

Your IP challenges your having spent so much time and effort on your argument by comparing the process of *becoming* a psychoanalyst with other specialist branches of medicine. He, the IP, says:

"[a]nyone who decides on this new specialised branch of medicine (i.e. psychoanalysis) will, when his studies are completed, take on the two years' training you spoke of in a training institute, if it really requires so much time".

"Really requires so much time". "Two years"? *Only* two years?

I alluded earlier to *your*, to us, relatively short analyses. Nowadays, training analyses themselves are much longer – from five to many more years. Candidates even borrow a term from you and joke about "Training analysis – terminable or interminable"! This is why the "time and money" issue is so real in the current economic circumstances faced by young (and not so young) aspiring psychoanalysts.

Your IP wonders why there is even a place for "lay analysts" in his (unrealistic) cosy scenario, where training for already medically qualified people exists, and they are merely seeking to take up your "new" specialty.

You take the opportunity to make abundantly clear your, as yet unasserted, major point: "Doctors have no historical claim to the sole possession of psychoanalysis".

Of course, not! But, you have to acknowledge that psychoanalysis was born of *your* efforts to understand what was then thought to be a medical (neurological) disorder – hysteria. Isn't that why you went to the Saltpetrière to study under Charcôt?

Then you grappled with what, to us now, seem momentous questions which had not occurred to anyone else before. You came to understand the *psychogenic* aetiology of some apparently neurological conditions and help mankind to subsequently look to the mind for explanations – and *not* the brain.

I consider that your struggles with "hysteria" indeed gave birth to our (impossible) profession.

So, you cannot deny that there is some – at least historical – justification for a residual link between "medicine" and "psychoanalysis".

You now take the opportunity to yourself challenge the use (mainly yours!) of the word "quack". You rightly say that "according to the law", a quack is anyone acting as a doctor (purporting to *be* a doctor) without the formal training qualifications to do so. Of course. But you then go on to redefine (so you claim) the word to mean "anyone who undertakes a treatment without possessing the knowledge and capacities for it".

This is no different *in principle* to your "legal definition". You assert that anyone without adequate and academically (university-based) formal qualifications to practice any treatment is by definition a "quack".

You then make what appears to be a shocking claim that many qualified *doctors*, "not only in European countries", are, according to you, *quacks*! You have cunningly made the point that *merely* being a medical doctor does not confer qualification to undertake psychoanalytic treatments. You even make the further disturbing assertion that a medical training may well be the opposite of what one will need to prepare for being a psychoanalyst (p. 230).

This Section VI of yours (pp. 229–238) is full of striking assertions, but if any reader of this letter to you has not already read your paper, he or she would do well to feast on almost every sentence of your comparing *and contrasting* psychoanalysis with medicine itself in these 10 pages of yours. I cannot do justice to them short of replicating the whole Section VI (you *will* find the paper reproduced at the beginning of this volume!).

Just a few points of yours: "every science is one-sided"; "physics does not diminish the value of chemistry"; "a sick person is a complicated organism"; "honesty compels me (you, Sigmund!) to admit that the activity of an untrained analyst does less harm than that of an untrained surgeon". You so persuasively argue – and at length – *against* incorporation of psychoanalysis in the medical sphere, that your IP seems to get impatient and interrupts you (p. 233) and calls you out for his perceived *hostility of yours* against the medical profession. He does finally come to agree that "if analyses are to be carried out, it should be by people who have been thoroughly trained for it".

He then wonders whether "with time" doctors who turn to analysis will do everything to obtain the necessary training. "I fear not" you almost shout and go on to further rail against medical schools and doctors.

Your IP – now himself perhaps despairing – asks, "Then what definite proposals have you to make?" . . . "I have not got so far as that yet; and I cannot tell whether I shall get there at all", say you.

You now spend a page addressing the situation in your Austria – where non-doctors practising analysis may be threatened (little did you know in 1926 exactly how they would come to be threatened!)

by laws against "quackery". They could easily emigrate to Germany, you write, "where no legislation will prevent them from finding recognition for their proficiency". (Full on irony again! "Recognition *for* their proficiency", maybe – but not, in the following 15 years, *of* their right to live!)

You then turn to yet another important question (p. 235): "Is the practice of psychoanalysis a matter which should in general be subject to official interference, or would it be more expedient to leave it to follow its natural development?" An important question indeed!

You immediately say you will not "come to any decision here and now" and "will take the liberty" of (merely?) outlining the issues. Furthermore, you say you will "not spare you (your IP) my unauthoritative thoughts on the subject". Unauthoritative, indeed! You, who have been for so long such an "authority" on topics psychoanalytical. Do you know how often you have been, and continue to be, quoted, with approval, in our psychoanalytic literature?

In the following three pages you argue as a very modern "small 'l' liberal" – an advocate for freedom of thought and progress in its most idealistic form. Your faith in human freedom of thought is pitched against authoritarian controls. You are most convincing – if somewhat unrealistic!

When you were writing these pages of your paper, were you not aware of the parallel struggles which you taught us about: the *id* against the *superego*? Are you not caricaturing "the authorities" – the makers of regulatory laws – as a harsh and punitive *superego*? In individual human lives – and in the societies in which they live – the battles between the freedoms of the *id* and the restraints of the *superego* are enacted all day every day (even at night, in our dreams, as you so notably led us to understand!) – throughout the ages. The forces of the *id* never rest – and the *superego* never ceases to be vigilant. Our individual *egos* are constantly called upon to keep the peace.

It is not different with psychoanalysis' legitimate *desire* to develop as it must and countries' need (in fact, obligation) to *regulate*, appropriately, what its citizens may or may not do to one another.

In modern times, individuals who may have been drawn to wanting to *practise* psychoanalysis as a result of positive personal experiences with it – but having *no* formal academic mental health qualifications – are very rare. They will be required to obtain some appropriate qualifications and experience prior to commencing training with any of the IPA-authorised taring institutes. You, yourself would not wish anyone to practise psychoanalysis *without* adequate training. (It is these, with or without, medical degrees, you call the "genuine quacks"!)

So, in modern psychoanalytic institutes, prospective candidates for training may come with academic qualifications other than medical ones, such as psychology or social work. The context of "time and place" with which you began your paper is now largely irrelevant – *but* – I will venture to assert – the issue of *freedom* vs *regulation* has been transplanted *into* the very psychoanalytic institutes which comprise your modern day International Psychoanalytic Association: if you want to see "regulations", you need go no further than look at the guidelines to admission and training of our very own candidates! I will not dare to canvass this issue any further – but merely draw your attention to it.

It occurs to me too, just now, that the history of development of psychoanalytic thought and practice has been full of similar "battles" between *authority* and *nonconformity*. A paper written by Martin Bergmann ["Reflections on the History of Psychoanalysis", *Psychoanal. Rev.*, (1993)] classified those who have proposed any "changes" in *your* concepts as *modifiers, extenders* or *heretics*. The many notable *modifiers* and *extenders* remain within "our fold" – but the *heretics* have (necessarily) either left us or been "expelled". You see, at least some regulatory defence of "the establishment" is usually required to keep the enterprise intact!

Getting back to your own paper, you conclude this important Section VI by acknowledging that you favour "a policy of *laissez faire*". I would say for admirably well-argued reasons – but, the realities of modern western countries and the running of professional societies (our own definitely included) require suitable regulations to keep vulnerable individuals (patients, clients, analysands) as safe as possible from the depredations of unscrupulous inadequately trained and qualified "*quacks*".

In your final **Section VII**, your by now very impatient IP exclaims "Yes, but the doctors! The doctors!" he begs you to get to your *real point*. He says, correctly, that the vast majority of your followers and pupils are "already" doctors and, in all likelihood, already meet your criteria of *not* being "quacks" – and that they agree with closing the practice of psychoanalysis to laymen.

You answer that most – but not all – are of this opinion. You proudly assert that your group of colleagues can survive having differences of opinion.

Your IP presses you further to justify your position.

You now go into an extended discussion of the importance of diagnosis and differential diagnosis – readily recognisable as the proper domain of *any* physician, of whatever specialty.

Regrettably, but again understandably for your time and clinical experience, you discuss this in what your modern colleagues would regard as (again understandably) in "old-fashioned" terms of "neurosis" and "feebleness of the ego".

A term which entered our literature in 1954 is "the widening scope" of psychoanalysis (Leo Stone, 1954). He intended this to describe what had in fact been occurring for some many years: the move away from confining psychoanalytic therapeutic attention to "neurosis" and including a variety of personality disorders and psychosomatic disorders as well as alcohol and drug disorders – and, you will be surprised to learn, even cases of "schizophrenia", which you had declared were *not* amenable to psychoanalytic efforts. The paper Stone presented was discussed at a Panel of the American Psychoanalytic Association – you will be proud to know – by your daughter Anna, who spoke of restrictions *she* experienced as a "lay analyst" in Britain at that time, referring to:

> certain principles which govern the selection of cases in the practice of a lay analyst, *even in a country like Great Britain* where authorities and public are extremely generous in their attitude to lay analysis (my italics).

In spite of widespread reservations as to questions of "analysability", quite a few of our colleagues in the mid-20th century bravely attempted to utilise *psychoanalytic methods* to *both* investigate – *and,* as a consequence – treat some *very disturbed* patients . . . to quite some good effect! It was *you* in fact who asserted that psychoanalysis was *both* a tool to investigate the mind *and* a method of treatment of mental illness. These admirable colleagues have enriched our field by doing exactly as you said – with severely ill analysands.

So, again, back to your own paper: you agree with your IP that basically it is imperative that a medical doctor be involved in the diagnosis and differential diagnosis of *all* patients who will "enter" psychoanalytic treatment. You even cover the eventuality that in the course of *any* psychoanalytic treatment, medical symptoms *may arise* which will require the cooperation of a medical doctor with the psychoanalyst. And, you surprise your IP with the statement "in such circumstances a medical analyst would not act differently". You follow with a very modern discussion of the interaction of psychoanalytic treatment with "physical medicine" and the importance of "the analyst" – medically qualified, or not – to *not* attempt to deal with the physical manifestations of mental illnesses without the support of a medical colleague.

You will not, of course, be aware of the extraordinary developments of, and advances in "psychotherapeutic agents" which have occurred since the 1950s. In fact, many such advances have threatened our own domain of having been "once upon a time" leaders in management of "disorders of the mind". There was a time when leading figures in psychiatry departments in universities, especially in America, were, almost *de riguer*, qualified psychoanalysts. No longer!

"Physical treatments" (mainly psychoactive medications) have replaced psychoanalysis as the "go to treatment" of mental disorder. This, of course, is to the detriment of many patients who are so often offered "the easy path" of taking medications – rather than the more arduous (and psychically threatening) path of self-knowledge as a way to overcome their symptoms of psychic distress.

Back to your paper again: on page 244, you state there are three groups of interests involved: those to do with patients, those to do with doctors and – importantly – those to do with science (and, so, in turn, the interests of *future* patients).

And, secondly, you now embark on a lengthy justification of your claim that, to the patient, "it is a matter of indifference whether the analyst is a doctor or not". It is only important that the analyst be well qualified.

You now (and, at last!) acknowledge that "the lay analysts who practise analysis today (are not) any chance collection of riff-raff, but people of academic education, doctors of philosophy, educationalists, together with a few women of great experience in life and outstanding personality". I am not sure whether today's *feminists* would praise you or lambaste you for this last part of your description of those whom you regard as the "lay analysts" of your times. (And, by the way, it is these *feminists* themselves who took great exception to many of your early theories – despite your pioneering interest in "what a woman wants".)

You then turn to the "interests of the doctors" and go on to assert that no one would gain by prolonging an already long medical training by incorporating psychoanalytic training into a medical curriculum. Probably so.

You go on to explore what is a very complex set of issues in your inimitable manner and you appear to conclude that "it is unjust to try to compel a person who wants to set someone else free from the torment of a phobia or an obsession to take the roundabout road of the medical curriculum". You develop an imaginative *metaphor* involving two paths up a mountain – one long and one short. Your upshot is: "I fear you will succeed in compelling the laymen to study medicine just as little as I shall be able to induce doctors to learn analysis". An impasse, indeed!

But your "list" of those practising "lay analysis" is not too different from a comparable "list" of today and, thus, most "potential" lay analysts (in your terms) have already acquired basic academic qualifications with which they could proceed to undertake psychoanalytic trainings with an "authorised institute" – authorised by your own IPA! So, the choice is made by each individual aspirant to becoming a qualified psychoanalyst, whether they be a medical doctor becoming interested in becoming a psychoanalyst – or another kind of professional with relevant qualifications also aspiring to psychoanalytic training.

Now let me introduce a (to me, important) "quibble" which appears to have been overlooked by your IP: I wish to examine the term "layman" itself (and, by implication, your term "lay"). A "layman" is defined in the dictionary as "a person who is not a member of a given profession, as in law or medicine". Surely, then, now that our own profession of psychoanalysis has been well established, anyone not a member of it now qualifies as a "layman" in respect of psychoanalysis! Individuals *become members* of the psychoanalytic profession by undergoing authorised trainings on the basis of coming to training with appropriate academic and clinical experience.

So, in order to not give further offence to current day colleagues, I would like to remove the term "lay analyst" from labelling *any* of our colleagues – whether medically qualified or not! The main criterion should be whether they have become qualified to practise as an analyst by an accredited IPA Component Society.

Now, finally, in your long paper, you come to the "third interest" – the interest of science.

I agree with you that

> we do not consider it at all desirable for psychoanalysis to be swallowed up by medicine and to find its last resting-place in a text book of psychiatry under the heading "Methods of Treatment", alongside of procedures such as hypnotic suggestion, auto suggestion, and persuasion, which, born from our ignorance have to thank the laziness and cowardice of mankind for their short-lived effects. It deserves a better fate and, it may be hoped, will be met with one.

(I can't help here exclaiming "Wow!!" What courage for you to have written such a sentence!)

You go on to argue persuasively for the role of psychoanalysis as a "depth-psychology" and it's becoming indispensable "to all the sciences which are concerned with the evolution of human civilisation and its major institutions".

Although I have been a psychoanalytic clinician for over 35 years and confined my efforts with my analysands to my consulting room, I have been sustained in a far broader professional and personal sense by the abiding truth of your assertion about the importance of psychoanalysis in the broadest sense which you just outlined on page 248, to which I just referred.

I wrote at the outset of this letter to you, that I would say a little more about Australia.

You may remember writing to your then-fiancée Martha Bernays, in 1882, that, because of money concerns, you both may have had to consider emigrating "to England or perhaps America . . . or Australia" (an afterthought?). Although your extended works *did* arrive in Australia – quite early in the 1900s, in fact – I cannot imagine that you, yourself, would have been "sustained" in the easy-going "outward looking" Australian culture of the times. We didn't look inward all that much then – perhaps we do more so now. There is in fact a volume titled "Freud in the Antipodes" by Australian historian Joy Damousi outlining the cultural history of psychoanalysis in Australia. Perhaps a librarian can get it for you – or try on Amazon via Google.

I mentioned at the beginning, too, that our public health insurance scheme *does* financially support patients in Australia undertaking psychoanalytically oriented psychotherapy with medically trained (!!) professionals – usually, psychiatrists.

So, psychoanalysis *has* taken root in Australia – as in all other Western societies. But we clinicians have to struggle in our Australian context against the preference among both mental health professionals and patients themselves for what you call "short-lived" effects derived from less arduous procedures than our psychoanalytically oriented methods involve.

I was, before digressing, referring to your "big picture" view of the role of psychoanalysis in human cultural development. You went on to assert, quite correctly, that for this to occur and continue, "analysts will be needed, for whom any medical knowledge will have particularly little importance".

You come toward concluding this Section VII – and, indeed, your whole paper – by writing "Our civilization imposes an almost intolerable pressure on us and it calls for a corrective". You hint that psychoanalysis itself may "be destined" for the task of preparing mankind for such a "corrective".

Your (I hope, tongue-in-cheek) reference to someone exclaiming about "a new kind of Salvation Army" by training a band of social workers in psychoanalysis, is your final "challenge" to your IP. Is this a "fantasy" of an ultimate application of psychoanalysis as "saviour of Mankind"? Perhaps a wry joke on your part after so seriously canvassing the important issues we – you and I – have been covering?

I will agree with your final sentence: "the things that really matter – the possibilities in psychoanalysis for *internal* (your italics!) development – can never be affected by regulations and prohibitions".

But I hope *you* will now agree – after this correspondence – that some appropriate *external* regulations *are* necessary for the appropriate establishment of relevant professional procedures and processes to secure the reputation of psychoanalysis as a clinical profession in modern times.

But wait!!

You have written a postscript in 1927.

Here you reveal your motive for having written your long 1926 paper "The Question of Lay Analysis" at all: a charge of quackery brought against your friend and colleague Dr. Theodore Reik, in the Vienna Courts. (We should here acknowledge that Dr. Reik *did* have a PhD in psychology and, thus, did in fact have appropriate academic qualifications as a practising mental health professional.)

You reveal that your "Impartial Person" was based on a *real* individual with whom you had discussed Reik's case. A man with some integrity, you write. Yet, you say, remaining unconvinced about your argument on the matter.

In your postscript you canvass many of the issues in your paper . . . but . . . you add some important personal detail: you write "I have never really been a doctor in the proper sense"! You admit to having been "compelled to deviate" from an earlier purpose in your life. I suppose you are acknowledging that you, yourself, have no reason to be committed to the medical profession – despite your being a member of it.

You claim that your personal "history" in this regard does not influence the basic issues you have addressed in regard to "lay analysis".

Au contraire! It is from you we have learned that personal history *always* is of relevance to manifestations of human behaviour – yours included!

Just as in the course of a long psychoanalysis, it takes time for the "original trauma" to surface – whatever form of trauma it may have been. I would have the temerity to suggest to you, dear Sigmund, that the court case brought against your friend and colleague, Dr. Reik, constituted one such *trauma* and stimulated your extensive defence mounted against the "assault" on both *his* and *your* professional standing, throughout your important paper – but only revealing this equally important fact in your "postscript" a year later.

This does not detract at all from anything you have written in your paper – least of all your statement on page 254: "I admit it. I only want to feel that the therapy will not destroy the science". All of us wish that!

The rest of your postscript raises many points to which you have alluded in your main paper.

But – finally – in your last paragraphs, you reveal knowledge of "the resolution passed by our American colleagues against lay analysts". You gave no indication in your main paper that you knew of this at all. You may well *not have known* of the major efforts of Dr. Robert Wallerstein about whom I told you, in having all this reversed – *but* you were evidently aware of the wholesale exclusion of "lay analysts" by the largest single Component Society of the IPA at the time from the beginnings of IPA-authorised psychoanalytic training in America.

Finally, finally, as in your final paragraph, "the possibility of receiving the approval of the medical profession" you had hoped for, for the lay analysts for whom you spoke, *was* achieved, and the formal inclusion of "lay analysts" (still a regrettable term) into the International Psychoanalytic Association has enriched our profession.

I remain, yours faithfully,

Dr. Ron Spielman
Sydney, Australia

References and further reading

Bergmann, M.S. (1993). Reflections on the History of Psychoanalysis. *Journal of the American Psychoanalytic Association*, 41: 929–955.

Bion, W.R. (1961). *Experiences in Groups and Other Papers*. London: Tavistock.

Fonagy, P. (2005). *An Open Door Review of Outcome Studies in Psychoanalysis*. London: International Psychoanalytical Association.

Fonagy, P. et al. (2002). *What Works for Whom? A Critical Review of Psychotherapy Research*. New York: Guilford.

Freud, A. (1954). The Widening Scope of Indications for Psychoanalysis – Discussion. *Journal of the American Psychoanalytic Association*, 2: 607–620.

Stone, L. (1954). The Widening Scope of Indications for Psychoanalysis. *Journal of the American Psychoanalytic Association*, 2: 567–594.

Wallerstein, R.S. (1998). *Lay Analysis: Life Inside the Controversy*. London: Routledge.

2

Wayward analysis

Ester Hadassa Sandler

Dear Dr. Freud,

In 1976, fifty years after you published the article "The Question of Lay Analysis", I welcomed to my office a lady about twice my age. My professional repertoire for a job of this nature is quite restricted, and, making matters more complicated, I still harbor strong memories from my galvanizing years of medical school, such a rich time in existential experiences: births, deaths, and the most varied and tragic forms of human suffering between these two extremes of life. Those were years filled with much study and work, when I witnessed spectacular cures and resounding failures; a time when every day there were new breakthroughs: ingenious techniques of organ transplants, and many other therapeutic resources which were being tested in their possibilities and limits. There was a vast amount of knowledge to learn, and an equally vast amount to discover; the encouragement for students to undertake scientific investigation led me to my own research project in the field of mental illness, with an epidemiological approach. But apparently, none of this is helpful for what I need now; quite the contrary.[1]

Unlike what you stated in the addendum to your text (1927), and as you had already written two years before in your "An Autobiographical Study" (1925 [1924], pp. 9–10), I felt great affinity for the whole universe unveiled by the study of medicine.

At the time when the woman came to my office, I was in the middle of the challenges, joys, and anxieties of mothering two young children, which in turn presented me with yet another of the three activities that you deem impossible in your "Preface to Aichhorn's Verw Ahrloste Jugend" (Freud, 1925, p. 273). *Wayward Youth* could be a good title for the stage in my life that I am trying to describe. The pressure of earning a living and contributing to support my family, added to the high material and emotional cost of both my personal analysis and the specialization course in psychotherapy of children and adolescents, heightened the uncertainties of the professional path I had chosen: psychoanalysis. It appeared as an even murkier and painfully uncertain path, especially when compared with the clearly established benchmarks (in appearance, at least) of a medical career for which I had trained, and where specialization studies themselves – residency – are considered remunerated work.

And if I allow myself to share these private issues with you, it is because you know, better than anyone, that it is not possible to separate our personal experiences from our choices, from our viewpoints, our repertoire, our limitations, and our very choice to practice psychoanalysis, as Money-Kyrle describes in his essay "Normal Counter-Transference and Some of Its Deviations" (1956, pp. 331, 333–334).

Meanwhile, I think about what to do with that lady who had been referred to me for analysis; to me because nobody else would take her. She had been an elementary-school teacher, and was now retired. Her CV as a mental patient included many years of fruitless treatment attempts with a variety of psychiatrists and psychoanalysts, culminating with an inpatient stay at a psychiatric hospital, where she received high doses of psychotropic drugs and electroshocks, and from where she had recently been discharged.

She is a hysteric, announces the colleague who had referred her to me, with the necessary reticence and undertones intended to reassure me – since he knows my reservations about accepting a patient without feeling fully prepared for it – but also to cool any enthusiasm I might have nurtured for my first adult psychoanalysis patient. Since such patient is a lost case, an untreatable person whose damages inspire little respect, I need not worry too much. My colleague, more or less like you, Dr. Freud, thought that if what I had to offer her were insufficient or innocuous, "However, if a doctor has been mistaken for a time over a case of this sort or has been in uncertaintyabout it, no harm [would have] been caused and nothing unnecessary [would have] been done. Nor indeed would the analytic treatment of this case have done any harm, though it would have been exposed as an unnecessary waste" (1926, p. 240).

It may surprise you, but by the mid-1970s the two or three years of personal analysis and theoretical study that I had, and which in 1926 you considered sufficient to prepare a novice analyst to start working,[2] meant very little, almost nothing from the institutional point of view. There was an ethical commitment, which I always respected, not to declare myself a "psychoanalyst" before being certified as such by an institute of psychoanalysis, which demanded many years of personal analysis, theoretical studies, supervision, and published scientific papers. A rather different situation from the one you present to your unbiased interlocutor in the text that inspired this dialogue; especially since the personal talents that you indicate as favorable for an analyst to do his job are not easy to find.[3] They demand a solid cultural and humanistic basis that only countless years of dedication, interest, and aptitude can build. And in this regard, I must agree with you, the training and preparation of a doctor are so absorbing that the damage to the area of general knowledge and culture is highly significant.[4]

In the daily life of the university hospital connected to the medical school that I enthusiastically attended – one of the best known and most respected in my country – there were serious and complex cases, cases of "real" diseases, and considered of scientific interest. People like Mrs. T, when they showed up, were considered screening flaws, and were often very harshly treated.[5] Her suffering, like that of so many other neurotic people, was not even considered "true" mental illness; anxiety attacks, neuroses in general, were called "hissy fits"; conversion neuroses, nicknamed "HY", were seen as pure faking, and stirred up even greater hostility, showing that the prevailing attitude in medical school in the face of issues of a neurotic nature had remained unchanged fifty years after your paper on lay analysis.[6] Neither was there a psychiatrist in the emergency room team, or at the disposal of the clinical outpatient centers for dialogue and guidance on how to understand and treat this type of suffering. Since my colleagues considered me to be a patient person – and this was not exactly a compliment – I was often called upon to deal with such nuisances. In fact, the emotional life of patients interested me as much as their physical issues, if we can even separate one from the others, but this was not yet clear to me.

Most medical students eagerly seek out all kinds of practical learning beyond what is offered in their regular curriculum; fortunately, in my medical school, there were some psychoanalysts who introduced psychoanalysis to interested students, in theory and practice; and so, searching here and there, I found a service for children with emotional and psychological problems, where I met Antonio, an eight-year-old boy who bit his nails and was very anxious. In the context of a medical school, students participate in various levels of patient care, accompanied and guided by more experienced colleagues. Patients are aware of this condition, and are in general very cooperative. So, it was quite natural to see Antonio without any preparation or prior knowledge, and without feeling that I lacked in ethics, or was a quack. But, suddenly, I've found myself alone with Antonio, who appeared to be not intimidated by my white uniform, he did not call me doctor, and did not even begin to cry. But I, much the opposite, felt very scared. He simply invited me to play and draw with him. My absolute ignorance made this experience a paradigmatic situation, a reference for the rest of my life. I discovered a new world, an area that interested me deeply and to which I decided to devote myself, because it had awakened in me a vocational appeal that I had not yet felt.

Working through my mourning for having renounced the activity for which I had prepared myself for years, and which had aroused so much interest in me, took a long time; the mourning process was intensified by the intellectual anxieties about entering a universe of hazy, chaotic, and continuously expanding knowledge, and for which I might not have aptitude. The psychoanalysis books I had erratically begun reading, by various authors and on multiple subjects, did not speak to me or to each other. There was a huge gap between the theories presented in those books and what happened in the everyday life of my practice.

One question kept returning to my mind, the same one asked by your interlocutor: "How and where can one learn what is necessary for practicing analysis?"(Freud, 1926, p. 228). You quote a warning by Mephistopheles that would have been illuminating: "it is vain that you range around from Science to Science; each man learns only what he can learn".[7]

When Mrs. T, the retired teacher, arrived in my office, I had already graduated from medical school, and I was accountable for myself and for my actions. My ignorance was not absolute anymore, but still unlimited. There was no one down the hall, a more experienced colleague or teacher whom I could consult before attending to the demands of my patient.

My work place was very simple: a couch, two chairs, and a small table. Until then, none of my patients had approached that couch, a sort of affirmation of my identity, since I no longer had on me the white apron, stethoscope, prescription pad, and other medical insignia that afforded me some credibility. And when Mrs. T finally arrived, nothing went as I had expected. She barely looked at me, did not ask any questions, did not request to see my credentials, and showed no sign of astonishment with my patently wayward youth. She immediately headed to the couch, laid down on it with familiarity, and began to "associate freely". For the next seven years, I learned the entire repertoire of psychoanalytic interpretations, theories, and jargon of that time, reproduced faithfully and at the same time caricaturally. The "teacher" T had found a "student" – and I had the proper *physique du rôle*. Anchored in this relationship, we talked and had a real connection. From what I was told, after we parted ways, Mrs. T had a less miserable life, and remembered me fondly. I started to receive other "difficult" referrals, and one day a supervisor said that I had the ability to work on transference. I thanked him for the compliment, although I did not dare ask what he meant by it; I continued to feel wayward, disoriented. Until I discovered, years later, that maybe it meant tolerating that my subjectivity would be destroyed at every new encounter with an analysand, as Ogden warns. Or, in the words of a poet:

> I am nothing
> I should always be nothing
> I can not wish anything
> Aside of that, I have within me
> all the dreams of the world.
> (Excerpt of the poem
> The Tobbaco Shop,
> Fernando Pessoa, 1928)

It still weighs upon me that the proficiency I sought to acquire would be attained at the expense of people whom I treated without being fully prepared to do it. As time went by, I was soothed by the notion that no experience can create or ensure an easier or safer path for the next experience. In this line of work, more than in any other, everything depends on the partnership established with the patient; suddenly, I understand the wisdom of your remark:

> it may perhaps turn out that in this instance the patients are not like other patients, that the laymen are not really laymen, and the doctors have not exactly the qualities which one has a right to expect of doctors and on which their claims should be based.
> (Freud, 1926, p. 184)

Now, more than forty years later, the memories and teachings of these inaugural experiences with the boy, Antonio, and with Mrs. T persist as a gold standard for me, not only because of my prejudice-free state of naiveté, which I can never recover, but because I surrendered to the experience that I consider essential in an analytical relationship; for the quality of the personal relationship that characterizes the analytical pair, for the possibility of jointly discovering a territory that is always unknown, abandoning – now, voluntarily – all the pre-established knowledge I had arduously acquired, and which I continue to try to acquire.

Rereading your article, I marvel at the clarity of the ideas, and the elegance of style with which you communicate them, synthesizing the main foundations of psychoanalysis theoretically and technically. I ponder whether my misadventures would have been smaller had I read this and other enlightening lessons[8] in psychoanalysis before beginning to explore my readings and consultations. Many of the things you observe, such as the personal conditions required to exercise psychoanalysis, the need to train more analysts who could care for more people and collaborate towards the scientific development of psychoanalysis, the respectable need of a beginning professional to work and earn a living – yes, you speak of all this frankly and naturally – these simple truths would possibly have appeased my conscience. The synthesis of the theoretical foundations of what you call profound psychology would have been an excellent study guide, and would have given direction to my readings.

But the fact is that it was not this article that introduced me to psychoanalytic literature, not even any other of your writings. My first psychoanalytic readings, due to my work with children, were texts by Klein and Winnicott suggested by my father-in-law, a wise and loving person who was also one of the first psychoanalyst in Sáo Paulo. Today, I believe that regardless of my starting point, the result would have been the same. To enter and orient oneself minimally within psychoanalytic literature, which Turilazzi Manfredi (1994, p. 9) compared to a "dense jungle of publications" (free translation)– an Amazonian jungle, I would say – was another hope I had to abandon as I approached psychoanalysis, as I studied it, practiced it, and to whose transmission I contributed, later, through the formation of new analysts: the hope of having some notion of how to acquire minimally systematic knowledge that could be articulated with other fields. Revisions, reformulations, contradictions, reservations, controversies forever came to inhabit my universe of readings and ideas, my scientific environment. Psychoanalytic trends, or vogue, as Bion (1979, p. 374) called it, in some places more than in others, in some periods more than others, went so far as to declare that Freud, i.e. your work, no longer had anything to teach to a psychoanalyst. This may or may not have been stated directly and clearly; in most cases it remained, and still does, implicit, manifesting itself as a tendency, a prevailing mentality. And to many it was enough to read summaries of your texts, or secondary literature by other authors about what you wrote, endorsing criticisms and reservations about your work without even bothering to read the originals. There were also those who did, and still do, a doctrinal reading of your texts, which I suppose you would not have appreciated.

In the postscript to your article, you describe the actual person who inspired your unbiased interlocutor as someone with a "friendly attitude and a mind of unusual integrity" (Freud, 1927, p. 251). Integrity of mind, cordial attitude, and tolerance of disagreement should be vital to scientific discussions in psychoanalysis, where the constant novelty, unpredictability, and uniqueness of clinical contributions contrast with theoretical attempts at abstraction and generalization, a profusion of them. All this makes the attempts to articulate the various conceptual points of view a constant challenge.

Your epistemological observation on the limits of each scientific field, and on the need to define the points from which we criticize a science for its limits, is so penetrating that I think it is essential to reproduce it here, applying it not to the confrontation of psychoanalysis by other fields of knowledge but to the relationship among the different streams of psychoanalytic contributions, which, when not engaging in rivalry and mutual antagonism, ignore each other:

> If it is described as one-sided, one must first discover the standpoint from which one is making that characteristic into a reproach. In itself every Science is one sided. It must be so, since it restricts to particular subjects, points of views and methods. It is a piece of nonsense in which I would take no part to play off one science against the other
>
> (Freud, 1926, p. 231)

In 1926, you mentioned that there were two institutes that trained psychoanalysts. Now, in 2016, ninety years later and considering only the IPA member organizations, there are about 136 institutes for the training of psychoanalysts distributed throughout most countries in Europe, Latin America, and North America; also in some Asian countries, such as India, Japan, and China, adding up to approximately 12,000 psychoanalysts, of which many, if not most, come from non-medical training.

Given this respectable contingent, would we then have arrived at a more favorable situation, quantitatively and qualitatively, to the growth of psychoanalysis in terms of scientific development? Psychoanalysis, in its longevity, faces a myriad of challenges and issues that need to be addressed so as to avoid a state of wayward longevity. Stefano Bolognini, in a text commemorating the hundredth anniversary of the IPA, divides these issues into questions of internal order to the psychoanalytic movement, such as the relationship among the multiple streams I mentioned previously, and questions of external order, that is, the relationship of psychoanalysis with the other sciences and culture in general:

> Concerning relations with the outside world I strongly believe that the IPA should also endeavor to be known outside its scope, and to ensure the presence and work of the analysts in various

> situations: therapeutic, cultural debate, scientific research. I simply think: "IF THE OBJECT IS NOT PRESENTED, THE SUBJECT (THE POTENTIAL PATIENT, THE MEDICAL, SOCIAL AND CULTURAL INTERLOCUTORS) CAN NOT RECOGNIZE AND ACHIEVE IT"; this is, from my point of view one of the basic problems of modern psychoanalysis, and that the IPA could at least partially remedy through a greater presence and self-presentation in the external world.
>
> (Bolognini, 2009, p. 149)

In your text, you observed a phenomenon that is increasingly true:

> Only psychiatry is supposed to deal with the disturbances of mental functions; but we know in what manner and with what aims it does so. It looks for somatic determinants of mental disorders and treats them like the other causes of illness.
>
> (Freud, 1926, p. 230)

However, psychoanalysis, in departing from medical education and from a dialogue with psychiatry, may have only exacerbated this situation of ignorance and denigration. In a way, from my point of view, very little progress has been made in medical terms towards clarifying the genesis and nature of mental illness. Biologically we remain in obscurity, with seemingly sophisticated but generic and imprecise explanations aiming at symptom relief and behavior control.

Unlike the time of my graduation, when people were ashamed to see a psychiatrist and worried about hiding this fact, psychiatry over the last four decades has become an attractive and almost glamorous specialty for both physicians and patients. A profusion of new drugs of dubious efficacy has come to be widely used by both psychiatrists and doctors, medicalizing people's emotional lives and their inherent suffering. Clinicians in all kinds of specialties use these types of medication widely, since most somatic complaints are of expressions of emotional suffering; and these, concomitant with organic diseases, apart from those admittedly psychosomatic affections.

Fewer and fewer young doctors have shown an interest in analytic training, a youth with very little curiosity, a youth that is almost not wayward at all, and that feels safe and satisfied to follow diagnostic protocols and statistical scales. There is no interest or curiosity in deepening the investigation of mental life and the factors involved in it. The old anguish neurosis, which you described so well (1894/95), now rechristened as "panic syndrome", inspires almost no one else, patient or doctor, to any further inquiry: What is the nature of these sufferings, what do they point to, and which aspects of mental life would they help us unravel? One of my analysands thus diagnosed, and medicated accordingly, could not part with his medication. He carried it with him everywhere, and held it in his hands in moments of terror; it was, according to him, his amulet. He never once opened the medicine container, never took a single pill. The psychiatrist, who continued to fill his prescriptions, never learned that. The same ignorance holds for other neuroses: hysteria, phobias, obsessions, current neuroses, and other organizations whose psychodynamics you and other leading authors have so richly and insightfully described. As you have noted, "The less such doctors understand about the matters, the more venturesome they become" (Freud, 1926, p. 232).

Bion drew attention to the issue of pain, electing it as an "element of psychoanalysis" (1963, p. 62). Mental pain differs from physical pain in several ways, and to detect it the senses are no longer sufficient. In psychoanalysis, as Bion points out, it is not enough for the physician to recognize the pain in his patient, the patient must also perceive it and be able to tolerate it and suffer it (Bion, 1970, p. 7). Nowadays, on the contrary, pain and suffering are enemies to be simply abolished.

This mentality is not restricted only to patients, who we can easily understand and forgive in their desire to obtain something that would not demand too much commitment from them, something that promised them relief without a huge investment; nor is it limited to psychiatrists, whose methods and goals would also justify this kind of short-range procedure. Unfortunately, this mentality has also reached and penetrated the activity and thinking of many analysts, who fail to recognize the material that is presented to them in this way, a material that can and should be treated psychoanalytically.[9] From my point of view, therefore, this frustrates the hope you suggest that

> in view of the intimate connection between things that we distinguish as physical and mental, we may look forward to a day

> when paths of knowledge, and let us hope of influence will be opened up leading from organic biology and chemistry to the field of neurotic phenomena.
>
> (Freud, 1926, p. 231)

Despite understanding your concern about the potential overload represented by inserting a subject like psychoanalysis in a medical school curriculum, I think everyone would benefit from this possibility, and everyone loses with this divorce between medicine and psychoanalysis: first and foremost, the patients; then, the physicians themselves, especially the generalists, to whom some fundamentals of what you call profound psychology could be very useful for purposes of diagnosis, management, and treatment. Last, but not least, psychoanalysis also loses, since fewer and fewer patients come to psychoanalysis, maligned as an old-fashioned, costly, and lengthy method, which yields few results. Or, in the words of Bolognini (2009, p. 148):

> The strong investment by health and university structures in biological-pharmacological therapies and superficial short therapies (cognitivists, behaviorists, etc.) that deceive administrators about the possibility of saving budgets, and patients about the possibility of achieving change fast, low-spending and almost no interdependence of an emotionally important object, as is an analyst (to whom the growing difficulty of motivating patients for authentic and genuine analytical treatment, currently being called "analysis" any kind of psychotherapeutic treatment and, "analyst" any therapist who has a couch (free translation).

Paraphrasing the title of your text, our question today is to find the "lay" patient, in contrast with the contingent of psychotherapists or people interested in analytic training: Who will those thousands of psychoanalysts analyze?

The experiences I had in medical school were central to me: a consideration for pain, the courage to make decisions and the need to take responsibility for them, arising from experiences I had in a medical school, although one could have such experiences in many ways, in other places. But I was also offered my first contact with psychoanalysis in medical school. Many of my colleagues, like myself, benefited from this, and devoted themselves to psychoanalysis.

Others exercise psychiatry and psychotherapy in a deep way, and based on psychoanalytic principles. Therefore, I believe that giving the conditions and tools for a future doctor to grasp the phenomena of mental life more clearly can decisively contribute to him or to her becoming a better physician, one who is more apt to perceive when a person might benefit from psychoanalysis.

Notes

1 "The first consideration is that in his medical school a doctor receives training that is more or less the opposite of what he would need as a preparation for psychoanalysis" (Freud, 1926, p. 230).

2 "A period of some two years is calculated for this training. After this period, of course, the candidate is only a beginner and not yet a master" (Freud, 1926, p. 228).

3 "On the other hand, analytic instruction would include branches of knowledge that are remote from medicine and that the doctor does not come across in his practice: the history of civilization, mythology, the psychology of religion, and the science of literature. Unless he is well at home in these subjects, an analyst can make nothing of a large amount of his material" (Freud, 1926, p. 246).

4 "A scheme of training for analysis has still to be created. It must include elements from the mental sciences, from psychology, the history of civilization and sociology, as well from anatomy, biology, and the study of evolution. There is so much to be taught in all this that it is justifiable to omit from the curriculum anything that has no direct bearing on the practice of analysis and only serves indirectly (like any other study) as a training for the intellect and for the powers of observation" (Freud, 1927, p. 252).

5 "It would be tolerable if medical education merely failed to give doctors any orientation in the field of neuroses. But it does more: it gives them a false and detrimental attitude" (Freud, 1926, p. 231)

6 "Neurotics, indeed, are an undesired complication, an embarrassment as much to therapeutics as to jurisprudence and to military service. But they exist and are a particular concern of medicine. Medical education, however, does nothing, literally nothing, towards their understanding and treatment" (Freud, 1926, p. 231).

7 *"Vereen's, dass ihr ringsum wissenschaftlich schweift, Ein jeder lernt nur, was er lernen kann." Goethe, Faust, Part I, Scene 4.* Quoted by Freud (1924–25, p. 9 n.2).

8 Particularly, Recommendations to Physicians Practising Psychoanalysis (Freud, 1912).

9 "It brings in the effect that if we are going to be landed with people like this, and we are going to be landed with them whether we like it or not, there's not good arguing about it's wrong to see patients of this kind (psychotic, seriously disturbed) because nobody else does. And sooner or later the

patient's revolt will take the form of demanding that people exist who can deal with their trouble. And the more progress we make as analysts, the more likely we are to be people who have to deal with that. Otherwise, we just fall back on drug treatment, ECT, and so on, which we are satisfied with, and obviously, the patients are dissatisfied with, or simply locking them up in hospitals from which they can't escape, and forgetting them" (Bion, 19 April 1967, in Aguayo and Malin, 2013, p. 86).

References

Aguayo, J., and Malin, B. (2013). (Eds.). *Wilfred Bion: Los Angeles Seminars and Supervision*. London: Karnac.

Bion, W.R. (1963). *Elements of Psychoanalysis*. London: Heinemann Medical Books.

Bion, W.R. (1970). *Attention and Interpretation*. London: Heinemann Medical Books.

Bion, W.R. (1979). April 1979. In: F. Bion (Ed.), *Cogitations*. London: Karnac, 1992.

Bolognini, S. (2009). Algumas idéias a respeito da IPA 100 anos após a sua fundação. *Revue Française de Psychanalyse* 43(4): 147–150.

Freud, S. (1895) The ground for detaching a particular syndrome from Neurasthenia under the description 'Anxiety neurosis'. *SE* 3: 90–116.

Freud, S. (1912). Recommendations to Physicians Practising Psychoanalysis. *SE*, 12: 11–20.

Freud, S. (1924). An Autobiographical Study. *SE* 20: 7–70.

Freud, S. (1925). Preface to Aichhorn's Verw Ahrloste Jugend. *SE* 19: 273–278.

Freud, S. (1926). The Question of Lay Analysis. *SE* 20: 179–183.

Freud, S. (1927). Post Script to the Question of Lay Analysis. *SE* 20: 251–258.

Money-Kyrle, R. (1956). Normal Counter-Transference and Some of Its Deviations. In: E. O'Shaughnessy and D. Meltzer (Eds.), *Collected Papers of Roger Money Kyrle*. Aberdeen: Clunie Press, 1978, p. 331.

Pessoa, F. (1928). The Tobacco Shop. English version by Richard Zenith. In *Fernando Pessoa and Co: Selected Poems*. New York: Grove Press, 1999.

Sandler, E.H. (2001). O nome do medo. In: *Psicanalise e Universidade* n.14 (pp. 95–109). São Paulo: Nucleo de Estudos e Pesquisa em Psicanálise. Programa de Estudos Pós-Graduados em Psicologia Clínica da PUC-SP.

Turilazzi Manfredi, S. (1994). *As certezas perdidas da psicanálise clínica*. Brazilian version by Fiorella Birolini. Rio de Janeiro: Imago Ed.

3

Who I think the layman is to Freud

Comments on Sigmund Freud's "The Question of Lay Analysis"

Jose Luiz Freda Petrucci

The "Question of Lay Analysis" was written when Theodor Reik was being prosecuted by Viennese authorities as a charlatan for practicing as a non-medical (lay) analyst. Freud advocated in defense of Reik. The paper is written in the form of a fictitious dialogue between Freud and the official responsible for the case against Reik, in an attempt to convince him that psychoanalysis can be practiced without the need for prior medical training. In doing so, he also reviews the principles of psychoanalytic methods. Here, I attempt another dialogue between Freud's legacy and the current psychoanalytic institution.

In the original text and the afterword, both from 1927, Freud reiterates his belief that a university degree does not qualify someone to be an analyst. Nevertheless, until recently, some institutes required a minimum of five full years of study at medical school. I am reminded of two cases that occurred during my training, when colleagues with degrees in psychology were required to study medicine in order to be accepted as candidates at an institute. In some cases, a graduate degree in psychiatry was even demanded, or at least advised. This, and other instances, are not in line with the thoughts or recommendations of Freud. In a study group I took part in some time ago to investigate the possibility of analyzing seriously ill patients, we became convinced that bringing the principles of psychiatry into psychoanalysis theory limited our ability to understand the emotional experiences that enable transference, and even more so what we referred to as "psychotic transference". The rational thinking required to consider the principles of psychiatry was a significant complicating factor in our efforts to direct our thoughts towards intuition (Bion, 1970, p. 24). In this respect, I became convinced that psychiatric diagnoses are becoming less and less useful in the psychoanalytic approach, once the therapeutic process has begun.

At one point in the paper Freud states emphatically that psychoanalysis is not a branch of medicine, or even medical psychology (in the old sense, of organismic psychology). At the time the paper was written, Freud was under intense pressure from the Viennese medical community, which sharply criticized his discoveries. Indeed, he puts forward a well-defined argument that this animosity implies the medical profession can have no current claim on psychoanalysis, except "from the point of view of the libido theory, upon the first or second of Abraham's substages – whether they wish to take possession of their object for the purpose of destroying it or preserving it" (Freud, 1927, p. 287). This brings me back to the old question regarding the relationship between power and psychoanalysis. Years ago I took part in a panel that discussed this relationship, which I will return to later.

Freud's opinion on lay analysis remains controversial and it is not my intention here to encourage it. I prefer to address a different issue that I imagine lies, at the very least, between the lines of "The Question of Lay Analysis": What qualities of psychoanalytic training truly qualify someone to practice psychoanalysis? And what personal qualities must someone have, or strive for, if they want to be a psychoanalyst and not merely a "lay" analyst? As such, I use the adjective "lay" here to reflect inadequate training in psychoanalysis.

- How many other things Freud said, apparently forgotten, are today hampering the development not only of psychoanalysis as a science, but the psychoanalytic institution itself, due to current conduct derived from ever-present "political correctness"? In my view, the "politically correct" often turns into something very similar to what Freud pointed out in his time: the repression of sexuality. Nowadays there is often an institutional repression of certain ideas that occurs, as Freud said, in service of the pleasure principle. I had some experience of this not long ago: when talking to a group of candidates from another institution, where I was a guest, they heavily criticized the way so-called educational analysis was performed: candidates began their personal analysis solely to comply with the regulations of the psychoanalysis institute, only to abandon it once their theoretical and clinical courses were over and the obligation had been fulfilled. Unfortunately, these assessments are rare among candidates, who will benefit most from receiving concrete psychoanalytical training.

- The dominance of "political correctness" over the quality of psychoanalytical training may be indicative of a tendency toward the formation of "lay" analysts. In other words, those who, regardless of their university qualification, do not receive adequate psychoanalytic training due to intolerance, for example, of evaluation procedures. As Freud wrote, feelings instead of arguments. Fortunately, a vice president of our institution emphatically stated in front of a large audience that the distortion of so-called training analysis is a major concern for psychoanalytical training. I refer to Freud here too: in "The Question of Lay Analysis", when referencing the resistance of political institutions to his discovery of child sexuality, he expresses regret that the institutions of the time were offended by the discovery. Freud recalls that this same sense of outrage also came to the fore whenever an institution was questioned about its mistakes. The reaction, as a whole, constitutes a large part of what I call "politically correct". Is this related to sexuality? Sexuality develops in phases, referred to as "stages" in psychoanalysis. One of the ways in which neuroses, or even more serious illnesses, take hold is by resisting the earliest stages of sexuality, forgoing evolution for more adult stages. Psychoanalytical institutions frequently see manifestations of this resistance, always in pursuit of the pleasure principle; Freud also makes reference to this as "resistance arising from the *id*". With respect to this issue, I have come to assume that many of the changes made in recent years with the stated intention of catering to "new social demands" in fact cover up, or avoid, dealing with issues such as negative or hostile transference.

- A question that Freud refers to, perhaps related to the previously mentioned point, are unsuccessful attempts at shortening analysis. This has been the focus of current concerns in pursuit of a review of psychoanalytical training. It has been clearly stated that the practice of starting therapy with the goal of satisfying institutionally imposed obligations has become commonplace. This resistance to training analysis needs to be considered in the selection process of candidates, which is often very superficial. I recognize that several institutions have tried to study the issue and establish more effective selection criteria, particularly as to whether applicants for psychoanalytic training are clearly aware of the importance of their decision. In any regard, we must agree with Freud that analysis is the best way to form an opinion regarding one's capability to practice psychoanalysis. Nevertheless, over time training analysis has become far removed from the evaluation of candidates. I have heard some analysts remark that applicants should only begin their psychoanalytic training after thoroughly exploring their capability in training analysis. Freud rightly insists that only the suffering of training analysis leads to knowledge of what it truly is.
- Let us consider what Freud writes about the possibility of an analyst's personal situation influencing the patient. This influence is the result of the analyst's personality, capable of generating admiration and even a certain measure of initial idealization. These conditions represent a powerful weapon of persuasion, since the intellectual content of explanations given to the patient will never be enough. The neurotic puts himself to work because he has faith in the analyst and believes in him because he acquires a special emotional connection with the figure of the analyst. This leads me to believe that psychoanalysis institutes should aim to provide psychoanalytic training rather than merely information on psychoanalysis. The activity of training psychoanalysts was already a concern for Freud, even at a time when he could influence the still fledgling psychoanalytic movement. Today, in the absence of Freud, the fundamental basis for the psychoanalytic institution is to represent the presence of Freud. At this point in my chapter, it is important for me to mention issues that are very much present: How are psychoanalytic institutions currently formed in terms of substituting the presence of Freud

and becoming capable of accomplishing all that Freud left us in his 1927 text? As mentioned previously, in "The Question of Lay Analysis", I feel that Freud went far beyond the professional origin of candidates for psychoanalytic training, focusing more specifically on what type of training they receive to no longer be "laymen" in psychoanalysis. This prompts me to mention a few things about the psychoanalytic institution.

- Some years ago I heard Christopher Bollas (Bollas, 2007) present the idea of a fourth active element in the Oedipal conflict. According to Bollas, in addition to the father, mother and child, the conflict also includes the family element. Based on his idea, I proposed elsewhere a fourth element, added to the triad of analytical training: in addition to training analysis, theoretical and clinical seminars and supervision, Namely, the candidate's participation (Petrucci, 2004), I feel that the psychoanalytic institution, and the candidate's participation in it, is the primary promoting element in the *training* of an analyst. Within the institution, candidates will have the opportunity to enrich their character, inasmuch as, in my view, the institution is a substitute for the presence of Freud himself. In this respect, I was encouraged to hear from an important representative of the board of the International Psychoanalytical Association that one of the current board's ideas is to improve the participation of psychoanalysis candidates in the institution as part of their training.
- The relationships between psychoanalysis and power were addressed at the 20th Brazilian Congress of Psychoanalysis[1]. My contribution to this panel was that what furnishes power to the psychoanalytical movement is the work of Freud (Petrucci, 2009). To discuss the issue, I chose the model that gives us the Oedipus conflict, since it is a universal invariant. The theory allows me to introduce a third element that, in my opinion, has a special connection both to power and psychoanalysis: the element of truth. This third element serves me well because, insofar as it does not exhibit characteristics of a thing-in-itself but rather represents a no-thing, it stimulates emotion and thought. On the other hand, within the psychoanalytical vertex, I intend to discuss non-truth, anything that aims to materialize as true but is not so. Since I exclude moral discussion, I categorize it as Column 2 on Bion's grid (Bion, 1977, p. 9).

- Column 2 signals, among other things, resistance, a well-known Freudian concept; in particular, I examined resistance to the inevitable psychic pain of psychoanalysis, both for the patient and analyst. In this I followed Bion in his article "Lies and the Thinker" (Bion, 1970, p. 107): the moral apex of a non-truth can be replaced by the scientific, psychoanalytic.
- I introduce truth because it is a defining element: outside the domain of truth, psychoanalysis does not exist. Truth and psychoanalysis are interdependent in a way that is painful because it is frustrating, but capable of promoting mental growth. My central discourse is between truth and psychoanalysis. Power is linked to one or the other at different times, with different consequences in one case or another. Following the Oedipus model created with the introduction of the third element, I have the triad Psychoanalysis-Power-Truth.
- Power should represent Freud but does not always do so. On one hand, Freud is an element I refer to as creative-persecutory. The volumes of Freud's work on our bookshelves are constantly pursuing us, accusing us of little knowledge. The power left by Freud is expressed far more in that which we cannot yet understand than in the theories we feel we do comprehend. Unlike Oedipus in the myth, who defeated the sphinx, Freud left it intact: that is the creative-persecutory power of Freud. He made us see that what we need to consider above all, therefore, is not what we know, but what we might never know. This is the model of Truth I use when pacing it as a participant in the relationship between Power and Psychoanalysis – something that will always be sought but never attained.
- When Psychoanalysis and Power combine they form a relationship in which Truth is excluded. Belonging to the universe of the abstract, Psychoanalysis only survives by tolerating frustration: Power does not tolerate it because it belongs to the domain of pleasure and feeds on this pleasure with the voracity of one seeking to possess, possess Psychoanalysis, since desire is its stimulus, but Psychoanalysis feeds on frustrated desire. Oedipus and the Sphinx come together to destroy the Sphinx, through arrogance. Truth is destroyed along with the Sphinx.
  - Evolution will be diverse when Power is dominated by Truth. This will not be a simple union, never involuntary: it depends on the attitude of those who have the Power and the

Psychoanalysis they were capable of acquiring. When searching for Truth they will be subjected to frustration and an active, conscious attitude will be needed to abdicate from desire and possession, since truth belongs to the universe of abstract things and cannot be possessed. In this space of frustration lies creativity, and Psychoanalysis can exist. The model is that of the child who, tolerating frustration, can learn from the experience of pain and tolerate the abstract, promoting mental growth, or the child that accepts frustration and exclusion, identifying with the loving relationship of his parents. In the myth the analogy would be Oedipus with Tiresias, preserving the Sphinx.

  - At this point I can formulate my thoughts in another way: Psychoanalysis as a creative act of Power subject to Truth creates a psychoanalytical movement that is equal to Psychoanalysis. However, if Psychoanalysis combines with Power and possession, the psychoanalytical movement will be without psychoanalysis.

- There have been discussions and decisions at many moments in the history of the psychoanalytical movement that serve as examples to illustrate my ideas on the training of psychoanalysts. It seems to me that Freud's "Lay Analysis" suggests, or at least that is how I interpret his work, that the real difference between a layman and a psychoanalyst is the training they were able to receive and not any instruction obtained beforehand.
- At times I came to think that the ideas I heard aimed to make psychoanalytic treatment more straightforward, less complex: when sessions become "low frequency" the assertion of less complexity is at least suggested. For example, it is said that psychoanalysis can be done with three weekly sessions, and I agree. For a truly "psychoanalytical" psychoanalyst, psychoanalysis will be so intertwined with his convictions that it will be difficult to do anything other than psychoanalysis. At this point in the somewhat sterile (in my view) discussion, I do not address "how many weekly sessions are needed" because the issue is far greater: the greater the frequency, the greater the chance of developing fundamental aspects of the psychoanalytic technique. As such, the assertion that one can do "low frequency" analysis is an affirmation that can be qualified under column 2 of Bion's grid. In other words, something we

know not to be true (Bion, 1963). In my view, it involves avoiding painful discussions for both patient and analyst: about the value of psychoanalysis; what type of gratification the analyst seeks in treating his patients; the value analysts attribute to their patients in terms of pursuing "health"; the personal availability of analysts in valuing their patients' need of them as opposed to unilaterally deciding they can facilitate treatment by resolving, also in a unilateral decision, that the patient does not need him "that much"; about how much suffering (inevitable, in order to use all the psychoanalytical instruments available today) the analyst is willing (or able) to endure.

- With respect to frequency, if proposals for amending the so-called minimum requirements for doing psychoanalysis are justified by "economic reasons", I once again appeal to Freud when raising my objections: How could he have ensured the survival of psychoanalysis through two wars that devastated Europe without suggesting that the psychoanalytic technique be "adapted" to those difficult times?
- Psychoanalysis subject to Power, according to my previously mentioned hypothesis, has allowed psychoanalytical institutions to exert significant influence on the training analysis of candidates in training. In pursuit of power, institutions tend to thirst for candidates, and the manner in which they satisfy this craving means many candidates become more committed to the institution than their self-analysis. This is the case of the situations described previously, where candidates admit to submitting to training analysis for the time required by the institution, and no longer. Certain institutional regulations, such as this one, often prompt "acting out" that is difficult to manage. This leads me to think of the range of "psychoanalyses" without psychoanalysis that this could lead to. As a colleague of mine said after I asked him to read and critique the work I cite here: "The institution and training analysts need patients more than those same patients need psychoanalysis". As such, many of the formats adopted in the so-called diffusion of psychoanalysis can become the diffusion of desire, the same desire that, without suppression, the oracle stimulated in Oedipus. In many cases, disclosure offers the easy yet inadequate and, consequently, vulgarization. It is not uncommon for institutions to base their worth on the number of candidates

they have and training analysts to judge their "prestige" according to the number of candidates they are analyzing.

- Based on the general opinion regarding qualification, the only person capable of qualifying, or not, as a psychoanalyst is the psychoanalyst himself, which significantly increases the need for adequate training analysis.
- In conclusion, I feel that psychoanalysis, the fruit of the desire to possess, obtains the thing-in-itself "qualification" or "supposed to know" from a theory not learned through the (emotional) experience. It stops being psychoanalytical psychoanalysis. The Sphynx is destroyed. Possession causes disaster. The psychoanalytical movement destroys psychoanalysis. It is strange that this is so rarely considered when attempting to understand why the demand for psychoanalysis has declined in most countries.

Note

1 Official panel on "Psychoanalysis and power": XX Congress of the Brazilian Federation of Psychoanalytical Socieities- FEBRAPI, Brasilia.

References

Bion, W.R. (1963). Elementos de Psicanálise. Brazilian version by Ester Hadassa Sandler and Paulo Cesar Sandler. Rio de Janeiro: Imago ed., 2003.

Bion, W.R. (1970). Atenção e Interpretação, Brazilian version by Paulo Cesar Sandler. Rio de Janeiro: Imago ed., 2007.

Bion, W.R. (1977). *Two Papers: The Grid and Caesura*. Rio de Janeiro: Imago ed.

Bollas, C. (2007). *Lecture in Jornada Annual do Centro de Estudos Luiz Guedes, Universidade Federal do Rio Grande do Sul, Sociedade Psicanalitica de Porto Alegre.*

Freud, S. (1927). The Question of Lay Analysis. *SE*, XX: 179–258.

Petrucci, J.L.F. (2004). O Tripé. *Paper presented in the Scientific Meeting of Sociedade Brasileira de Psicanálise de Porto Alegre*, August 3, 2004 (recorded in tape).

Petrucci, J.L.F. (2009). Psicanálise e Poder, *Revista de Psicanálise de Sociedade Brasileira de Psicanálise de Porto Alegre*, 11: 135.

4

Some notes about alike applications of psychoanalysis

Irina Panteleeva

The main object of this chapter is a single quotation from Freud's *A Question of Lay Analysis*, or to be more exact, from his *Postscript* to it. This quotation has had high probability to remain in the peripheral area of Freud's heritage, but also there is some evidence in support of its being just an ugly duckling among his ideas, and the time has come for it to develop into a beautiful swan. Our aim is to draw attention to a possibility of application of scientific psychoanalysis to various fields of human activity, with *all* those applications being of similar value and prestige. In other words, it seems like an interesting intellectual exercise to think of reasons why Freud's idea that "the true line of division is between scientific analysis and its applications *alike* in medical and in non-medical fields" (Freud, 1926, p. 257, italics added) still resides mainly in the realm of logical truths, and does not attract a substantial amount of energy to become a vigorous practical endeavor.

To explore this idea of psychoanalysis as a science with *alike* applications, especially with the view of the role of lay analysis and analysts in mind, we start with comparing it with some other definitions of psychoanalysis. Freud's well-known statements of what psychoanalysis is could be difficult to integrate into a single notion, as they might show psychoanalysis from rather incompatible points of view. In his *Lay Analysis*, for instance, Freud gives us a picture of the profession in which there are not many reasons for domination of medical specialists, as "doctors have no historical claim to the sole possession of analysis" (1926, p. 229) and moreover, "doctors form a preponderating contingent of quacks in analysis" (p. 230). However, in his *Postscript* to this work, a year later, he significantly softens his expression of desirability of doctors as analysts, saying that people with an education in medicine "are the best material for future analysts" (p. 257). And then, almost at the end of his *Postscript* and seemingly in parenthesis follows the statement that the habitual distinction between medical and applied analysis was made only for practical reasons, but "that is not a logical distinction" (p. 257), and then Freud introduces his vision of "the true line of division", around which our current interest centers.

It is not suggested here that we may discover how much weight Freud himself ascribed to this distinction and to the possibility of *alike* of application and whether it was for him of some profound importance or just a minor comment he would make among other things. In favor of exploring this particular statement's context and implications there are at least a few arguments. First of all, seemingly light-weighted and peripheral comments happen too often to be the most revealing and emotionally charged. Freud himself advised as early as in 1913 against disregarding as something less meaningful what is said outside of "an official portion" of the session (p. 139). It is highly probable that addressing this text to an analytically literate audience Freud might have expected them to read his parenthetical comments with such analytical attention. Besides that, another attempt to put together different partial views of what psychoanalysis is or should be has good chances not to harm psychoanalysis but to make a contribution to integrity and maturity of the profession.

We will look in some detail at different implications of Freud's messages concerning lay analysis with the purpose to compare how this message can be read differently by medical analysts, lay analysts, or their patients. The initial hypothesis is that there must be a deeper and more complex play of forces besides the obvious division into a group of medical analysts who favor the idea that they are "the best material for future analysts", a group of lay analysts, who believe that " doctors form a preponderating contingent of quacks", and their patients, whose transference is inevitably influenced by their own and their therapist's reading of the message. Based on this discussion of the message itself, we will compare two lines of historical development in psychoanalysis: one that exemplifies the division between lay and medical analysis, favoring either of them, and one that tends to conform to the notion of the division between psychoanalysis as a science and its *alike* applications, with the aim to demonstrate the advantages and promising nature of the second one.

Freud's message about alike applications

Let's take a closer look at our central figure's background. It's origin is quite humble: it belongs to a work written, according to Freud himself, as "a piece of polemics written for a special occasion" (Freud and Pfister, 1963, p. 105); and it resides at the end of *Postscript* between a cynical joke about women and a couple of final paragraphs discussing practical reasons of American rejection of lay analysis. However, it's wording is ambitious, aspiring to give us a rare and succinct statement of the essence of psychoanalysis:

> For practical reasons we have been in the habit – and this is true, incidentally, of our publications as well – of distinguishing between medical and applied analysis. But that is not a logical distinction. The true line of division is between scientific analysis and its applications alike in medical and in non-medical fields.
>
> (Freud, 1926, p. 257)

We cannot say that this dictum was totally neglected in psychoanalytical literature, but there is an impression that it did not have enough or proper attention, especially when the authors dealt specifically with the question of either lay or applied analysis. For example, we do not find it in Wallerstein (1998), which is probably the most detailed narration of the history of lay analysis. This quotation also cannot be found in Esman (1998), which may be the most discussed paper about applied psychoanalysis besides Freud's works because it was selected for an open Internet discussion on the IJPA's website. Reading Esman (1998) does not make clear if the author will use or comment on this quote at all until the very end of his paper, when he concludes it with an earlier and less peripherally placed passage from Freud (1926):

> the use of analysis for treatment of neuroses is only one of its applications; the future will perhaps show that it is not the most important one.
>
> (p. 248)

Other authors, for example Bell (1999), Camden (2009), Oyer (2016), do cite it in various contexts, but without making it their main focus. The author who does start his paper directly with this quotation (Pigman, 1992), seemingly uses it to stress that he does not share Freud's optimism at least about the near future of applied analysis. Bell (1999), however, makes a point that psychoanalytic treatment is "an *application* of psychoanalysis and is not coextensive with it" and calls this distinction crucial (p. 3), which give us some support in our interest in this particular statement of Freud's.

Even if it is probable that Freud himself did not give much weight to the passage under discussion and did not think of it as something important, it still may be an interesting and productive investigation to look at its context and implications. Firstly, Freud himself would hardly discard something as unimportant just because it looked like a parenthetical comment to the main discourse, in the same way as he recommended to integrate into the session the patient's "informal 'friendly' portion" of communication with his doctor just before or after the session (Freud, 1913, p. 139). He might have also kept in mind and addressed that big part of his readers who would have some acquaintance with psychoanalysis and psychoanalytical situation and an ear tuned to such nuances of partitioning of the discourse. Secondly, even if this was not Freud's intention mainly or at all, the wording of this passage seems so deep and beautiful and it's positioning in the text is quite intriguing, that we cannot help but proceed with exploring its meaning further.

As for the position of this quote, it may be worth mentioning that this is not the only work of Freud's where he puts a quite important statement somewhere at the end of the work and seemingly in parenthesis, or without a strong overt connection with the main topic of the work or its concluding part. At the end of *The*

Future of an Illusion, Freud starts a very short paragraph of only two lines saying that "no, our science is no illusion" (1927, p. 56). As the work is commonly perceived as showing *religion* as an illusion, it is a rather unexpected conclusion. The more predictable would be something of "yes, religion is an illusion etc.", and it makes us wonder if the question of whether *psychoanalysis* is an illusion (and what its future is) was the main issue that bothered Freud that time as well as the main but undisclosed topic of his work which we tend to read as a paper about the illusory nature and the future of religion. Freud wrote to Pfister about a secret link between these too works:

> I do not know if you have detected the secret link between *[The Question of] Lay Analysis* and *[The Future of an] Illusion*. In the former, I wish to protect analysis from the doctors and in the latter from the priests. I should like to hand it over to a profession which does not yet exist, a profession of lay curers of souls who need not be doctors and should not be priests.
>
> (Freud and Pfister, 1963, p. 126)

Dufresne, as he put it, "have taken pains to expose the textual and thematic connections between *Lay Analysis* (and its 'Postscript') and the *Future*" (2017, p. 58). Here we add an additional link between these two works, which is a stylistic device of unexpected concluding remarks that retrospectively change the reading of the whole preceding text.

Another rhetorical device used by Freud in his addressing the problem of lay analysis is worth mentioning as well. The main question of *Lay Analysis* is apparently if lay analysts should be allowed to practice it at all and whether they can be good enough analysts. Let's repeat here a condensed version of Freud's answers to these questions throughout the text of *Lay Analysis*, which read as follows:

1 "doctors form a preponderating contingent of quacks in analysis" (p. 230)
2 doctors "are the best material for future analysts" (p. 257)
3 distinction between medical and applied analysis "is not a logical distinction" (p. 257)

The peculiarity of this sequence of arguments is better seen in comparison with other descriptions or definitions of psychoanalysis made by Freud in many different ways. There is an academic definition, which he wrote in *Two Encyclopedia Articles* (1923), where he states that the name of psychoanalysis refers to an investigation procedure, a method of treatment, and a collection of information (p. 235), with each part of this threefold definition in no contradiction to each other. In other cases, Freud gives us definitions that on the surface look quite incompatible with each other, but usually he writes them in different places, and does not put them together in one piece of work. For example, Szasz (2004) lists eleven quotes from seven different works of Freud's that speak of psychoanalysis as a medical procedure, and again eleven quotes but from only four different sources that say that psychoanalysis is not a medical procedure (pp. 28–30). In *Lay Analysis* and its *Postscript*, Freud used rather incompatible arguments in one and the same place. He gives the main place to the first argument, then adds the second argument in *Postscript* to soften the first one, and then right after it or even in the middle of it comes our statement under discussion about the logical distinction between scientific analysis and its applications. Adding the latter statement shifts the whole line of reasoning to resemble the kettle logic from one of Freud's favorite jokes. To the accusation of teaching analysis to lay people (returning a damaged kettle), we have three different answers. First, lay analysts are not a preponderating contingent of quacks (the kettle was returned undamaged); second, doctors, not lay people, are our best material (the kettle was originally damaged); and finally, it's not logical to separate analysis into medical and non-medical (the kettle was not borrowed at all).

We understand that we may never know if Freud enjoyed this rhetorical analogy with a purpose in mind and if he himself considered the above reading as a valid intellectual exercise. We hoped that such exercise in reading a piece of a classical text might be productive and interesting by itself, as it draws attention to the subtle complexities of Freud's thought, as well as might provide us a ground from which we can go further and discuss some underlying phantasies in reading and reacting to Freud's message of either lay or applied analysis in relation to different categories of its readers, such as medical doctors, lay specialists, and their patients.

Freud's message about alike applications: how it is read

Doctors' resistance to psychoanalysis and lay analysis as a part of it has been scrutinized and discussed almost as comprehensively as resistance of their patients to the psychoanalytical process. In the early days of psychoanalysis, as Freud put it, they "met it with everything possible that could damage it" (1926, p. 229). Then, from Theodor Reik's being sued by his former patient in 1926, to the heated debates with the following lawsuit against the American Psychoanalytic Association in the 1980s, this resistance attracted more and more attention. In the light of the lawsuit the main interest focused on whether the reason for doctors' resistance to lay analysis was their financial interest or genuine care about high standards of the practice. The controversy started to lose its importance when the settlement agreement was signed, and seems to have become a historical fact some years after that. Initially, the views were highly polarized. Freud expressed his concern that the demand that only doctors can practice analysis can be "after all only a slightly modified derivative of the earlier attitude" (1926, p. 183). Summarizing Freud's position, his biographer Gay (1988) says that Freud "did not hesitate to question his opponents' motives; resistance to lay analysis, he charges, was really resistance to analysis in general" (p. 493). Gay, however, calls such verdict "facile and tendentious", and appeals to the "stature, and the arguments, of psychoanalysts on the other side" (p. 493), who had to "decisively distance themselves from all charlatans" (p. 497).

Returning to our three parts of Freud's message, we may say that however questionable it is to equal lay analysts with charlatans, we can leave this issue more or less peacefully in the past, as well as hope that nowadays there are not many "quacks" among doctors to make a real difference. Also, the difference between logical and practical distinction of different kinds of analysis may not be of high relevance to the majority of practitioners. The second point of the best material and doctors' attitude to it seem to be still relevant nowadays and in lack of due attention. There is an old Russian saying about the guelder rose that boasts that it is good with honey, with honey's answer that it is good itself, without any guelder rose. When psychoanalysis is not allowed to be an independent and independently taught discipline without necessary or highly recommended medical (or even psychological) education, it becomes a guelder rose of therapy. Such restriction undermines its independent value. Besides, a medical diploma never was a guarantee of highest moral standards. We should not forget that Freud illustrated his point of "best material" by a joke about women, in which they were called "the best thing of the kind" (1926, p. 257). Recalling that Freud's attitude to women in general was rather condescending, we may see an ironic connotation of his "best material" remark. Linking psychoanalytical education with initial medical training exemplifies ambivalence towards psychoanalysis: on the one hand, it should be protected from intruders as something of great prestige, on the other hand, it is not encouraged to be taught and subsequently practiced without support of preliminary therapeutic background as if it cannot be substantial and productive by itself. And even if doctors can be "the best material", it does not follow that they automatically become the best analysts.

Motives of lay analysts as a *group* seem to be never scrutinized with such vigor as doctors' motives, which is quite surprising. They are presumed to be straightforward and sincerely willing to make an honest living or express their passion for psychoanalysis by making it their job. At least in Wallerstein (1998), we were not able to find mention of a discussion of their motives, in full contrast to the debates about lay people's fitness or desirability to be allowed to study and practice. It does not make their way in psychoanalysis less free from hidden pitfalls compared with that of doctors. As there is not much research in this area done until now, we can only list some of the underlying problems that may stem from the complexity of Freud's message to them. The first problem is that Freud might have unwillingly projected his personal unresolved problems in relation to the medical profession or academia into the group of lay analysts. In many instances, he defined analysis as a medical procedure (Szasz, 2004, pp. 28–29), but at the same time he encouraged non-doctors to be his followers, and legally it is one thing for a doctor to practice a new treatment, and it is absolutely a different thing for a non-doctor to declare that he or she has learned the new method and it gives them the right to treat patients. Promised by stimulating the interest and ambitions, but limited in availability, legally or organizationally, the "forbidden fruit" of the profession becomes more attractive than it may be in case of a general agreement about their role in psychoanalysis. Additionally, excessive energy is spent, apart of dealing with legal issues, on competing with doctors in the diagnostics and treatment of symptoms as well as in trying to adjust to marginalized research positions and areas designated to them in established academic institutions, energy that can find better use if lay analysts concentrate on their own ways to be successful in their practice and research.

Patients' fantasies about their analysts have been studied thoroughly, but, again, it does not seem that there has been enough research done in the area of their initial choice of medical or non-medical analysts. Freud does not make the choice between medical or non-medical analysts an easy one for a prospective patient. If the patient chooses the medical one, he risks to be treated by one of the "preponderating contingent of quacks in analysis", but if he is inclined to choose a lay analysts, he may fear that his analyst will not be one of the "best material". Those who favor the idea of lay analysis could use Freud's argument that "the possession of a medical diploma does not impress them [patients] nearly so much as doctors believe" (1926, p. 255). Their opponents' general idea is that "the person who walks into the consulting room of a psychoanalyst with the problems we see in daily practice cannot be properly diagnosed or treated by anyone lacking medical and psychiatric training" (Wallerstein, 1998, p. 282). Their position seems to agree with Freud's one in relation to diagnosis, as he insisted "that in every case which is under consideration for analysis the diagnosis shall be established first by a doctor" (1926, p. 243). However, nowadays several authors speak either of limits to the utility of diagnosis (for example, McWilliams, 2011, pp. 18–19) or express a more critical warning that "the power to give names to our pain is a mighty thing and easy to abuse" (Greenberg, 2013, p. 4). Among patients there are, of course, those who still come to analysis to be cured from a symptom, but also there are others, and their number seems to have a tendency to grow, who come into analysis not with a feeling that they need to be cured but with a wish to understand better themselves and the world around them, and already as early as in 1912 Freud spoke about "more than one advantage" of becoming a psychoanalytic patient "without being driven to it by illness" (1912, pp. 116–117). For a practically healthy person, diagnostic skillfulness may not be a priority quality of their analyst, and even may go against their conscious or unconscious image of an ideal analyst who, among other things, does not pathologize patients.

Another interesting development may result from Freud's way to present in *Lay Analysis* the main theoretical tenets of psychoanalysis. He does it by using his theory of psychosexuality. For the theoretical introduction to a highly controversial topic of lay analysis he picks up his no less controversial sexual theory (instead of, for example, less objected interpretation of parapraxes and dreams, as he did in his *Introductory Lectures* (Freud, 1916–17)). For his contemporaries, this brave disclosure to the impartial reader of the existence of transference-love and a technique of resolving it for the purposes of treatment helps Freud to persuade his readers to believe him that a person who has learned the technique of dealing with the transference is "no longer a layman" (1926, p. 228). As for the future generations of his readers, this focus on transference-love could be misleading. While specialists are aware of many other forms of transference, an ignorant prospective patient may believe that this transference-love not only "happens in every case" (Freud, 1926, p. 226) but must and needs to happen. Such belief is illustrated by a comical and at the same time sad situation described by Greenson (1967), in which a patient asks when she was "supposed to fall in love" with him (p. 285). Among many forms of transference, to the question of lay analysis is rather relevant the one when a patient "finds the analysis of the doctor more interesting than his own" (Freud, 1912, p. 118), that is, the patient wants to analyze or cure his analyst. Searles (1979) advances a hypothesis that "in transference terms, the patient's illness is expressive of his unconscious attempt to cure the doctor" (p. 381). Expecting an erotic transference to be the main vehicle of the treatment puts the transference in the form of wishing to analyze the doctor or to become an analyst in danger of being overlooked and insufficiently analyzed as a valuable transference, both in medical or non-medical patients, with probably different consequences though. Without proper analytical attention, a transferential wish to cure might push lay specialists towards healing jobs for the wrong reasons or at least their healing energy would be impaired by the transference resistance to its full undistorted use. In medical analysands, this transference wish to cure has even more chances to be overlooked, as their healing aptitude might be taken for granted as something one hundred percent healthy, and thus its unanalyzed part will reappear again and again in countertransference with some adverse effects for their patients.

Another peculiarity of Freud's message may be called a psychoanalytic Barber's paradox. It could affect all categories of his readers, but the analysands who read his *Lay Analysis* could be more prone to misinterpret it. Here we are speaking about Freud's ideas of training analysis as prerequisite of becoming an analyst. Hardly anyone can disagree with this requirement, which Freud repeated in many instances, including his *Lay Analysis*, if we are right that his notion of "particular training" (1926, p. 233) which he demands implies having a personal training analysis. However, it is obvious that Freud himself, being the first analyst ever, could not have been analyzed by someone else in proper training analysis, and we do not encounter any of his published texts where he discussed how this lack of personal analysis hindered his work with a patient, but in spite of that he still remains our indisputable model analyst. To identify with the father of psychoanalysis in an easy shortcut way, it might be quite tempting at least to think that breaking a rule would bring a long-desired cure. That tendency was discussed in psychoanalytic literature (for example, Gabbard, 2003; Sandler and Godley, 2004), but the importance of alertness to this temptation is difficult to overestimate.

With all these nuances discussed we may say that neither of the preceding categories of readers in general has motives or interest in taking Freud's comment of equality of application of psychoanalysis more or less seriously into their consideration. It's logical truthfulness does not seems to correlate either with the conscious or unconscious picture of what psychoanalysis is or what they can do with it. However, we should not be discouraged yet but look at what is going on in the practical area, and whether this notion of alike application of psychoanalysis is as peripheral or alien to it as it is to the conceptual domain. First, we will have a look at the practical ways of its unequal application, and then explore some quite rare but very promising attempts to apply it in agreement with Freud's statement of possible and desirable equal application.

Inequality in application

To evaluate the weight or amount of an application, it would be reasonable at this point to clarify application of what and what kind of application itself we speak here of. In the quote under discussion, Freud wrote about "scientific analysis and its applications alike" (1926, p. 257). For our purposes, the question of what kind of science psychoanalysis is or whether it is a science at all would be both rather irrelevant here and too distracting in its complexity. In order to narrow down our use of the term "scientific analysis" we propose to mean by it mainly whatever Freud himself meant by it. Bell (1999) comments to this quote that "[b]y 'scientific' Freud is referring to the theoretical structure of that body of knowledge that constitutes psychoanalysis" (p. 3) and we can use it as our working definition for the present purposes.

As for the type of application, we will try to avoid using the term "applied psychoanalysis" as it has undesirable connotations of superiority of psychoanalysis over the areas it is applied to and superiority of "pure gold" clinical psychoanalysis over the less valuable "alloy" of applied one, as well as associations with the division between pure theoretical and applied practical sciences. Further, we will avoid as irrelevant here the question of the direction of the application, that is, if psychoanalysis really is applied to another science, or vice versa. Instances of this opposite direction of application are discussed, for example, by Bell (1999) when he speaks about Freud's application of group psychology *to* psychoanalysis (p. 4), or in Esman (1998), with a similar view of application of data of Freud's own dreams to the theory of psychoanalysis, as well as a number of other illustrations. Making the meaning of "to apply" as "to have relevance or a valid connection" (Merriam-Webster online dictionary) our main meaning of the work would allow us to eliminate at least this terminological potential of inequality.

Even with this possibility of equally directed application, it is reasonably safe to say that clinical psychoanalysis prevails in prestige in the eyes of both psychoanalysts themselves and of general public, as well as in number of its practitioners and profoundness of its work. It is still firmly associated with "pure gold" (Freud, 1919, p. 167). At least, we would hardly imagine a paper in psychoanalytic literature devoted to a topic of necessity or urgency to return to clinical offices and to spend less energy on interdisciplinary research or other extra-clinical activities, while there is a number of papers encouraging clinical and extra-clinical research (for example, Kernberg, 2006; Leuzinger-Bohleber et al., 2006). It is true that "fewer and fewer practice long-term psychoanalysis characterized by frequent sessions" (Eisold, 2005, p. 1183), and in this way tend to shift from the area of psychoanalysis to psychotherapy. Formally these therapists shift from the area of pure analysis to less elitist psychotherapy, but it does not seem to reduce dramatically the number of psycho-dynamic psychotherapists who would still and with valid reasons name themselves psychoanalysts. As for profoundness of clinical work accompanied by theoretical advances of psychoanalysis, of course, there are works of different level and importance in this domain as everywhere, but as a whole it has surely come a long way since its early days and achieved admirable results. Applied published works were criticized rather severely though. There is an opinion that the further psychoanalysis "strays from the clinical situation, the more problematic it becomes" (Pigman, 1992, p. 299), or that "psychoanalytic literary criticism has always been something of an embarrassment" (Brooks, 1987, p. 334). A book on applied topics, despite the importance of the aspects discussed in it, was not recommended by an official reviewer to general public because, among other things, the parallels between the studied area and clinical practice "are faintly drawn" (Thomson, 1984, p. 395). One of the answers to such critical attitude is given by Rustin (2017), who suggests that instead of focusing on "sociologists who might have developed a psychoanalytic perspective, but who didn't", the authors of the book he reviews could discuss "the work of the leading sociological figures who did successfully achieve this synthesis" (p. 5). Rustin suggests several names of the prominent thinkers of the past and present, and concludes that "all these writers have had a major impact on social thought" (p. 5), and his optimistic attitude give us a strong impression that the number of good works in the areas where psychoanalysis is applied is not that big as in the clinical area, but there are a few of them that make the whole idea of connecting psychoanalysis with other disciplines worth the efforts.

Besides unequal application of psychoanalysis as a whole to different other areas, there are also some interesting aspects of unequal distribution of forces among psychoanalytic human resources. In spite of Freud's overt support of lay analysts in his *Lay Analysis*, as Schröter (2004) suggests, the early lay analysts entered clinical sphere "contrary to the original intentions of Freud" (p. 164) who wanted them to be university lecturers (p. 166) or psychoanalytic researches in non-medical areas (p. 165). Freud supported their analytical careers only when it was clear that it was difficult for them to secure their living with other jobs and thus they "must not be left out in the cold" (p. 164). For medical analysts it was a matter of fact that they could and were welcomed to practice analysis, but for non-medical ones it was more an exception due to special circumstances. While neither of them was either interested in or able to secure a position as a researcher or full-time lecturer, only lay analysts' way to clinical practice was perceived as their failure in other areas. Medical analysts felt at home in clinical analysis from the beginning, but lay analysts had to put additional efforts to go against different forces pushing them away from it.

Related to it is another inequality of distribution of patients which are considered proper for lay and medical analysts, respectively. Again, since the early days, the analysis that lay analysts were allowed to practice with the least reluctance was child and didactic analysis. For some reasons "pedagogic child analysis" (p. 168) did require less medical knowledge that analysis of adults, and for many years "didactic analyses were viewed as non-therapeutic, i.e. non-medical" (p. 165). It was the case not only in Freud's time, but much later in America, when, according to Wallerstein (1998), in the middle of the last century a number of non-medical training analysts were not allowed to become members of the American Psychoanalytic Association, but were allowed to analyze candidates and treat wives and children of its members (p. 103), and even in their local institutes they obtained membership "only with the stipulation that they only teach and do training analysis" (p. 104). In other words, as Wallerstein put it, they were not eligible to join the national association "which was open to their students" (p. 104). A particular restrictive pressure was exerted on the lay analysts' choice of patients, either supposedly belittling them by limiting their load of patients to children or elevating them to teaching status only, but one way or another pushing them away as much as possible from a prospect of equal status with medical analysts.

Ways of alike application

Besides the main application of psychoanalysis to medicine in the form of its clinical practice or "pure psychoanalysis" or its diluted variant of various psycho-dynamic psychotherapies, there is one more and quite promising way of its medical application, namely Balint groups. We do not know whether Michael Balint himself was interested in the equality in application of psychoanalysis in accordance with the quotation under discussion here, but for sure he was "a keen exponent of the value of the application of psychoanalytic principles and insight to other fields of medical and social practice" (Haynal, 1988, p. 92). Balint was "one of the pioneers of the positive use of the counter-transference" (Elder et al., 2003, p. 84), and his "premise was any emotion felt by the physician in treating a patient should be considered a symptom of the illness" (Haynal, 1988, p. 92). He wanted to create "a training to general practitioners that would bring about limited though considerable change in doctor's personality, allowing a better understanding of the doctor-patient relationships" (Haynal, 1988, pp. 92–93). His seminars and workshops in the 1950s and 1960s evolved in establishing a number of Balint groups all around the world, united by such organizations as the International Balint Association, the Balint Society in the UK, the American Balint Society and many others. There is no need to idealize this particular way of applying psychoanalysis. Its implementation has its own difficulties. For example, "the use of Balint groups attenuates significantly after physicians graduate from residency" (O'Sullivan et al., 2016, p. 42). However, these difficulties, properly analyzed, seem to make the idea of Balint groups even stronger and a perfect illustration of what Freud might have wanted to see as an equal application of psychoanalysis to various other disciplines.

Another important application of psychoanalysis, which looks like the most promising among equals, is the application to education. Freud himself stressed its importance and possible fruitfulness. In his lectures (Freud, 1933), he says that the application of psychoanalysis to education "to the upbringing of the next generation" is "so rich in hopes for the future, perhaps the most important of all activities of analysis" (p. 146). In particular, he speaks of prophylactic analysis "as a measure for safeguarding his health"

(p. 148), which should be combined with "a certain amount of analytic influencing of his parents" (p. 148). However, he stresses that "the analysis of teachers and educators seems to be a more efficacious prophylactic measure than the analysis of children themselves, and there are less difficulties in the way of putting it into practice" (p. 150).

With this optimistic outlook we opened the volume of *Journal of Applied Psychoanalytic Studies* (July 2002), which was a special issue devoted to the topic of psychoanalysis and education of children. It includes a presentation of three programs with their discussion. It is stated that these programs "provide fine examples of psychoanalysis as applied to the field of education" (Golland, 2002, p. 281). The first program "provides consultation for teachers in dealing with children with behavioral problems", the second one gives "a specific intervention aimed at preventing violence in inner-city youngsters" and the third one "provides a curriculum and a training program for interested teachers" (p. 281). They are reported to be successful "with different populations, in different states" (p. 279), with the third program being a more successful "than most in selling itself and that fact deserves applause" (p. 279). However, the discussion of these programs by Golland, published in the same volume, contains rather disturbing points. The title of Golland's paper is "What Do Teachers Want (From Psychoanalysts)?", and the answer we receive there is "that what most teachers want of applied psychoanalysis" is "free, long-term consultation and support for exclusion" (p. 277) and that "many teachers are unlikely to agree to additional professional development without immediate and concrete incentive" (p. 279). It is unclear why such an oversimplified picture of teachers became the result of the implementation of these programs and whether such vision influenced the teachers' reluctance to implement them in the first place, as well as why the programs were not addressed specifically to the teachers who had less cautious interest in psychoanalysis. Another disquieting feature of these programs is that they deliberately omit "talking about sex and death", because it "would risk wearing out the welcome of psychoanalysis in schools" (p. 280). Firstly, we agree with Freud's warning against partial use of psychoanalysis and the "buffer-layer" between analysis and its opponents, which "consists of people who allow the validity of some portions of analysis" but "on the other hand reject other portions of it" (Freud, 1933, p. 138). Secondly, from that discussion it is not clear whether the authors of the programs tend to at least partly equate using, for instance, the theory of Oedipus complex as the operational instrument of the educators involved in application of psychoanalysis and speaking about it directly with their students.

In the same volume of the *Journal of Applied Psychoanalytic Studies* we also feel lucky to find an interesting case presentation, as such presentations of applied cases seem to be published in less abundance than vignettes from the work of clinical psychoanalysts. Kusché (2002) illustrates the work of one of the programs by an example of how, according to the author, "the teacher modeled an analytic process" (p. 288). We discuss it here in an attempt to overcome our problem that we have difficulties in seeing that it was psychoanalysis and not something else that was applied there, even if it was "a delightful experience" (p. 287) and the author concludes that all children, with the teacher and the author as well, learned a lot from that experience. We understand that there is a general difficulty in presenting the subtlety of therapeutic work. Sandler and Sandler (1984) called it the "major task for future researcher to discover why the transcribed material of the other analysts' sessions often makes one feel that they are very bad analysts" (p. 396). It seems that this difficulty is quite persistent and applied to descriptions of applied psychoanalytic cases as well. Thomä et al. (2012, p. 27) addressed this problem in relation to clinical practice, and hopefully there will be some research dealing with the same issues in applies analysis. For the time being, we just make some remarks about this vignette with a view to increase interest in discussing such cases and related research work.

The example presents the work of a therapeutic preschool classroom. The lesson starts with the following incident:

> On that particular day, the lesson was "Proud and Ashamed". This was also Bobby's turn to be the PATHS Kid. He was excited and had hidden a secret toy in his sock as a surprise for his fellow classmates. Bobby had shared his secret with Jerry, with his explicit instruction that he not tell anybody else. Jerry, however, immediately disclosed the secret aloud to the teacher, which was heard by the entire class. Bobby's feelings were hurt and he

> left the group with the announcement that he no longer wanted to be the PATHS Kid. Jerry looked pleased.
>
> (Kusché, 2002, p. 287)

Then we are given a brief story of what happened next. The teacher "explained the dynamics", that is that Jerry hurt his friend's feelings, "showed the class 'ashamed face' ", "read the definition of ashamed", and as a result Jerry "began to empathize with Bobby" (p. 287). The author concludes that Jerry learned to control better his impulses and Bobby learned to talk about his experience instead of running.

The author starts her discussion of the example and what is psychoanalytic with a definition of the psychoanalytical mode of therapeutic action by Cohen, according to which it is "the revival of unrecognized meanings and structures that yield new integrations" (p. 288). However valid, productive and substantiated this approach may be, we still have an impression that this presentation could give us in this case of applied psychoanalysis more evidence of psychoanalysis in its more traditional sense and less resemblance with the usual, non-therapeutic, and non-psychoanalytic approach of a teacher. From this vignette we cannot understand what were unconscious motives or intrapsychic conflicts of two boys. Was Bobby unconsciously projecting his unwillingness to be a PATHS Kid into his friend by telling him the secret? Why did they acted out these scene right at the beginning of the lesson called "Proud and Ashamed"? Was it their enactment of the anticipated topic of the lesson and in this way Jerry unconsciously tried to help the teacher? Why did the teacher stress only "ashamed" part of the topic and what happened with the "proud" part? Was Jerry initially proud of himself and maybe supported silently by his classmates and was their unspoken pressure the very factor that made it so difficult for Jerry to control his impulse and why did he have that impulse to betray his friend in the first place? Could the teacher have worked with suppressed generosity and playfulness of Bobby, who might have seen the incident as his initiation trial and learned to be proud of his kinder approach to his friends accidental loss of impulse control? Were Jerry's actions a part of a children's hazing ritual? Was Bobby expected to react tougher to his friend's misconduct? What was the group dynamics at the class? And what was the meaning of that secret toy? Young doctors can write a research paper (for example, O'Sullivan et al., 2016) to deal with their feelings in a Balint group, but children use less sophisticated means like their toys. It is possible to continue the list of questions if we are to speak about other "unrecognized meanings" of that case and wonder why the teacher chose this strategy of putting stress exclusively on the shame of only *one* boy. Of course, we can say that we have no reasons to believe that the program is not as successful as reported by its authors. However, we are afraid that it might harm "the cause of psychoanalysis" in the way the early wild analysts did more harm to it than to their patients (Freud, 1910, p. 226) by presenting such a one-dimensional picture of psychoanalysis and its application.

Discussion and conclusion

When we picked up a single sentence from Freud's work and made it the center of our investigation, we were aware that it was quite a risky enterprise. On the one hand, it was tempting to think of what Freud might have said if asked about this sentence, because of the idea that psychoanalysis is mainly Freud's "creation" (Freud, 1914, p. 7) and nobody else knows what he meant better than he does himself, and so we would never know his real investment in the sentence. On the other hand, there is a way to look at psychoanalysis as something that was not created, but discovered, by Freud. According to Bion (1970), "psychoanalysis, the thing-in-itself, existed. It remains for Freud to reveal the formulation embedded in it. Conversely, once formulated by Freud it remains for others (including Freud himself) to discover the meaning of the conjunction bound by his formulation" (p. 117). From his second point of view, "the conjunction" of Freud's formulations is what we have to explore. We consider both approaches as valid and productive and we tried to do our work with due respect to both of them. What we wanted to avoid, and hope that we managed to do it, is to pick up a certain aspect of Freud's work and build our own theory or conclusions on it with total disregard to the context and Freud's thinking as a whole in all its complexity.

We believe that Freud's remark about "the true line of division" between scientific analysis and its applications "alike in medical and in non-medical fields", which was the main object of our attention, in spite of its being parenthetical and maybe even due to it, is rich in meaning and practical value. Its complexity can be partly explained by the specifics of Freud's attitude to medical profession and scientific establishment, as well as the wide range of readers he addressed in his *Lay Analysis*, including his contemporaries and future generations. Initially, for many years, this idea was mainly overlooked and each party used other quotations from *Lay Analysis* to support their position, and application of psychoanalysis was replete with inequalities of various kinds some of them we discussed here. Mainly it was characterized by predominance of medical analysts in number and status. In early years of psychoanalysis, such tendency was justified by the necessity to protect still young profession, and training people with medical diplomas to be psychoanalysts was the most reliable way to secure survival and prosperity of psychoanalysis as a profession and a scientific discipline. However, with time this attitude looked more like an infantile defense that was not appropriate to the professional and scientific entity with more than a hundred-year history, and the tendency to undo these inequalities is getting stronger and stronger. As applications of psychoanalysis look younger or at least less mature than clinical psychoanalytic practice itself, several problems related to their growths may be observed. There are several prominent thinkers such as mentioned by Rustin (2017, p. 5) and a number of others whose work can be considered as a successful example of applied psychoanalysis, but their achievements look even more impressive in comparison with many other attempts to do similar work. Here we tend to have some level of agreement with Pigman (1992) in estimation of the current state of applied psychoanalysis, as he says that "recent developments in the theory and practice of clinical psychoanalysis make applied psychoanalysis a more questionable enterprise than even before" (p. 299). However, we cannot share his regret that applied psychoanalysis will not "cease" in response to his arguments (p. 310) and in spite of some difficulties appropriate to the age and developmental stage of the discipline we believe that it may have a great future in accordance with Freud's predictions. For the academics who want to do applied psychoanalysis, Pigman (1992) suggests to seek clinical training or at least psychoanalytically informed treatment and to avoid overgeneralizing from personal experience (p. 310), but we have not encountered some study of what be advisable for psychoanalysts who want to do applied analysis in addition to their clinical practice.

In the early days of psychoanalysis, Jones outlined three possible attitudes towards place of laymen in it. He said that there seemed to be three general opinions among his colleagues on this issue, namely: "(1) only medically qualified analysts should conduct psycho-analyses, (2) it is irrelevant whether the analyst is medically qualified or not, and (3) it is desirable that most analysts be medically qualified, but there is no good reason why selected lay persons should not conduct analyses under certain definite conditions" (Wallerstein, 1998, p. 24). If development of psychoanalysis goes in the direction of its science being equally applied in medical and non-medical fields, the peculiarity of the lay analysis question may become obsolete. Firstly, there would be a valid place for analysis of patients with non-medical purposes and aims; secondly, there would be "certain definite conditions" for medical analysts to be trained to work in other than clinical applications of psychoanalysis. All these applications can be united by a psychoanalytic thinking or attitude, which we would name psychoanalytic *Weltanschauung* if we did not know that Freud did not favor the idea that psychoanalysis can form a *Weltanschauung* of its own (Freud, 1933, p. 158). They also may result in a family of areas of psychoanalytic application, in the sense of Wittgenstein's notion of family resemblance (Wittgenstein, 1953, p. 36, §66), when each area of application is unique and there is no single set of obligatory features that they all should have in common, but they still undoubtedly belong to one family. Simonelli (2012) advances the idea of family resemblance among different clinical and theoretical schools of psychoanalysis, and French (1997) argues that "a strong 'family resemblance' exists between teaching and psychoanalysis in terms of setting, role, transference and underlying notions of human development" (p. 483). We would combine these ideas into a proposal to think of all applications of psychoanalysis, including non-medical ones, as a family of alike representatives of a big psychoanalytic family. It will still be necessary to define those common fundamental features that will let all these applications bear the name of psychoanalytical ones, but there is a hope that it is a rather good way to go from the situation where, from the one hand, some analysts are doomed to be of lower status just because of their lack of medical education or, on the other hand, psychoanalysts feel themselves as intruders to other areas rather than welcomed collaborators or risk to be an embarrassment to their strictly clinical colleagues or specialists from other areas. Such convergence of practical and logical truths may represent an even higher stage of maturity of psychoanalysis as a living creature, as well as pay a long-delayed tribute to Freud's vision of the lay analysts' place and the future of psychoanalysis in general.

References

Bell, D. (1999). Psychoanalysis a Body of Knowledge of Mind. In: D. Bell (Ed.), *Psychoanalysis and Culture: A Kleinian Perspective* (pp. 1–24). London: Duckworth.

Bion, W.R. (1970). *Attention and Interpretation*. London: Tavistock.

Brooks, P. (1987). The Idea of a Psychoanalytic Literary Criticism. *Critical Inquiry*, 13(2): 334–348.

Camden, V.J. (2009). 'My Capital Secret': Literature and the Psychoanalytic Agon. *International Journal of Psychoanalysis*, 90: 1123–1137.

Dufresne, T. (2017). *The Late Sigmund Freud: Or the Last Word on Psychoanalysis, Society, & All the Riddles of Life*. Cambridge: Cambridge University Press.

Eisold, K. (2005). Psychoanalysis and Psychotherapy: A Long and Troubled Relationship. *International Journal of Psychoanalysis*, 86: 1175–1195.

Elder, A. et al. (2003). *Balint: Object Relations, Pure and Applied*. London: Routledge.

Esman, A.H. (1998). What Is 'Applied' in Applied Psychoanalysis. *International Journal of Psychoanalysis*, 79: 741–756.

French, R. (1997). The Teacher as Container of Anxiety: Psychoanalysis and the Role of Teacher. *Journal of Management Education*, November, 21: 483–495.

Freud, S. (1910). "Wild" Psychoanalysis. *SE*, 11: 225–226.

Freud, S. (1912). Recommendations to Physicians Practicing Psycho-Analysis. *SE*, 12: 111–120.

Freud, S. (1913). On Beginning the Treatment. *SE*, 12: 121–144.

Freud, S. (1914). On the History of the Psychoanalytic Movement. *SE*, 14: 7–66.

Freud, S. (1916–17). Introductory Lectures on Psycho-Analysis. *SE*, 15–16: 243–462.

Freud, S. (1919). Lines of Advance in Psychoanalytic Therapy. *SE*, 17: 167–168.

Freud, S. (1923). Two Encyclopaedia Articles. *SE*, 18: 235–259.

Freud, S. (1926). The Question of Lay Analysis. *SE*, 20: 177–258.

Freud, S. (1927). The Future of an Illusion. *SE*, 21: 1–56.

Freud, S. (1933). New Introductory Lectures on Psycho-Analysis. *SE*, 22: 5–182.

Freud, S., and Pfister, O. (1963). *Psychoanalysis and Faith: The Letters of Sigmund Freud & Oskar Pfister*. New York: Basic Books.

Gabbard, G.O. (2003). Miscarriages of Psychoanalytic Treatment with Suicidal Patients. *International Journal of Psychoanalysis*, 84: 249–261.

Gay, P. (1988). *Freud: A Life for Our Time*. New York: W. W. Norton and Company.

Golland, J.H. (2002). What Do Teachers Want (From Psychoanalysts)? *Journal of Applied Psychoanalytic Studies*, 4: 275–281.

Greenberg, G. (2013). *The Book of Woe: The DSM and the Unmaking of Psychiatry*. New York: Blue Rider Press.

Greenson, R.R. (2016) [1967]. *The Technique and Practice of Psychoanalysis*. London: Karnac.

Haynal, A. (1988). *The Technique at Issue*. London: Karnac.

Kernberg, O. (2006). The Pressing Need to Increase Research in and on Psychoanalysis. *International Journal of Psychoanalysis*, 87: 919–926.

Kusche, C.A. (2002). Psychoanalysis as Prevention: Using PATHS to Enhance Ego Development, Object Relationships, and Cortical Integration in Children. *Journal of Applied Psychoanalytic Studies*, 4: 283–301.

Leuzinger-Bohleber, M. et al. (2006). What Is Conceptual Research in Psychoanalysis? *International Journal of Psychoanalysis*, 87: 1355–1386.

McWilliams, N. (2011). *Psychoanalytic Diagnosis*. New York: Guilford.

O'Sullivan, M. et al. (2016). Where Teaching Meets Therapy: An Exploration of the Experiences of General Practice Trainees Participating in Balint Group Discussions. *The Journal of the Balint Society*, 44: 40–50.

Oyer, M.W. (2016). *Let Fall: Hysteria and the Psychoanalytic Act*. New York: CUNY Academic Works.

Pigman, G. (1992). Applied Psychoanalysis Today. *Criticism*, 34(3): 299–315. Retrieved from www.jstor.org/stable/23113549.

Rustin, M. (2017). The Unhappy Divorce of Sociology and Psychoanalysis: Different Perspectives on the Psychosocial Edited by Lynn Chancer and John Andrews Palgrave. *International Journal of Psychoanalysis*, doi:10.1111/1745-8315.12619.

Sandler, A.-M., and Godley, W. (2004). Institutional Responses to Boundary Violations: The Case of Masud Khan. *International Journal of Psychoanalysis*, 85: 27–43.

Sandler, J., and Sandler, A. (1984). The Past Unconscious, the Present Unconscious, and Interpretation of the Transference. *Psychoanalytic Inquiry*, 4: 367–399.

Schröter, M. (2004). The Early History of Lay Analysis, Especially in Vienna, Berlin and London: Aspects of an Unfolding Controversy (1906–24). *International Journal of Psychoanalysis*, 85: 159–177.

Searles, H.F. (1979). The Patient as Therapist to His Analyst. In: H. Searles (Ed.), *Countertransference and Related Subjects: Selected Papers* (pp. 380–459). Madison, CT: International Universities Press.

Simonelli, T. (2012). What Is Psychoanalysis? https://thsimonelli.blogspot.ru/2012/07/what-is-psychoanalysis.html

Szasz, T. (2004). What Is Psychoanalysis? In: A. Casement (Ed.), *Who Owns Psychoanalysis?* (pp. 25–39). London, New York: Karnac.

Thomä, H. et al. (2012). *Psychoanalytic Practice: 2 Clinical Studies*. Berlin: Springer Science & Business Media.

Thomson, D. (1984). Review of the Book *The Emotional Experience of Learning and Teaching* by I. Salzberger-Wittenberg, G. Henry and E. Osborne. *Journal of the Royal College of General Practitioners*: 395.

Wallerstein, R. (1998). *Lay Analysis: Life Inside the Controversy*. Hillsdale, NJ: Analytic Press.

Wittgenstein, L. (2001) [1953]. *Philosophical Investigations*. Oxford: Blackwell.

5

Theodor Reik

The analyst of silence and surprise

Avedis Panajian

This chapter is about Theodor Reik. There is no theory or school of thought named after him. There are no Reikian analysts. Regretfully, he has not been given the recognition that luminaries such as Bion or Klein have received. In this chapter, I attempt to shed some light on the life and work of a gifted analyst and explain why his work has remained unexamined in psychoanalytic texts.

Reik was a morally courageous and an intellectually independent man who believed that systemizing psychological work leads to rigidity, compulsion and incoherence. He said that the mechanical application of psychological knowledge in analytic work is a criminal act against an embryonic thought. His interests were broad and included primitive tribes, culture, ritual, primary process, symbols, literature, poetry, music, love and sex, murderous urges, and hard sciences. Reik was more interested in listening to the primary process communication within himself and with his patients than the verbal communication.

Reik identified himself as Freudian. He considered silence the most essential aspect of psychoanalysis and agreed with Freud's first model of the mind, the topographical model. He followed Freud's understanding of the unconscious processes and the repressed unconscious. Both Freud and Reik strongly believed in the role of unconscious fantasies in contributing to one's personality development. Reik believed in and expanded upon Freud's "free floating attention" and suspending judgment. Reik was strongly Freudian in believing in the Oedipal complex, symbolism, and primary process. He also believed that real change and the unconscious manifest themselves in surprises.

Reik didn't always follow his master. He differed from Freud in the concept of transference and on what Freud meant by interpreting the transference; he did not believe in the death instinct, and he continued to base his work on the idea that we are driven to pursue pleasure and satisfaction. His view on masochism differed significantly from Freud (more will be said on this later). Reik anticipated some of the major ideas of Wilfred Bion and some of the contemporary analysts such as Thomas Ogden and Antonino Ferro. His methods share similarities with Intersubjective analysis; however, there are major differences between the two perspectives. This chapter illuminates these ideas.

As we know, Freud's self-analysis was the cornerstone for the development of psychoanalysis. However, his written work on his internal processes was limited. Freud viewed countertransference as an obstacle. He initially recommended that the analyst could overcome his blind spots regarding unconscious feelings triggered by the patient's transference through self-analysis. Two years later, in 1912, Freud, under the influence of Jung and the Zurich group, recommended that further analysis was the way to overcome such blind spots. Freud also believed that the appropriate mental stance of the analyst with his patients was an "evenly-hovering attention." By this he meant a mental attitude that received all the patient's associations with equal attention. Freud did not systematically examine what an evenly hovering attention entailed.

Reik viewed the analytic process as consisting of a series of "shocks" experienced as the patient deeply understands his repressed processes. When such an understanding is a lived moment, the effect – the shock – will be felt long afterwards. It is the moment of *surprise* during analysis that leads to experiencing shocks. Reik stated,"surprise is the expression of our struggle against any call upon us to acknowledge something long known to us which has become unconscious" (1959, p. 2). He said that the analyst needs to approach psychic material with total openness of mind. He believed that we cannot investigate the unconscious processes with any clear and definite ideas of what we may find. Such ideas are often derived from theoretical knowledge, and felt that they had no use in the investigation of the unconscious processes and the repressed. He said,"let me commend the deliberate discarding of order and forced regulation in our technique, the lack of all system, the absence of every definite plan; let me be permitted to declare myself the opponent of any and every mechanization of analytic technique." The only governing principle is to be surprised. He added, "to discard conscious directing ideas in analytic work and to surrender themselves without resistance to the guidance of the unconscious" (1959, p. 7).

Surprise in analytic work has multiple determinants. Some determinants are unique to a specific analyst while others have common generic meanings and forms. Determinants lead to unconscious conflicts between seeing something in us and in the patient or not seeing, between discovery and curiosity, courage and fear, known and unknown. Determinants shift from expectations to surprise. The analyst's unconscious responses are often in dynamic tension with the patient's unconscious and repressed material. Analyst and patient may unconsciously collude in order to diminish surprises to avoid discovery and mental pain and suffering. Other times, patients experience sadistic pleasure in fueling the analyst's surprises to continue to deny and repress their violent feelings and wishes for punishment for having such feelings. An analyst without the ability to experience varying levels of surprise in relation to the patient will have blind spots in making new and subtle observations and correcting his hypotheses regarding the analytic situation as it shifts from one moment to another.

Freud advised that the analyst to proceed "without any purpose in view, allows oneself to be taken by surprise by any new turn in view, and always meets them with an open mind, free from any presuppositions" (1912, p. 114). Surprise was the engine that moved the analytic process.

Reik believed that it is essential for an analyst to pursue self-analysis. In reading Reik, we get to know his literary, artistic and musical rhythm. His work inspires, evokes and stimulates us. He makes suggestions instead of teaching. He shares the literary style of Freud and strongly believes that one's background and education played a major role in evolving one's style of working and being in the world. Analysis requires of analysts an ongoing, deep, sincere and thoroughly honest knowledge of themselves as the instrument of psychoanalysis. In reading his work, we join him as he listens, feels, assimilates, waits, understands and interprets the unconscious.

Reik's early years

It is helpful for us to learn about the sociocultural milieu that influenced Reik's early years. Reik was born in Vienna on May 22, 1888. He was the third son of Max and Caroline Trebitsch Reik. The family lived in a Jewish middle class district, a short walking distance from the street where Freud had lived as a boy.

Reik's father was a kind, flexible and proud man, but also demanding, strict and valued achievement. He was an outspoken atheist. When Caroline's father came to live with the family, being a Talmudist, Reik's father and grandfather argued constantly about religion. This impacted Reik's interest in religion and ritual.

Reik's mother was a patient but morose and depressed woman who was devoted to her family and provided comfort to them. She loved music and occasionally sang or played the piano for the family.

Reik had two older brothers who both impacted his life. Hugo was fifteen year older, and Otto, thirteen. Reik reminds us about how he made Freud a father substitute since he lacked more affection from his own father. He also informs us that his rivalry with his brothers reminded him of his rivalry with Hans Sachs and Otto Rank.

Reik was not a good student in early school years. He was interested in playing football and was active in a gang of boys who fought with other gangs of boys. In adolescence, he became an insatiable reader, devouring many novels. Reik was devoted to the music of Beethoven, Haydn, Mozart, Schubert and Schumann. He worshipped Gustav Mahler.

At eighteen, Reik experienced the first great tragedy of his life. He was preparing to enter the University of Vienna when his father died of arteriosclerosis at the age of 66. The doctors attending to his father instructed Reik to go the nearest drugstore and obtain a life-saving medicine. When he returned to the house his father had already died. What followed was a lifelong tormenting question: "Could I have saved my father's life if I had run more quickly" (1951, p. 12). A similar disappointment repeated when Freud died before Reik could show him his finished work on "Masochism in Modern Man". Reik wanted the affirmation of these two cherished men in his life.

His father's death impacted the family greatly. The mother became very depressed and remained melancholic almost until her own death four years later. The family had limited money. Reik tutored students in German and Latin while attending the University. He states how his father's death drove him to study compulsively all the works of Goethe, whom his father greatly admired.

It was in 1910 that Reik first met Freud and began to attend the lectures and meetings of the Vienna Psychoanalytic Society. He wrote many articles, reviews for scientific journals, as well as a book dedicated to Freud, on Arthur Schnitzler. Freud felt the young Reik was gifted with psychological insights and understanding. He advised Reik to go to Berlin to get analysis with Karl Abraham.

In 1914, Reik married his childhood sweetheart and one year later had a son, Arthur, who was named in honor of Arthur Schnitzler. While the young married couple lived in Berlin, Freud visited them and awarded him the first International Prize in Applied Psychoanalysis for his study "The Puberty Ritual of the Primitives." Reik continued his work with Abraham until he was called into service during the First World War. While he was in the army, Reik was awarded the medal of bravery and achieved the rank of lieutenant. After the war, he returned to his wife and child and began practice in Vienna. It was during these years that he frequently met with Freud and received consultations. He was eventually elected secretary of the Vienna Psychoanalytic Society. In 1928, he went to Berlin to teach and established a thriving practice.

On July 19, 1926, Reik was sued in Vienna for "quackery" by one of his patients. He was charged with not being a proper analyst because he was not a physician. This marked the first open attack on lay analysts. Freud was very upset and responded by writing his booklet "Lay Analysis", which he described as being "very outspoken." The case against Reik was eventually dropped (Jones, 1957, p. 126).

In 1934, Reik and his wife fled Nazism and went to the Hague in Holland, where he became a member of the Dutch Psychoanalytic Institute. His wife Ella, who had been suffering from a heart ailment for many years, left to visit their son Arthur in Palestine. Soon upon her return to Vienna she died.

Reik continued to practice in Holland, where he married Marija and had his first daughter, Theodora. In 1938, he again felt the threat of the Nazis and sailed to the United States.

Reik arrived in New York at the age of 50 with his wife who was about to give birth to their second child. Although Reik had already been an analyst for twenty-five years and authored seventeen books and hundreds of articles, he had little money to live on. The New York Psychoanalytic Society would not accept him as a full-fledged member because of a regulation that restricted membership to those holding an MD degree. This wounded Reik deeply and for many years "he suffered from bitterness and disappointment of the rejection" (Gustin, 1953, p. xii).

Reik's second daughter Miriam was born six weeks after his arrival in the United States. A survivor of many paradoxes, Reik felt discouraged by the New York Psychoanalytic Society, but at the same time, he found in himself not as much of a stranger in the United States as he thought. As many times in his life following severe disillusionment, Reik discovered unknown resources in himself. He became enormously creative. Several of his most respected books were chosen by Book Find Club. These included: Listening with The Third Ear; Fragment of Great Confession; and The Secret Self. In 1948, Reik became the founder and president of the National Psychoanalytic Association for Psychoanalysis. This became the first non-MD training institute in the United States (Gustin, 1953).

Reik's thoughts about poised attention

Reik spoke about "tiny signals, the faint stimuli which slip past and attain such suggestive significance for the conjecture of unconscious processes. In face of such differentiated data so hard to grasp, one assumes that the keenest attention is called for" (1936, p. 31). Not so. Reik cautions us that the analyst should not practice such keen attention because it will create a tension that would be difficult to maintain for hours. He recommends, following Freud's "free-hovering attention," poised attention. Freud reminds us that if we focus our attention to a fixed point we tend to follow our own expectations. The outcome often becomes one that we find will satisfy our expectations. Reik reminds us that the practice of poised attention is much more difficult. In poised attention, it is only afterwards that we find out the significance of things to which our attention was directed. In analytic work, we shift our attention from external to internal and vice versa. Attention directed inwards is much more difficult to grasp. Our voluntary attention, even when directed inwards tends to protect us from both the dangers and the advantages of surprises. Reik recommends the withdrawal of attention that leads not to inattention but rather to freedom and mobility of attention. Such mobility of attention helps us become ready to receive a variety of stimuli from our unconscious. Rigid attention distracts us from turbulent experiences that are essential in facing transformations and developing faith in facing the unknown and the emerging stimuli from our unconscious. Inability to be attentive and/or dominated by rigid attention often involves repressed unconscious fantasies that are fighting to keep from becoming conscious. In fact, in such situations, patient and analyst are unable to liberate themselves from specific disturbing unconscious fantasies. Reik makes a valuable argument that by withdrawing our attention as analysts from what is immediately before us, we open an unusual path toward the psychic process of conjecturing. By such withdrawing of attention, we foster the emergence of sudden ideas that help prepare us to understand unconscious processes. Ability to shift our attention rewards us later in evolving our capacity for self-analysis in areas that we had never dreamt about. Reik makes it very clear: It is the active, forced, and voluntary attention that has the potential to interfere with the process of receiving the unconscious data and hinders progress in scientific knowledge.

Reik, listening and silence

According to Reik, Freud did not like music much (Freeman, 1971). He described Freud as "entirely visual" and described himself as entirely auditory. Reik gives the example of how he and Freud would go collecting mushrooms. Freud always knew where they were and Reik could never see them. Reik said of Freud, "his glance was very sharp and observant, while mine was not. Freud did not much like art or painting. He mostly liked sculpture" (Freeman, p. 8).

In reading Reik, one gets the impression that Reik and listening are one and the same. Those who knew Reik would agree that he had sincerity, honesty, and moral courage that was evident in his ongoing self-analysis.

What factors are involved in listening to unconscious processes in oneself as an analyst and in one's patient? Listening becomes seriously hindered when we are preoccupied with comprehension. In listening, pacing is essential. What is the pace of listening? And how does listening lead to comprehension? In listening, the analyst turns inward and activates all his senses, thus leading to unity and total presence. To listen is to face that which appears and disappears and, yet, leaves its impact. To listen, is to be in the transition such as facing the transient nature of truth. To listen is to continuously allow oneself to be formed and reformed. It is to tolerate meaning that is not yet accessible. It welcomes the pressure of the present sense beyond the sound of listening. To listen is to allow sound and meaning to vibrate. Listening requires spacing, and resonance. To listen is to enter a relationship with one's self and a relationship with the other's self. To listen is to be open to registering of the sonorous and the resonance. Sonorous time takes place all at once and not in simple succession. It is present in waves and expands. It envelopes or separates; stretches or contracts. Sonorous is the result of space-time. It opens its own space, spread through its resonance, expands and reverberates. To listen is to enter that space where one is also penetrated. To listen is to become open inside oneself and around oneself. It is to share inside/outside and separation/participation. In the opening presence and in acoustic spreading, "listening takes place at the same time as the sonorous event" (Nancy, 2007, p. 14). In listening, we pause to listen to the rhythm. In rhythm, we are both separated from ourselves and waiting to come back in unity with ourselves.

In listening, the analyst waits. In waiting, he becomes frightened. Frightened of awareness of time and absence of time. In waiting, there is fear of the infinite. It is only in silence that we listen to the past, present and future at once. Without waiting, there is an interruption in listening. In waiting, we listen to something new. We are taken by new words and ideas. New questions are raised. In silence, boundless knowledge reveals the depth within the analyst and simultaneously shocks him by its boundlessness. In waiting, the unexpected arrived meanings also confront us with questions. In silence, we listen to the fear of the return of the unthinkable. Without silence, meaning is searched as a protection from the dread of madness. In silence, the return of memories breaks things apart; disturbs silence and defies efforts at meaning. In pausing, we beckon the unknown, but we don't welcome this unknown. We think we call for forgotten memories, when in fact forgotten memories pull us towards themselves. Forgetting is more primary than remembering. We forget what we never knew; but we think we could have known. They had never become a memory. What we could have known was never a memory and needs to be mourned as a loss.

In listening and in silence, the analyst reaches the deepest levels and listens to his voice at these levels, and in reacting to his patient, he can reach the patient's deepest level and the patient's unconscious voice.

Reik's *Listening with The Third Ear*

Reik's book *Listening with The Third Ear: The Inner Experience of a Psychoanalyst* (1948) is a superbly honest autobiographical study of his process as he listens to the patients' and his unconscious repressed process. His listening is much based on beat, time, rhythmic sensitivity and having sharp musical ears. His listening is unique in appreciating musicality of language and in marking clues that were defensively hidden and unconscious. He had a way of following clues leading to scientific testing and rational thinking.

Reik said, "The third ear is the kind of instrument of perception for the unconscious and especially for the repressed" (1968, p. 2). I am reminded that in primitive tribes, a man would lie on the ground and place his ears toward the ground and listen to what he hears and understands. Is that just listening to what is going on around him, or is he trying to reach a level within himself so that he could listen to his own voice? How we listen determines what we hear.

Reik's approach to psychoanalysis is both an art and a science. He wonders what helps the analyst in the understanding of the patient and what really helps the patient. Is it the analyst's silence, listening, honesty, integrity, inner freedom, moralistic values or courage? Is everybody a psychologist because he has an unconscious? How can we train a psychologist to be a good analyst? Reik avoids using the term "intuition" and prefers the word "conjecture", which eventually leads to comprehension. Conjecture is felt as surprise. He said, "the most vital knowledge obtained by the analyst of the unconscious-repressed is, for him too, a surprise" (1948, p. 246). It is therefore a confirmation of an unconscious expectation. He continued: "It develops from the truly starling to the startlingly true" (p. 247). Conjecturing is our initial process, our initial impressions. He uses the analogy of a crime, the unknown culprit leaving some clues at the scene of the crime; he loses a piece of a personal belonging, and the detectives follow the clues and pick up the suspect. The interrogation, taking the suspect's statements, all these are part of a psychological conjecture. The reconstruction of the crime and the conviction of the culprit is an intellectual process called "comprehension." In the preliminary stage, the analyst behaves like a detective and preserves the clues for clinical use later. It is essential that he not follow a logical proof of his impressions nor be concerned about contradictory trains of thought. Reik said it is even desirable to entertain wild ideas in the initial stage. Bion, decades later, spoke about the courageous analyst who "dares to have wild thoughts." Dare to let the wild thoughts take their time and let them evolve into new paths without rushing to drown them with known ideas and logical deductions. Furthermore, Bion distinguished decades later between imaginative conjectures and rational conjectures. By analytic comprehension for Reik meant looking at one's history, results are tested and testing must be performed carefully, clearly, consciously and logically. Conjecture must unconsciously pass through intellectual comprehension.

I recall one of my male patients and noticed several clues about him that I always remember: his shirt had no wrinkles, he placed his keys in the same place under a lamp in my office, his tie matched his shirts elegantly, he walked in the same way, he gave me the same look, he lay on the couch in the same way, and he made sure his hair was not messed up. After the sixth session, I said to him, "You remind me of the best car salesman that I had ever seen. You are utterly put together with such style and elegance." He got up from the couch, looked at me with rage and smiled, and said, "I don't know whether I should thank you or kill you." He then lied back on the couch. It took many months and years of analysis for my initial conjecture to be tested, examined, re-examined and logically and carefully followed up with his history until one day years later he told me, "The first few sessions when you told me that I reminded you of a beautiful car salesman has always been with me. Now, I learned so much how all my life I lived out of guilt and for others. I have always been a side kick. I never felt that you hated me nor that you were angry at me when you told me about what I reminded you of." The movement from conjecture to comprehension was felt to be of great value for this patient.

Reik regarded moral courage as the most important quality for an analyst. By moral courage, he meant "inner truthfulness", and in this, the analyst needs to be superior to his patient. Reik valued the intellectual independence that he embodied in his character. He felt that an analyst needs less theoretical and practical knowledge but more expansion in intellectual independence. In his opinion analytic training should be geared to help the candidate develop intellectual freedom, sensitivity, honesty and courage. Candidates in training are taught rigid systems and theories that insulate them against taking risks and facing the turbulence needed to develop sensitivity, courage and independence. Reik also emphasized that the training of analytic attitude and the understanding of the language of primary process are crucial for becoming a good analyst.

Reik makes it clear that his association with Freud taught him the appreciation for silence and how to remain silent in psychoanalytical work. He goes on:

> The analyst hears not only what is in the words; he hears also what the words do not say. He listens with the "third ear", hearing not only what the patient speaks but also his own inner voices, what emerges from his own unconscious depths. What is spoken is not the most important thing. It appears to us more important to recognize what speech conceals and what silence reveals.
>
> (1948, pp. 125–126)

Reik describes the analytic process as the "work shop." He refers to it as the "analytic atmosphere, magic situation, or impossible situation." He prefers not to use Freud's concept of transference. Psychoanalysis is like imagination and cannot be rote learned. The whole technique must be lived. He describes the wealth of the analytic experience in the following way:

> I have been blessed and cursed a thousand times, killed and kissed in thought, annihilated and royally rewarded in fantasy, and all because I sit unseen in a chair behind a woman or a man and listen to what he thinks or feels-simply because I am an analyst. So powerful is fantasy working in broad daylight.
>
> (1948, p. 111)

Reik considers the unconscious an independent "sense organ" through which one could resonate with the unconscious of the patient. He speaks about "context," "tact" and "timing" and how to reach the depth of the changing truths. He is not simply analyzing transference and resistance. For him, how to listen was much more important than what to listen to. His aim was to convey in detail the phenomenological experience of the listening attitude. His personality is his instrument. As such, artistic, literary associations, patterns, storylines, universal and personal myths, poems, primary process language, all weave together to create rhythm and music.

The Compulsion to Confess and the Need for Punishment

In 1924, Reik, at the age of thirty-five, lived in Vienna and had an established career as an analyst and writer in clinical and applied psychoanalytic areas. Furthermore, he enjoyed a warm and professional relationship with Freud, his master. The same year, Reik gave a series of lectures at the Teachers Institute of the Vienna Psychoanalytic Association titled "The Compulsion to Confess and the Need for Punishment." This was published in German in 1925 and not in English in the United States until 1959. Reik believed that "instinctual expression was subjected to a transformation under the influence of guilt and self-punishment. Most symptoms also have the character of an unconscious confession and that their purpose is to mitigate the pressure of guilt feeling" (1959, pp. ix–x).

In 1941, Reik published his major work *Masochism in Modern Man*. This book elaborated unconscious guilt and punishment issues of masochistic character structure. When instinctual urges are inhibited or modified by the environment, the infant experiences violence or rage. If modification is applied with patience, kindness and love, the infant's psychic development will be characterized by minimum guilt and little need for punishment. These are called "benign repressive experiences". If the infant is exposed to anger, impatience, lack of warmth and love, the infant is likely to experience stronger feelings of guilt and greater need for punishment (e.g. withdrawal or difficulty being soothed). These are called "hostile repressive experiences". The manner and nature of the repression as experienced by the child and as applied by the mother determine the direction and development of the child's character development. Reik incorporates his concept of the unconscious compulsion to confess within Freudian theory of the Oedipus complex (1959). He states that "The Oedipus complex and the feelings of guilt resulting from it are the cause of the inhibition of the child's urge for expression and for its later transformation into the compulsion to confess" (1959, pp. 223, 224). The strength of the need for punishment is dependent on the relative benign or hostile nature of superego. Confession occurs through symptoms and those symptoms provide both satisfaction from guilt and anxiety as well as pain and suffering. This work of Reik was mainly based on the Freudian model of instinctual drives and the Oedipus complex. However, what was significantly different from Freud was its explanatory power. Reik believed that our social, cultural and religious institutions were all based on an unconscious compulsion to confess and the need for punishment. Furthermore, he emphasized that man's destiny for survival as a race is determined by reducing these unconscious forces (p. x).

A forty-year-old married woman was a patient of mine. She had a traditional father who believed that the man in the house is the leader and the rest of the family needs to honor and listen to him. He was a hard-working man who provided for his wife and their three daughters. The patient's mother was rather submissive and compliant to her husband. The patient is the oldest daughter in the family. In her current marriage, the patient developed a dread of aging and became very competitive toward younger, attractive females. She had conscious fantasies that she and her husband were going to be famous and make a handsome couple that everyone would admire. In reality, she viewed herself and her husband as losers, without jobs, and dependent on their parents' help. The patient developed many physical symptoms and had several cosmetic surgeries to avoid getting older. She isolated herself and often did not want to be seen by people. She fought with her husband for failing her idealized fantasies, and at times, told him that she regretted marrying him because without him she could have been a "famous" person. Her ongoing physical and psychological symptoms provided her both pain and confession for her unconscious feelings of rage at her parents now directed at her husband. Oedipal issues with her father are denied; cruel and harsh superego quickly turns into hostile feelings. This patient continues to expect and believe that life is punishing her and that her current marriage is part of that punishment.

Masochism in Modern Man

In the beginning of psychoanalysis, Freud viewed masochism as a component of the libidinal drive and as sadism turned inward against the self. In *Beyond the Pleasure Principle,* he viewed primary masochism as present from the beginning of life. Sadism was the projection of masochism and was equated with the death instinct.

Reik did not agree with Freud's death instinct and the repetition compulsion in masochism. Reik remained very close to Oedipal formulation and saw a masochist as unconsciously wanting to be defeated and humiliated at the manifest level. Behind the suffering, there are unconscious wishes for gratification. Reik was a Freudian in placing emphasis on unconscious fantasies. However, in masochism, he viewed pleasure seeking and relentless seeking for internal satisfaction as the goal. He did not integrate the role of real or fantasied traumas during infancy and childhood with playing a major role in many addictive types of masochism. A masochist, according to Reik, robs the punisher of his power and frustrate him by defeating himself. He seeks the satisfaction of defiance, mockery and subtle aggression.

According to Reik, masochism originates in infancy as the unconscious fantasy of violence and murder against inhibiting parental authority. The infant masters his fear of retaliation by turning his hostility against himself. The excitement in anticipating punishment serves as a way of lessening the pain of punishment and gaining gratification through endurance. Masochism originates in exaggerated guilt regarding one's own aggressive thoughts. However, the pride in exaggerated guilt provides an ideal view of oneself as the superior sufferer. Reik's view of masochism provides us valuable insights regarding a patient who suffers from Oedipally based masochistic power and pleasure. His view, however, falls short in explaining how a masochistic individual who endured chronic parental abuse and humiliation gets stuck in repeating self-injury, self-defeat, and humiliation.

The following example provides some insight into one of my patient's unconscious processes through Reik's model of masochism. A male patient in his mid-fifties denied hostile and murderous feelings toward his father who had been tyrannical and physically abusive toward him. He was able to entertain intellectual insight as long as they were separated from experiential understanding. He was skilled in making himself physically and psychologically ill. He had been in and out of therapies and consulted medical doctors for numerous physical and psychological symptoms. He exaggerated his symptoms and anxiety and found himself fighting in anguished, helpless, petrified ways that no one could help him. He felt defeated and lived in an ongoing agony and dread. He had moments of peace after each dramatic event. Underlying his feelings of defeat, were feelings of being powerful and victorious. He felt he had exhausted those who wanted to help him. This gave him deep satisfaction and temporary relief. He obsessively looked for different types of cures. He felt himself to be superior in his ability to research and lecture and intimidate the helping professionals who were the authority figures. The murderous feelings toward his father are indirectly satisfied by defeating and feeling victorious toward those who have power and authority. In fact, after each dramatic and traumatic event, he walked around as all-knowing, prideful and powerful. The patient denied feeling guilty and projected his hostility and guilt feelings onto people in authority whom he believed were irresponsible and neglectful of their duty.

Reik's understanding of masochism did not include the role of early trauma in understanding repetitive masochistic patterns of self-injury and self-humiliation. Addiction and identification with an early abusive, absent, or depressed mother and father was not integrated with the Oedipal model in understanding masochism. In understanding my patient's unconscious process, it was essential to integrate his identification with the tyrannical father whom he hated, yet struggled to differentiate himself from.

An interview with a former patient of Theodor Reik

Betty is a ninety-seven-year-old woman to whom I was introduced by a former student of mine named Mary. I met Betty at her home once in March 2017 for eighty minutes. What follows is a partial transcription of the interview with Betty. Betty had been told that I was writing a paper on Theodor Reik; she agreed to meet me and record the session, and gave me permission to use it for this project. Since Betty's memory was not ideal, I have selected areas that illustrate both when Betty's memory was very intact and other moments in the interview when she was struggling with her memory. Betty was pleasant, kind, and eager to meet me. I experienced her as very engaging; she was pained when her memory failed her. In fact, she wanted so much to remember more about her time with Theodor Reik.

Panajian: Thank you very much for seeing me and for agreeing to be interviewed by me about your time with Dr. Reik.

Betty: My memory is, you know.

Panajian: Yes, of course, I understand. As Mary had told you, I was her teacher and it was very kind of her to introduce me to you.

Betty: Yes.

Panajian: There is going to be a book on lay analysts and I wanted to write a chapter on Dr. Reik.

Betty: Yes.

Panajian: What is the impact on you years later since you saw Dr. Reik? What is your memory of how he impacted you? What stays with you as you think of him?

Betty: You'll have to guide me, because I'm losing track.

Panajian: Sure, in New York, approximately when did you see him?

Betty: It was just at the end of the war.

Panajian: He came to U.S. in 1938.

Betty: I saw him in the forties.

Panajian: In the forties?

Betty: Mm-hmm (affirmative).

Panajian: Okay, 1940s, you saw him.

Betty: I think it was around 1947.

Panajian: What is your memory as far as how long you saw him?

Betty: How long?

Panajian: How long do you think you saw him in treatment, approximately?

Betty: Maybe about a year.

Panajian: About a year.

Betty: Mm-hmm (affirmative).

Panajian: Uh-huh. That was once a week or several times?

Betty: Two times and sometimes three times.

Panajian: Twice or three times.

Betty: I was working and going to college at the same time.

Panajian: Uh-huh.

Betty: It was $10 an hour.

Panajian: Was it?

Betty: Uh-huh (affirmative).

Panajian: I am sure he needed the money those days, because he was not an MD and was not recognized with his PhD as an analyst.

Betty: Yeah.

Panajian: The literature says that in the beginning Freud helped him quite a bit be sending him some money.

Betty: He what?

Panajian: Dr. Reik struggled to make it in practice because he was a PhD analyst. He had difficult time to making a living and Freud helped him for a while.

Betty: Yeah. He lived on the . . . had an apartment on East 48th Street. It was a good area in New York.

Panajian: You were going to college, and you were working?

Betty: Mm-hmm (affirmative).

Panajian: How did you get to him? Who referred you to him?

Betty: I was dating, whom I married, a young scholar who had heard of him.

Panajian: So, your date referred you to him?

Betty: Yes. He felt that everybody needed analysis. He was interested in analysis.

Panajian: Uh-huh.

Betty: He recommended Theodor Reik. Theodor Reik had a very good reputation.

Panajian: You started seeing him.

Betty: Mm-hmm (affirmative).

Panajian: Was he a friendly person?

Betty: Very.

Panajian: Very friendly.

Betty: Very warm, yeah.

Panajian: Very warm, very friendly.

Betty: Mm-hmm (affirmative).

Panajian: He was not stuck up.

Betty: No. He wasn't Germanic.

Panajian: Humble?

Betty: Very humble.

Panajian: Professional?

Betty: Yeah.

Panajian: But very kind?

Betty: Yes. At the time, he was treating a young playwright who became very famous, who had in fact a play on Broadway at the same time. I'm trying to think of the young man's name now, and I can't, but it was at the time when All My Sons was playing. It was a play that was similar to that, and Theodor Reik said, "I wrote that play."

Panajian: Did he?

Betty: He felt that he had invested so much in that patient.

Panajian: I am sure I can find out who was at that time based on the information that you gave me.

Betty: Yeah, because it was on Broadway.

Panajian: Did Dr. Reik have humor?

Betty: Yes.

Panajian: He did have humor.

Betty: Very much so. I was dating a young man who was interested in analysis who constantly accused me of seeing other men, having affairs. Reik said, "Well, if you have the name, you should have the game."

Panajian: He did have humor.

Betty: Yes, very much so, yes.

Panajian: "You have the name. You should have the game." I like that. He was in a way pretty quick with his responses.

Betty: Yes.

Panajian: Very sharp?

Betty: Yeah, very.

Panajian: Was he pretty direct?

Betty: Pardon me?

Betty: Yes.

Panajian: If he had something to say, he said it.

Betty: Yes.

Panajian: What if you got hurt about something he said? What would he do?

Betty: No. He was very sensitive.

Betty: Yes, but a good sense of humor. He was very warm, very kind.

Panajian: Would he shake your hand in each session? Or just in the beginning of treatment? Do you remember?

Betty: I don't remember.

Panajian: How was his office, do you remember?

Betty: Hm?

Panajian: How was his office?

Betty: He lived there. It was his apartment.

Panajian: It was in his apartment.

Betty: Mm-hmm (affirmative). It was a walk-up apartment, no elevator.

Panajian: Did he have photographs of Freud? Pictures of Freud?

Betty: No, I don't remember.

Panajian: Did he say anything about Freud? Did he talk about him to you? He knew Freud very well.

Betty: I know.

Panajian: He did not talk about his days in Vienna?

Betty: No. He could not talk about his personal life.

Panajian: He was there more for you.

Betty: Yes. I'm trying to think of who . . . I was very young, so I wasn't . . . It was a world that I wasn't familiar with, but it was very . . . he was very warm, very friendly, so the atmosphere was conducive to being relaxed and talking easily about yourself.

Panajian: Go ahead, I'm sorry.

Betty: Every once in a while I would try to get, because he was very . . . sitting in the chair behind the couch, he was very quiet, and so every once in a while I would try to think of something outrageous to get a response from him, and I'd get an "Oh."

Panajian: He was pretty quiet?

Betty: Yes. It wasn't conversational therapy at all.

Panajian: Yeah, silence . . . I did read that silence was very important for him and that he learned it from Freud.

Betty: Mm-hmm (affirmative). Yes.

Panajian: Was he interested in dreams?

Betty: Yes.

Panajian: He was?

Betty: Mm-hmm (affirmative).

Panajian: He was interested in your dreams.

Betty: Mm-hmm (affirmative). He was untidy in his appearance. The shirttail was always sticking out in the back. He didn't have any. . . . He had no concern about his appearance, but he was very clean.

Panajian: He was a pretty confident man.

Betty: Yes.

Panajian: Was he his own person? Did he have his own mind?

Betty: Very much so, yeah.

Panajian: Did he ever accept any gifts? Did you ever give him any?

Betty: No. I was a poor student.

Panajian: Uh-huh.

Betty: I remember it was $10 an hour.

Panajian: How can you forget $10 dollars an hour?

Betty: That was a lot of money.

Panajian: Yeah.

Betty: I was going to all-girl college in New York.

Panajian: What were you studying?

Betty: Child psychology.

Panajian: You were?

Betty: Yes. I was one of six children, and so finding your place in a family of six kids not easy.

Panajian: Reik had two older brothers.

Betty: I never knew that.

Panajian: They were much older than him.

Betty: Did they come to the United States?

Panajian: No, they did not. Reik did not like much rules place on him. He tried to test the limits.

Betty: I had that feeling about him. He was not rigid.

Panajian: Yes, that is a very good point.

Betty: He was very open and warm.

Panajian: It comes through in his writing. Would you say also creative and intuitive?

Betty: Yes.

Panajian: Intuitive?

Betty: I used to try to shock him, because nothing. . . . I'd get a response from him like "Oh."

Panajian: You had to interrupt that silence.

Betty: Yes.

Panajian: New York Psychoanalytic did not accept his diploma.

Betty: I know. You had to be a doctor, which is ridiculous.

Panajian: I feel the same way. It is psychology and not medicine.

Betty: I know, right? Strange.

Panajian: Did you know anything about how he started to find his own institute?

Betty: I had left. I think I had left New York. When was it?

Panajian: 1948.

Betty: That is when I left.

Panajian: Did he talk to you about all the political war surrounding institutes, MDs, PhDs etc.?

Betty: No. It was professional.

Panajian: You found that year that you spent with him helpful to you.

Betty: Very helpful, yeah. It was helpful in my relationship with the man I was dating. He was very jealous of my seeing other men. I was pretty attractive in those younger years, and in fact, I got most of my jobs where I worked on my looks.

Panajian: What kind of work did you do?

Betty: Modeling school in New York, receptionist in Saks 5th Avenue, in the beauty salon.

Panajian: So, he was helpful for you to really take care of you with your date?

Betty: Very helpful. I tried to read his [Reik's] books, too technical. He said to me, "You're in it."

Panajian: He meant he learned from you.

Betty: I don't know.

Panajian: He had sense of humor.

Betty: Very much.

Panajian: Did he smoke in the session.

Betty: No.

Panajian: What did he wear?

Betty: Casual, regular jacket, shirt and pants, never in a suit.

Panajian: Did you know that he lived in New York with his second wife and two daughters?

Betty: No. I never saw his wife. I knew he had a wife. I did not know that he had children.

Panajian: He also had a son who went to what was known those days as Palestine. His first wife had died and Freud was very helpful in giving him support.

Betty: He was a very unassuming man. He had a lot of integrity. I am glad that his reputation is getting revived again.

Panajian: I hope so.

Betty: Medical training is rigid. You don't have the freedom to . . . I am trying to think of the word.

Panajian: Not expansive and reaching other fields? Such as mythology, poetry, novels, etc.

Betty: Yes, not expansive. That is the word.

Panajian: Dr. Reik was very well read in so many areas. He also loved music.

Betty: What is the book going to be called?

Panajian: Lay Analysts.

Betty: Have you met any other patients of him?

Panajian: No. I would not know how to find any. Thanks to Mary that I found you. I am so, so appreciative.

Betty: I keep thinking about that playwright that I kept seeing him coming out of the apartment. I cannot remember his name.

Panajian: I will try to find his name or names and let you know which one it is?

Betty: Good.

Panajian: After you moved away from New York, did you marry your boyfriend.

Betty: Yes. He was a very difficult man. I eventually left him. He was shocked. He was an intelligent man and he would let you know it. But he was not as intelligent as he thought. He was shocked when I divorced him. I had two wonderful children from him.

Panajian: So, you had the confidence and the strength to do what you thought was best for you. (Here, Betty became a bit somber and waited a bit.)

Betty: Theodor Reik helped me believe in myself.

Betty thanked me for the flowers that I had taken for her. Two days after the interview, she called me. She was clearly happy and said, "I remember the playwright's name, Arthur Laurents. That was him. I just read about him and it was him."

Indeed, when I did my search about Arthur Laurents he clearly states that his analyst while he was in New York was Theodor Reik. Arthur Laurents was a highly regarded playwright.

Discussion and conclusion

One of the main reason for writing about Theodor Reik is my concern that his valuable contributions to psychoanalysis, culture and mankind have been fading. Indeed many legends' contributions to psychoanalysis have been fading. A major exception is Freud and, lately, the work of Wilfred Bion. Even some significant contributions of Wilfred Bion are fading. I can only raise possible reasons for this: Is it due to our personal and collective envy, superiority and laziness in studying the work of Reik? Is it due to our ignorance and narcissism, which are shaken up when confronted by the enormous literature that Reik grasped, and as a result, we reject his work in order not to be reminded of the richness of his mind and the narcissistic injury that we might face? Is it due to our anxiety and dread that reading Reik triggers by activating our unconscious guilt and need for punishment that we rather not think or feel? Do we identify with the crimes of which we are unaware when studying Reik? Is it our tendency to stay away from the basic mysteries of mankind with which Reik was preoccupied? Is it due to Reik being an unassuming, down-to-earth human being who never lost his principles, duties and humanness? Is it because he is a person who faced tragedies and disillusionments while at the same time, transformed such experiences wisely to find his inner resources, becoming a better person, and understanding the human essence in general? He continued to become a person who faced his duties and responsibilities with courage, honesty and humility. Are we looking for another type of hero whom we can idolize? Perhaps down-to-earth, a person who has a sense of responsibility as a man, father, and professional does not fit our current definition of a cultural idol? Are we neglecting such a person and, in doing so, evading the same qualities in ourselves? And finally, and perhaps most significant, is it due to the spotlight that Reik focuses on the analyst's unconscious mind?

Reik, just like Bion, believed that true analysis starts when formal analysis stops. He reminds us, like Bion, that the mind needs truth the way the body needs food. Unlike Freud, Reik's focus is on the ongoing self-analysis in and outside the session. Self-analysis throughout one's life. Self-analysis by facing one's internal dread to allow surprises to shake our personality structure at its core. The kind of surprises coming from our infinite unknown that leads us to states of depersonalization and disorientation. The kind of surprises that lead us to be shaken up from the core of our narcissism. Self-analysis requires moral courage – not understanding, explaining, organizing, intellectualizing, connecting, insight or seeking solutions. Self-analysis that is capable of waiting, tolerating, suffering and allowing the unknown to reveal itself. Only then, new learning becomes possible.

Reik, Bion and Searles are among the few who placed the spotlight on the analyst's character. Psychoanalysts and analytic training institutions avoid placing the spotlight on the analyst. The narcissism, suffering, humility, mourning and the acceptance of narcissism and self and other idealizations continue to dominate the field. Reik reminds us of our humanity. He begins as an artist and then continues as a scientist. His work is utterly personal. Analysts tend to stay away from the personal that shakes our core. His work does not let the co-construction hide by acting out through enactments. His co-construction focuses on unconscious fantasies that preceded the dyad. Reik's work cautions us that co-construction is valid up to a point. Revival of unconscious fantasies in the present is crucial. Co-construction needs to be taken in context. If it is over emphasized, then what preceded gets lost. No individual is responsible for the other's basic personality make up. Analysts' split-off aspects and analysts' ongoing fantasies need to be looked at as a re-enactment from his past. Acting out of countertransference is too often confused with co-construction. Chronic countertransference especially with severe disorders requires self-analysis outside the session.

In addition, by patiently waiting in silence and letting his subjective private experiences enlarge, Reik invites and detects unconscious fantasies that preceded the dyad. The analyst who cannot be alone and wait in the presence of the other will not be able to study his private mind not find clues about the patient's unconscious fantasies and how they are acted out instead of suffered. Reik reminds us that analysis is both a personal and an impersonal process. The analyst moves from one to the other. Without being personal and impersonal, the analyst cannot study his own mind and allow the proper distance from experiencing the patient's associations as personal attack and as a result, unconsciously retaliating against or punishing the patient.

References

Freeman, E. (1971). *Insights: Conversations with Theodore Reik*. Englewood Cliffs, NJ: Prentice-Hall, Inc.

Freud, S. (1912). Recommendations to Physicians Practicing Psychoanalysis. *SE*, 12. The Hogarth Press, London.

Freud, S. (1920). Beyond the Pleasure Principle. *SS*, 18. The Hogarth Press, London.

Gustin, J. (1953). On Theodor Reik. In R. Linder (Ed.), *Explorations in Psychoanalysis: A Tribute to the Work of Theodor Reik* (pp. ix–xiii). New York: Julian Press, Inc.

Jones, E. (1957). *The Life and Work of Sigmund Freud*. Vol. 3. New York: Basic Books.

Nancy, L.J. (2007). *Listening*. New York: Fordham University Press.

Reik, T. (1936). *Surprise and the Psychoanalyst*. London, New York: Routledge Taylor & Francis Group.

Reik, T. (1941). *Masochism in Modern Man*. New York: Farrar and Rinehart, Inc.

Reik, T. (1948). *Listening with the Third Ear*. New York: Farrar, Straus and Company.

Reik, T. (1951). New Ways in Psychoanalytic Technique. *Psychoanalytic Review, 46C*(3), 51–65.

Reik, T. (1959). *The Compulsion to Confess and the Need for Punishment*. New York: Farrar, Straus and Company.

Reik, T. (1968). Theodor Reik Speaks of His Psychoanalytic Technique. *American Imago*, *25*(1): 16–21.

6

From word to deed

Why psychoanalysis needs laypersons?

Bernd Nissen

With his comment on lay analysis Freud entered the "Tageskampf der Meinungen" (Daily Battle of Opinions) which Simmel formulated so splendidly in his contribution to the discussion (1927, p. 192) (inadequately translated as "engaging personally" in the *International Journal of Psychoanalysis*) (1927, p. 259). He tries to convince an Impartial Person, probably the physiologist Durig, that non-physicians can work responsibly in psychoanalysis. As is well known, Freud never departed from this position, despite all the crass differences of opinion that erupted (see the controversy in the Internationale Zeitschrift für Psychoanalyse and the *International Journal of Psychoanalysis*, 1927). Freud presents the psychoanalytic method to this imagined layperson in great detail.

Freud's paper about lay analysis shows his mastery: great scientific rigour without concealing open questions and problems, on the highest theoretical, clinical, human (note the dignity/respect with which Freud describes patients' symptoms in the first section) and linguistic level. Authorities of the time acknowledge this mastery.

Strachey wrote in his editor's note to "The Question of Lay Analysis":

> Freud presented in the following pages (lay analysis; BN) what was perhaps his most successful non-technical account of the theory and practice of psycho-analysis, written in his liveliest and lightest style.
>
> (1926, p. 181)

And E. Jones acknowledged in his (very critical) review of Freud's contribution:

> About the first part, which occupies more than two-thirds of the whole, there is little to be said except to marvel once more at the ingenuity with which Professor Freud can expound a familiar theme over and over again with constant freshness and novelty. He has perhaps never written a better description of what psycho-analysis is, its theory and practice, than in the present exposition. It is one that every analyst will read with profit.
> (1927, p. 87)

Yet Freud draws from his exposition only the conclusion that lay analysts can work responsibly in psychoanalysis. At the same time, his argumentation reaches beyond this narrow, professional-political minimum position: "It is argued that psychoanalysis was after all discovered by a physician in the course of his efforts to assist his patients" (p. 253). Yet from this one cannot draw the conclusion that psychoanalysis is a branch of medicine, which Freud illustrates with a comparison: "The whole theory of electricity had its origin in an observation of a nerve-muscle preparation; yet no one would dream today of regarding it as a part of physiology" (p. 253). Freud makes it clear that "psycho-analysis is not a specialized branch of medicine. I cannot see how it is possible to dispute this. Psycho-analysis is a part of psychology; not of medical psychology in the old sense, not of the psychology of morbid processes, but simply of psychology" (p. 252).

However, the implication and in my opinion inevitably resulting consequence that psychoanalysis substantially needs lay analysts, Freud does not state explicitly (possibly out of respect for the contrary positions). It is my thesis that psychoanalysis must unite the most diverse academic trends so as to do justice to the complexity of its subject and to the "inseparable bond between cure and research" (p. 256).

I would like to trace and deepen some selected meta-psychological and clinical-theoretical lines from Freud's argumentation in order to demonstrate that only by joining different scientific perspectives can the psychic be understood psychoanalytically as an independent scientific reference system.

The magic of the word

We find the perhaps most important comment related to treatment and theory on the issue of lay analysis in the first chapter. Employing an informal and elegant style, Freud touches on the fundamental basis of psychoanalysis, and it is interesting to note that he substantiates it with three quotations from Shakespeare and Goethe. Freud may be aware that ultimately this fundamental basis as the human condition can only be tackled using the presentative symbolism of the greatest art.

The Impartial Person has been showing signs of impatience while Freud has unfolded neurotic symptoms and asks, "what the analyst does with the patient whom the doctor has not been able to help" (p. 187).

> Nothing takes place between them except that they talk to each other. The analyst makes use of no instruments – not even for examining the patient – nor does he prescribe any medicines. If it is at all possible, he even leaves the patient in his environment and in his usual mode of life during the treatment. This is not a necessary condition, of course, and may not always be practicable. The analyst agrees upon a fixed regular hour with the patient, gets him to talk, listens to him, talks to him in his turn and gets him to listen.
>
> The Impartial Person's features now show signs of unmistakable relief and relaxation, but they also clearly betray some contempt. It is as though he were thinking: 'Nothing more than that? Words, words, words, as Prince Hamlet says.' And no doubt he is thinking too of Mephistopheles' mocking speech on how comfortably one can get along with words – lines that no German will ever forget.
>
> 'So it is a kind of magic,' he comments: 'you talk, and blow away his ailments.'
>
> Quite true. It would be magic if it worked rather quicker. An essential attribute of a magician is speed – one might say suddenness – of success. But analytic treatments take months and even years: magic that is so slow loses its miraculous character. And incidentally do not let us despise the word. After all it is a powerful instrument; it is the means by which we convey our feelings to one another, our method of influencing other people. Words can do unspeakable good and cause terrible wounds. No

> doubt 'in the beginning was the deed' [Goethe, Faust; BN] and the word came later; in some circumstances it meant an advance in civilization when deeds were softened into words. But originally the word was magic – a magical act; and it has retained much of its ancient power
>
> (p. 187f.)

For the issue of lay analysis, a deeper understanding of these remarks is imperative. Analyst and analysand talk to each other and listen to each other, no other medical procedures are applied – Freud is perfectly clear and unequivocal in this matter, unlike other critics of lay analysis. Shakespeare and Goethe are Freud's chief witnesses, words that are only words do not help, they need the link to the origin, to the beginning – and there was the deed.

Yet how is the link between word and deed to be imagined/thought? What is more: Freud speaks of the word as a magical act and that it has retained much of its ancient power. Does this not mean that there is not only a link between word and deed but also a development in the use of the word in which the word becomes a name and symbol?

To understand these complex processes, it is in my view necessary to consider both the basic theoretical and clinical-theoretical dimension.

Basic theoretical model

From the perspective of basic theory, Freud in my view draws up the following model (see the seventh chapter of the Interpretation of Dreams; the central meta-psychological writings between 1914 and 1917). A baby is confronted with internal stimuli, which he experiences with unpleasure and which we call hunger. The mother breastfeeds him; an experience of satisfaction occurs. When further sensations of hunger occur, he switches to the "hallucinatory cathecting of the memory of satisfaction" (Freud, 1900, p. 598), he sucks his thumb or comforter. This hallucinatory cathecting is for him being breastfed, hence indistinguishable from the real, experienced event of satisfaction. The hardness of reality will teach him, unpleasure increases. A tension between the experience of real satisfaction (at the breast) and a hallucinatory replication arises. "Such hallucinations, however, if they were not to be maintained to the point of exhaustion, proved to be inadequate to bring about the cessation of the need or, accordingly, the pleasure attaching to satisfaction" (1900, p. 598). The first crossroads is reached: Can he bear the hardness of the reality of anticipating the breast (mother) or does he turn away?[1]

It is necessary to expand on this model, which Freud considers from different perspectives (see for example sections C and E in the seventh chapter of the Interpretation of Dreams). In my interpretation, the moment in which the baby is confronted with hunger stimuli a primal fantasy of expectation of a breast is activated. The primal fantasy is one of Freud's central meta-psychological speculations, showing his philosophical bond with Kant. The primal fantasy is like Bion's notion of a pre-conception (see Bion, for example, 1963, p. 93; Grotstein, 2007, p. 63, n. 2). The a priori primal fantasy, as a categorial organizing schema, takes charge of accommodating life impressions, and at the same time confers the expectation of an object on the elements that are expelled to the outside. This has two implications. First, at *intrapsychic* level, the primal fantasies perform significant constructive functions of accommodation, which Freud describes precisely: "wherever experiences fail to fit in with the hereditary schema, they become remodelled in the imagination [. . .]. We are often able to see the schema triumphing over the experience of the individual" (Freud, 1918, p. 119). Second, in *interpsychic* terms, impressions and pre-mental elements are pre-conceptionally addressed to an object, so that they become recognizable to the object and a shared relational space can potentially arise. I.e. to the baby's crying, which is also a motoric discharge of unpleasurable tension, objectal expectations are added that do not yet have any conceptional quality; for the experience of satisfaction, the realization of the primal fantasy has not yet occurred. These objectal additions enable the object to hear the cry as a call (the motoric discharge becomes projective identification) and thus to orient itself to the child. In this orientation the primal fantasy breast of the mother is also activated.

The moment at which the primal fantasy breast of the baby and mother meet with its realization is a presence moment. Bion speaks of O. This presence moment is an event in which the primal fantasy is there in order to become (paraphrasing Winnicott [1971]).

I.e. the primal fantasy "breast" should be understood as a mother-child encounter. Mother and child are there in order to become. This presence moment is devoid of a reflexive subject, devoid of me and you, not conscious and not unconscious. Doing and wanting are not divorced. And yet everything is "there." For Bion, O cannot be known. He writes: "My reason for saying O is unknowable is not that I consider human capacity unequal to the task but because K, L, or H are inappropriate to O. They are appropriate to transformations of O but not to O. . . . Transformations may be scientific, aesthetic, religious, mystical, psycho-analytical" (1970, p. 140).

O can be experienced, "its presence can be recognized and felt, but it cannot be known" (Bion, 1970, p. 30). Any form of description is on this or the other side of O. Therefore, Bion speaks of O-becoming or O-being (see e.g. 1970, p. 27). We can experience O, but we cannot think in K at the same time. Word comes later. What does this mean? In my view we have to dissect Freud's experience of satisfaction: it has its origin in the presence moment, must then be transformed to K in order to become finally a preconception (no hyphen; see Grotstein, 2007). Bion speaks of the transformation $O \rightarrow K$, hence a transformation to knowing.

Bion attempted to describe this process, which is so difficult to understand. According to Bion (1970), in the sinking presence a "constellation" forms; Bion uses this term to "represent the process precipitating a constant conjunction" (1970, p. 33, n. 1). He continues: "The facilitation of 'constellation' must in turn be seen as a step in the process of at-one-ment (the transformation $O \rightarrow K$). In practice, this means not that the analyst recalls some relevant memory, but that a relevant constellation will be evoked during the process of at-one-ment with O, the process denoted by the transformation $O \rightarrow K$" (1970, p. 33). We have seen that the relational pre-conception finds its realization in presence (O). That means that in the oneness (at-one-ment) of presence, duality exists in order to become. The pre-conception is to be thought of as a relational connection that meets its realization in oneness, but then urges the development of duality, thus initiating the constellation. Oneness is therefore only oneness because it carries in itself the duality that leads to the differentiation of subject and object and to the differentiation of preconscious and unconscious (see Nissen, 2015).

I.e. the primal fantasy breast becomes in the experience of satisfaction a scene in which mother and child meet – and this applies to mother and child at the same time. The memory-trace is thus a scenic *gestalt* but of a different kind in mother and child. For the child – in Bion's language – the pre-conception breast becomes the conception, for the mother it becomes a (psychic) thought that has a name and can be used.[2] The mother takes on a containing function for the child.

"'in the beginning was the deed' and the word came later." But for the mother word and deed are linked by the presence event. This is why the word as a name has its magical power.

With the baby it is different. The constellation transformed from O to K has not yet found its psychic equivalent in the word. It is there as a memory-trace but not yet suitable for thinking. It is therefore suitable in a further increase of stimuli for the hallucinatory cathexis of the experience of satisfaction in which wanting (sucking at the breast) is again equal to doing.

Until, as we have already heard, hard reality claims its right (see 1900, p. 566). If the emerging frustration can be tolerated, a thought may emerge about the difference between the hallucination failing and the reality that the mother can breastfeed. In this thought both the experience of satisfaction and the reality are sublated, hence the primal fantasy breast is preserved as a scenic *gestalt* and the factualities of dependence and separation installed for development. Under acknowledgement of reality, deeds were softened into words – but words are connected with the deeds and retained much of their ancient power.

Clinical model

In essence, the basic theoretical considerations are in my opinion reflected in Freud's clinically theoretical models. For without magic no treatment technique can work. But, as mentioned, this magic is not suggestion or not devoid of substance.

Freud captured one of the most central features of psychoanalytical effectiveness in his wonderful phrase that a neurosis cannot be slain in absentia or in effigie (1912, p. 108, or 1914b, p. 152). The neurosis must show itself in statu nascendi, as Freud had already stressed in the "Studies on Hysteria" (Breuer and Freud, 1893–95,

p. 6). That means the neurosis must show itself at *the moment of coming into being*. *Statu nascendi* is not a simple revival of the past, or of constructions of the past, but a process of creation by which neurosis comes into being in the analytic space (see Nissen, 2015).

But what does this mean? It is well known that one of Freud's basic assumptions is that of the primary and secondary process: "The primary process endeavours to bring about a discharge of excitation in order that, with the help of the amount of excitation thus accumulated, it may establish a *'perceptual identity'* [with the experience of satisfaction]. The secondary process, however, has abandoned this intention and taken on another in its place – the establishment of a *'thought identity'* [with that experience]" (1900, p. 602). In the secondary process the Pcs. "*can only cathect an idea if it is in a position to inhibit any development of unpleasure that may proceed from it*" (1900, p. 601). Yet this is precisely what fails in neurosis in which repression has become pathogenic:

> Among these wishful impulses derived from infancy, which can neither be destroyed nor inhibited, there are some whose fulfilment would be a contradiction of the purposive ideas of secondary thinking. The fulfilment of these wishes would no longer generate an affect of pleasure but of unpleasure; *and it is precisely this transformation of affect which constitutes the essence of what we term "repression."*
>
> (1900, p. 604)

If now the repressed, unconscious wish persists and is reinforced, it pushes into the Pcs., there is "a defensive struggle" (1900, p. 605), finally to a formation of symptoms. "But from the moment at which the repressed thoughts are strongly cathected by the unconscious wishful impulse and, on the other hand, abandoned by the preconscious cathexis, they become subject to the primary psychical process and their one aim is motor discharge or, if the path is open, hallucinatory revival of the desired perceptual identity" (1900, p. 605). The Pcs. can therefore no longer work with signals of those complexes and be of use for the thought activity.

Freud goes on to illuminate these dimensions with other concepts; he speaks of word and thing presentations. The thing presentation "consists in the cathexis, if not of the direct memory-images of the thing, at least of remoter memory-traces derived from these" (1915c, p. 201).

The thing presentation appears here as a cathected memory-trace which is thought as a branched out association complex (see 1891). Word presentations on the other hand are linked with consciousness, verbalization and with psychic quality (see 1891, 1895, 1915c, 1923).

> [T]he conscious presentation comprises the presentation of the thing plus the presentation of the word belonging to it, while the unconscious presentation is the presentation of the thing alone. The system Ucs. contains the thing-cathexes of the objects, the first and true object-cathexes; the system Pcs. comes about by this thing-presentation being hypercathected through being linked with the word-presentations corresponding to it. It is these hypercathexes, we may suppose, that bring about a higher psychical organization and make it possible for the primary process to be succeeded by the secondary process which is dominant in the Pcs. Now, too, we are in a position to state precisely what it is that repression denies to the rejected presentation in the transference neuroses: what it denies to the presentation is translation into words which shall remain attached to the object. A presentation which is not put into words, or a psychical act which is not hypercathected, remains thereafter in the Ucs. in a state of repression.
>
> (1915c, p. 201f.)

The thing presentation is assigned to the primary process in which perceptual identity prevails. The thing presentation may thus become hallucinatory wish fulfilment in which the hallucination of sucking at the breast cannot be distinguished from real sucking. Only with tolerance of the absence of the needed object can a thought emerge that becomes a word presentation. With the linking of word and thing presentation a conscious presentation of an object can emerge. A name is created (i.e. it is a creative process), which, as Bion explains, assumes two functions in the psychic: to bind interrelated phenomena, thus to save them from disintegration, and to enrich them with new meaning (see Bion, 1963, p. 87ff.). In this name, however, the thing presentation is always included, i.e. the magic of the word, the deed.

The aim of the psychoanalytic treatment process must therefore be to link word and thing presentation so that a name can emerge that becomes a presentative symbol (Langer, 1942), allowing the formation of new symbols.

I now see the linking of word and thing presentation as a presence moment, as an O. At this moment wanting and doing are not separated, the deed is there without it taking place. The neurotic conflict or the trauma that has actually remained in presence are there to be sublatedby transformation into the name, to K.

To really understand the force of this dynamic it is necessary to explore the thing presentation more deeply. Let us stay with the example of breastfeeding. I had already explained that the thing presentation (as a cathected memory-trace) should not be seen as a memory of a partial object (such as the breast) or of a nutritional-physiological process, neither should it be conceptualized as an engram (see also Laplanche and Pontalis, 1972). The idea of having sucked at the breast, of having experienced love, should therefore be seen scenically as a mother-child encounter. It occurs in different associative complexes. A complex relationship is thus realized at the presence moment and recorded as a branched out memory-trace. For Freud hardly any sensuous-emotional traces are still contained in the memory-trace. Using Kant's words, we might describe this memory-trace as being void.[3] So what are the "intuitions" in the psychic? It will be the psychic factors that appear sensually and are qualified. Bion describes this process as follows:

> Suppose ψ represents a constant, (ξ) an unsaturated element that determines the value of the constant once it has been identified. We may use the unknown constant ψ to represent an inborn pre-conception. Employing a model to give temporary meaning to the term 'inborn pre-conception' I shall suppose that an infant has an inborn pre-conception that a breast that satisfies its own incomplete nature exists. The realization of the breast provides an emotional experience. This experience corresponds to Kant's secondary and primary qualities of a phenomenon. The secondary qualities determine the value of the unsaturated element (ξ) and therefore the value of ψ (ξ). This sign now represents a conception.
>
> (1962, p. 69)

I.e. in the mother-child encounter as an emotional experience quality/affect and presentation/idea are united. We had already heard that for the mother with her developed psychic apparatus this experience becomes a thought, thus word and thing presentation are linked. For the child on the other hand the emotional experience, which is a conception in the presence of the object, becomes a memory-trace which, when it is cathected, pushes as a thing presentation for satisfaction. According to Freud, unconscious presentations/ideas are devoid of quality, or, more precisely, we should say devoid of differentiated qualities.[4] Yet, and that is important, the thing presentation pushes for satisfaction – and it was saturated sensually and emotionally (and will be different and more differentiated in the new experience of satisfaction). I.e. in the thing presentation the *anticipation/expectation* of a sensually and emotionally saturated relationship is as a scene inherent. For Freud it makes little sense to speak of unconscious affect (see 1915d, 1915e). The qualification of this discharge process is performed by the consciousness that Freud and Bion see as the sensory organ for the perception of psychic qualities (see Freud, 1900, p. 615; Bion, for example 1962).[5]

We can thus see the thing presentation as a kind of preconception (no hyphen) pushing for 'actual' satisfaction. If this direction is later rejected by the preconscious (the ego) for factual, moral, aesthetic or other reasons, this may lead to a transformation of affect or suppression.

Short clinical vignette[6] – part 1

A patient of mine began treatment because of, among other things, violent outbursts (lack of impulse control) towards his wife and persistent infantile conflicts with his parents. After we had spoken for many months about his warded-off love for the mother, he "suddenly" recounted a scene from his childhood with such intensity that it cannot be reproduced in words, of how he was walking in the spring sunshine that was breaking through the gentle green with his mother holding his hand wearing a cream-coloured dress that slightly billowed in the wind to fetch milk. All was present: the beautiful mother, her tender touch, the perfusion with oedipally, orally saturated love and happiness, the light, the colours, the sun, the wind, the milk (jug).

At the centre of this little presence moment are the psychogenetically shaped primal fantasy "breast" and that of the oedipal which, though a (screen) memory, become sensually present. These sensory impressions are psychically qualified elements which in their arrangement, similar to a painted picture, give expression to the satisfied (breastfed) love. We can easily recognize the circular conditionality of primal fantasies and elements: The primal fantasies first make the specific psychic elements out of the sensory ones; the constellated elements first allow the primal fantasies to emerge. At the same time, it becomes clear that the primal fantasies as a non-sensual schema have receded into the background again, eluding the explicit and discursive purpose. The tension between elements and conceptional schemata that confront the analytic pair in the presence now needs a name which in its determination has primarily a presentative quality – and as a presentative symbol becomes the starting point of symbol development.

At the same time the scene of this brief presence moment was a part of a scene between the patient and me which was included in the presentative interpretation. For I said to the patient: "That's the way you loved your mother." For months we had spoken about his love for his mother, which he was always defensive about – that it was there was irrefutable, only what it was like, he concealed. This quality and thus what was real about this love were guarded like a secret, the picturesquely drawn scene was therefore something like a revelation – and like a confession. The name of the presence picture was the love for the mother, in the "that's the way" the enactment is captured in the transference.

Psychic disorders

In the example, the boy's almost heavenly love for his mother seems to have been successful, but it was pushed into the abyss of defence – word and thing presentation were separated until the presence moment. I.e. there must have been a psychic conflict which compelled this love to remain hidden.

The rifts in the neurotic illness are located in early childhood, namely at a time in which the child's ego was still undeveloped. Freud expounds his opinion of psychic illness and its emergence origin to the Impartial Person.

Freud sees the ego modified by the influence of the external world, since reality claimed its right with the failure of the hallucinatory wish fulfilment. Nevertheless, the ego is "first and foremost a bodily ego, it is not merely a surface entity, but is itself the *projection* of a surface" and continued in a footnote: "I.e. the ego is ultimately derived from bodily sensations, chiefly from those springing from the surface of the body. It may thus be regarded as a mental projection of the surface of the body, besides, . . . representing the superficies of the mental apparatus" (Freud, 1923, p. 25; italics BN).

So it is a fragile thing, the ego: it is the part of the id that is turned towards the external world, attempting to control the instinctive needs and constituting via physical projective processes the self. At the same time, it is the mediating authority

> between the claims of the id and the objections of the external world. It carries on its activity in two directions. On the one hand, it observes the external world with the help of its sense-organ, the system of consciousness, so as to catch the favourable moment for harmless satisfaction; and on the other hand, it influences the id, bridles its "passions," induces its instincts to postpone their satisfaction, and indeed, if the necessity is recognized, to modify its aims, or, in return for some compensation, to give them up.
>
> (p. 201)

From the pleasure principle to the reality principle.

But negative psychic developments occur during the years of childhood when the ego is still frail: "A small living organism is a truly miserable, powerless thing, is it not? compared with the immensely powerful external world, full as it is of destructive influences. A primitive organism, which has not developed any adequate ego-organization, is at the mercy of all these 'traumas'" (p. 202).

I.e. Freud fully acknowledges the role of the external world, seeing in the failure of primary objects traumatic potential. Yet the ego can learn to avoid via signals of anxiety to avoid assaults from overstimulation by fleeing or changing the external world.

For Freud, however, localization of the pathogenic potential in the external world is not enough. On the contrary, he focuses primarily on the instinct, i.e. the inner urge. To many this may appear unfamiliar/strange since psychoanalysis is getting more and more lost in the interpersonal, but for me Freud's argumentation was a wake-up call not to lose sight of this dimension.

For Freud the tiny little helpless person is first of all an instinct-driven creature:

> Well then, we assume that the forces which drive the mental apparatus into activity are produced in the bodily organs as an expression of the major somatic needs. You will recollect the words of our poet-philosopher: "Hunger and love [are what moves the world]." Incidentally, quite a formidable pair of forces! We give these bodily needs, in so far as they represent an instigation to mental activity, the name of "Triebe" [instincts], a word for which we are envied by many modern languages. Well, these instincts fill the id: all the energy in the id, as we may put it briefly, originates from them. Nor have the forces in the ego any other origin; they are derived from those in the id. What, then, do these instincts want? Satisfaction – that is, the establishment of situations in which the bodily needs can be extinguished. A lowering of the tension of need is felt by our organ of consciousness as pleasurable; an increase of it is soon felt as unpleasure. From these oscillations arises the series of feelings of pleasure-unpleasure, in accordance with which the whole mental apparatus regulates its activity. In this connection we speak of a "dominance of the pleasure principle."
>
> (p. 200)[7]

These instinctual demands press forward again and again and become dangerous both when the environment fails and also when prohibitions from the external world are feared or occur.

> Imagine now what will happen if this powerless ego experiences an instinctual demand from the id which it would already like to resist (because it senses that to satisfy it is dangerous and would conjure up a traumatic situation, a collision with the external world) but which it cannot control, because

> it does not yet possess enough strength to do so. In such a case the ego treats the instinctual danger as if it was an external one; it makes an attempt at flight, draws back from this portion of the id and leaves it to its fate, after withholding from it all the contributions which it usually makes to instinctual impulses. The ego, as we put it, institutes a repression of these instinctual impulses. For the moment this has the effect of fending off the danger; but one cannot confuse the inside and the outside with impunity. One cannot run away from oneself. In repression the ego is following the pleasure principle, which it is usually in the habit of correcting; and it is bound to suffer damage in revenge. This lies in the ego's having permanently narrowed its sphere of influence. The repressed instinctual impulse is now isolated, left to itself, inaccessible, but also uninfluenceable.
>
> (p. 202f.)

A human being's instincts, which should be thought psychosomatically (see Freud, 1915a), initiate de facto the pathological spiral, regardless of whether there is or is not a failing environment (it can, but does not have to exist!). Let us take a closer schematic look at this dynamic. At first we assume an early disorder, a newborn baby in a failing environment, for example, a mother incapable of love. The baby, who does not yet have a developed ego, expects a nourishing, i.e. in the mental area: a loving breast so that the primal fantasy is realized as a mother-child encounter. The baby now encounters a "bad" breast, i.e. an event occurs in which (from the observer's perspective) no positive realization of expectation occurs, the emotional experience is traumatic. It is important now that the baby feels with what is understood – where there is nothing to understand! It believes it is the loving mother who makes life and development possible, even though it is the failing one who does not make life possible. At the same time the somatic experience is devastating confusion (basal thought disorder). I write somatic experience here deliberately since what Bion calls emotional experience is in this case almost only experienced as somatic tension states. Perhaps the baby tries to evade this external threat by (motoric) obviation, it turns its head away, no longer drinks, struggles. But before this there is the instinct! Before it comes to the breast the next time, the instinct has already made an impact. The first memory-trace, driven by the instinct to become a thing presentation, is 'there' in the cathexis as a hallucination (perceptual identity). Then the instinct becomes a source of danger. That is why "the ego treats the instinctual danger as if it was an external one." Then, fatally, the real breast, even if it is 'good,' is often treated like the 'bad one.' The consequences of such an early disorder can be devastating. In addition to the repressions described by Freud, traumatic, actual (Baranger et al., 1988) processes may emerge or even breakdowns (Winnicott, 1974) may occur, leading to the abandonment of hope of a containing object (see Bion, 1970; Meltzer et al., 1975) and finally ending in autistoid organizations.

Yet even though the ego has become more mature, the instinct's primacy continues to exist in psychopathological dynamics. Considering our clinical example, we assume there is a boy in an oedipal conflict. The patient loved his mother, orally, phallically, oedipally, while disappointment and anger appeared in the anal area in domination, control and ejection (cf. Abraham, 1924) of the object. Here, too, we have to understand that in the id (in the unconscious) the love for his mother means that he sensually enjoys the oral delights, is phallically beamed at by the mother and interacts with her oedipally. Thus, in urging a libidinous excitation polymorphous love is 'there' in the cathected thing presentation, hallucination and reality are not definitely separated/ distinguishable! The force of this hallucinatory yearning became evident in the outlined moment of presence. And it found its phallic-oedipal realizations, as the (screen) memory "fetching milk" showed. Sexual instinctual excitations therefore lead unconsciously to the certainty of being the mother's "man" and must be cut/honed by reality.

If the parental object is now not able to offer the oedipal primal fantasy adequate realizations with a clear demarcation, no idea can emerge in which the oedipal exclusion is the same as the inclusion in the relationship and its safekeeping. The spectrum of negative psychopathological developments is wide, ranging from negative, destructive realizations to low frustration tolerance towards inherent disappointments. It is important, however, in all cases that the instinct begins to work in the unconscious and that perceptual identity prevails there – and all attempts to escape the instinctual danger will lead to disaster. A word can no longer be created, so any ways of defusing the conflict by change, symbolically and/or subliminally, are thwarted. The connection between word and thing presentation must emerge in the analytic process in statu nascendi and be settled in presentia. I.e. the impact of the deed, which is preserved in the primary process, must become real in the treatment – in the presence moment.

Clinical vignette – part 2

In the presentative interpretation: "That's the way you loved your mother" the neurotic conflict remained unsublated. It was irrefutable that understanding the mother's love was a fundamental fact. Yet why was it so difficult for him to communicate this spherically beautiful love? Why the outbursts (lack of impulse control) against his wife when he can love like that after all?

The "that's the way" is a presentative presentiment, but not yet a presentative name. It indicates that the primal fantasies of the love for the mother are a part of a complex that is pressing for enactment. And this was to be sought in the oedipal area which though shimmering in the milk fetching scene has not been given its final form.

In the following months we tried to grasp the disappointment with the mother and the idealization of the hated yet secretly loved father. This was followed by a similarly dense and intensive scene. He remembered as a little boy being held by the nanny and the parents all dressed up to go out for the evening. He then said dejectedly: "My father gripped my mother and tugged her along with him. He held her arm. They walked along the hallway, then my mother turned round, waved to me, and then she looked at my father, laughing and radiant . . . silence. . . . You see, she loved him!"

So the father didn't make off with the mother, didn't abduct her to late-night parties and delights, but the mother loved him, left the boy behind in order to enjoy the pleasures of the night. A disappointment he never forgave her for and which he acted out towards his wife (the slightest associative things would lead to aggressive outbursts). The father was crudely idealized for fear of castration, thus kept at bay, at the same time protected against his own aggression.

In this process primal fantasies evolve that are to be understood as a scenic relationship. The primal fantasy breast should be thought of as a scenic encounter between mother and child, which with its realizations is given an elementary form and in this patient was condensed in a very sensual screen memory (milk fetching image). The oedipal primal fantasy is by definition a complex relationship scene. In our patient, however, the realization of the oedipal truth led to a disappointment shock which made its further processing difficult and even impossible – too great were the anger and disappointment, too little did the objects help to acknowledge this mental truth.

The complex "love for the mother" exists in the patient in a differentiated, evolved form; it seems as it is not per se pathogenically conflictual. The neurotic conflicts emerge only through the oedipal truth that the patient experiences as castration, as a narcissistic slight or insult and unbearable disappointment. With each new, instinctual surge of love it is 'there' in the unconscious and must be warded off. Anal-sadistic control and domination channel the affects, leading in failure to anal-sadistic ejection. The destroyed objects are reintrojected as remnants of the Oedipus complex, creating a form of the superego shadow (Freud, 1917b).

The effect of the treatment

The psychoanalytic treatment must therefore reach the point in the (transference) process at which the neurotic complex or the traumatic event appears in presentia, i.e. when the deed included in the thing presentation is 'there.' In our example the desire for the mother is really to love her phallically oedipally, the wish cannot be separated from the deed. Hatred of the father is really wanting to remove him, here too the wish cannot be separated from the deed. Only when this impact appears in the presence moment (in O) can a word be found creatively, a link between thing and word presentation be established that can lead to finding a name and symbol formation. This is the magic of the word.

In analytic treatments it is therefore necessary to wait for the kairos in which the O appears. Freud also indicates this to the Impartial Person: "You must wait for the right moment at which you can communicate your interpretation to the patient with some prospect of success. . . . You will be making a bad mistake if, in an effort, perhaps, at shortening the analysis, you throw your interpretations at the patient's head as soon as you have found them" (p. 220). Freud emphasizes that the analysis must succeed in reproducing the kernel of his intimate life history as though it were actually happening (p. 226). Then transference can be interpretatively sublated. "The only possible way out of the transference situation is to trace it back to the patient's past, as he *really* experienced it or as he pictured it through the wish-fulfilling activity of his imagination" (p. 227; italics BN).[8]

In my interpretation of the Freudian theory and argumentation the "really" can also be understood beyond the dispute over memory, construction, reconstruction. The "really" has its foundation in the instinct (Trieb). The instinct "as the psychical representative of the stimuli originating from within the organism and reaching the mind" (1915a, p. 122) and as "the nucleus of the Ucs" (1915c, p. 195) fulfils the primal fantasies (pre-conceptions), which in their realization contain the kernel of his intimate life history, hence the individual psychical truth that is revealed in O in which the reflexive subject is absent. As already described, the thing presentation presses for "actual," for real satisfaction. Only the evoked presentation, which revives the original affect, is therapeutically effective. This applies to both the conflict and to the trauma which has remained actual. With the transformation to K this "really" is again concealed, but as a deed it was indeed 'there.' This "really," which is revealed in the testimony of the transference, thus sublates the neurotic conflict, the traumatic event.

The role of sexuality

Freud had already developed the concept of the death instinct at the time of writing his defence for Reik. In lay analysis he refers again with recourse to Schiller to the duality of ego and sexual instincts ("hunger and love") which preceded the period of ego and object instincts (see Freud's own overview of the instinct theory at the end of Chapter 6 in "Beyond the Pleasure Principle"). In his argumentation with the Impartial Person he refers de facto only to sexuality. There may be political reasons for this, and it seems that he uses this paper to finally put an end to all the ignorance, arrogance and stupidity that is hurled against psychoanalysis. Here the text takes on almost dramatic proportions: The Impartial Person:

> "I shall venture, for once in a way, to take sides on that point. It strikes me as extremely bold to assert that sexuality is not a natural, primitive need of living organisms, but an expression of something else. One need only take the example of animals."
>
> That makes no difference. There is no mixture, however absurd, that society will not willingly swallow down if it is advertised as an antidote to the dreaded predominance of sexuality.
>
> I confess, moreover, that the dislike that you yourself have betrayed of assigning to the factor of sexuality so great a part in the causation of neurosis – I confess that this scarcely seems to me consistent with your task as an Impartial Person. Are you not afraid that this antipathy may interfere with your passing a just judgement?
>
> (p. 208)

Yet what could the scientific reasons be for Freud to give sexuality the most prominent position?[9] Without a doubt "The libido has the task of making the destroying instinct innocuous" (1924, p. 163); without such making innocuous there would be no life. Yet that cannot be the reason. It must lie in Freud's understanding of sexuality.

The sexual instincts are based on the vital instincts, the pleasure in sucking is for example 'socialized' with food intake, as Freud calls it (1905). Yet despite this dependence (anaclisis) and despite the "'diphasic onset' . . . of sexual life" (p. 211) the sexual instincts are not secondary but independent and psychically primary; "sexual instinctual impulses accompany life from birth onwards" (p. 209). These polymorphic-perverse aspirations quickly detach themselves from the physiological functions, may find auto-erotic satisfaction and develop erogenous zones. "The sexual function, from its beginnings to the definitive form in which it is so familiar to us, undergoes a complicated process of development. It grows together from numerous component instincts with different aims and passes through several phases of organization till at last it comes into the service of reproduction" (p. 210). This shows that the object of the instinct is not biologically determined but variable and diverse, and that its aims are variable. Sexuality is, as Laplanche and Pontalis (1972) describe it in their discussion of the keyword "sexuality," in its genesis not exclusively biological and neither is infantile sexuality a retrospective illusion.

But what is included in sexuality, what is the catalytic moment that makes the self-referential process of sexual organization possible? And why does Freud insist that sexuality play a powerful pathogenic role (he even warns in "Group Psychology and the Analysis of the Ego" (1921) against softening the sexual with the term Eros.

Laplanche and Pontalis answer the first question with recourse to the primal fantasy, which has phylogenetic roots and as a categorial schema assumes an organizing function in the mental area. It is interesting to see that Freud in conversation with the Impartial Person again and again refers to cultural history and mythology. What is dealt with in these original writings of mankind are the original themes of human life, indeed of human being. These "primal scenes" are therefore inscribed in human life, or more precisely: utilize sexuality as a medium. But then what is subject to repression, in more general terms: defence, is not the biological sexual instinct but the psychic scenes which become conflictual or are overwhelmed traumatically by reality. These psychic scenes or primal fantasies are therefore sublated in sexuality. As sexual lust as an instinct recurs rhythmically pressing for satisfaction, the primal fantasies also press for realization – and that with the sexual instinct deprived of the ego's sovereignty. That is not a problem as long as these emotions are in harmony with the instances and the external world. But if they encounter a failing environment, traumas emerge, if they encounter internal and external disapproval, conflicts emerge. Since these traumas and conflicts are coupled with the sexual instinct, the conflicts or traumas always occur intrapsychically if the instinct presses for satisfaction. This is why, I believe, Freud attaches such great importance to the instinct and the goings-on of the unconscious; this is why he emphasizes the role of sexuality. Sexuality is pleasurable, can never be completely killed and recurs rhythmically, following the laws of the unconscious, again and again.

In the unconscious the desire for the object is already the deed, the turning to the object already seduction – mysteries that cannot be solved but can be sublated in the word.

Laypersons in psychoanalysis

With such an interpretation of Freudian criticism and theory it is evident that "psycho-analysis is not a specialized branch of medicine" and also not one of academic psychology with its different branches (cognition, motivation, etc.). Psychoanalysis aims at understanding the psychic truth and reality of the individual in their complex dynamic and structure. To this day the linkage between healing and research applies that all basic theoretical, theoretical and treatment innovations, the number of which is myriad, hail from the psychoanalytic treatments. It is unquestionable that findings from related disciplines such as infant research and attachment theory, neuroscience, psychiatry, perception psychology, cultural history, mythology, linguistics and so on are important for psychoanalysis. But psychoanalysis has its own scientific reference system, however, namely the psychic. Other sciences could not be recommended as its leading system.

Now the conclusion might be drawn (as was frequently the case as early as in the discussions in 1927) that psychoanalytic universities should be established. I think that this is wrong. Psychoanalytic training cannot take place at universities. The substantial core of the education is the training-analysis and is psychoanalytic treatment under supervision. The psychoanalytic treatment is the highly frequent meeting of two people with no time limit who in the relationship work on the mysteries, conflicts and traumas and create words for them so that they become thinkable. This process is complemented by a canon of scientific literature that is explored in seminars. Psychoanalysis as the science of the human being, however, needs a wide range of different educational backgrounds in its ranks, since the subject of psychoanalysis can be intuited from a wide range of different perspectives (Bion, 1965, 1970). Even divergent positions enrich analytic thinking: artists, on the one side of the spectrum, know more about the inherent laws of creative processes than most social and natural scientists; mathematicians, on the other side of the spectrum, teach us for example something about points, lines, areas and spaces which are helpful for gaining an understanding of many pathologies (for instance two-dimensional flattening in autistoid or severe depressive disorders). But they profit, as Bion showed, from psychoanalysis as well.

All sciences have developed from the mind, from human being's unconscious. Psychoanalysis is the science of the unconscious – which is why it needs a variety of scientists in its ranks.

Notes

1 Here it becomes clear why Bion attaches so much importance to the tolerance of frustration.

2 It may also be asked if a distinction between word and name should be introduced. The word (word presentation) can be detached from the thing presentation and thus no longer be a mental signifier; the term 'name' should include this connection.

3 "Gedanken ohne Inhalt sind leer, Anschauungen ohne Begriffe sind blind. Daher ist es ebenso notwendig, seine Begriffe sinnlich zu machen, (d.i. ihnen den Gegenstand in der Anschauung beizufügen,) als seine Anschauungen sich verständlich zu machen (d.i. sie unter Begriffe zu bringen)" (Kant, 1787). In English (translated by J.M.D. Meiklejohn): "Thoughts without content are void; intuitions without conceptions, blind. Hence it is as necessary for the mind to make its conceptions sensuous (that is, to join to them the object in intuition), as to make its intuitions intelligible (that is, to bring them under conceptions)."

4 Freud ascribes to the unconscious two basal qualitative states: pleasure and unpleasure (see for example 1900, 1915c). Even when he brings qualitative factors into play in "Beyond the Pleasure Principle" (1920) and in "The Economic Problem of Masochism" (1924), he tries to define them observably, e.g. rhythm and the like.

5 In "The Unconscious" Freud concludes: "The whole difference arises from the fact that ideas are cathexes – basically of memory-traces – whilst affects and feelings correspond to processes of discharge, the final manifestations of which are perceived as sensations. In the present state of our knowledge of affects and feelings we cannot express this difference more clearly." (1915c, p. 178). In "The Neuro-Psychoses of Defence" (1894a) Freud compares the quota of affect with an electric current. This means that the qualification remains coupled with the consciousness.

6 The clinical example is taken from Nissen (2014).

7 It is interesting that Freud again refers back to a writer (Schiller), and at a time when the concept of the death instinct was already developed, calls self-preservation and sexual instincts a duality.

8 In German the sentence has a more precise meaning: Instead of 'pictured' Freud uses 'gestalten.'

9 He writes at the end of his life: "Theoretically there is no objection to supposing that any sort of instinctual demand might occasion the same repressions and their consequences; but our observation shows us invariably, so far as we can judge, that the excitations that play this pathogenic part arise from the component instincts of sexual life" (1940, p. 186).

References

Abraham, K. (1924). Versuch einer Entwicklungsgeschichte der Libido auf Grund der Psychoanalyse seelischer Störungen. In: *Karl Abraham: Gesammelte Schriften Bd. II*. Frankfurt am Main: Fischer Taschenbuch Verlag.

Baranger, M., Baranger, W., and Mom, J.M. (1988). The Infantile Psychic Trauma from Us to Freud: Pure Trauma, Retroactivity and Reconstruction. *International Journal of Psycho-Analysis*, 69: 113–128.

Bion, W.R. (1962). *Learning from Experience*. London: Tavistock.

Bion, W.R. (1963). *Elements of Psycho-Analysis*. London: Heinemann.

Bion, W.R. (1965). *Transformations*. London: Tavistock.

Bion, W.R. (1970). *Attention and Interpretation*. London: Tavistock.

Breuer, J., and Freud, S. (1893–95). Studies on Hysteria. *SE*, II.

Freud, S. (1891). *Zur Auffassung der Aphasien: Eine kritische Studie*. Wien & Leipzig: Franz Deuticke Verlag.

Freud, S. (1894). The Neuro-Psychoses of Defence. In: *The Standard Edition of the Complete Psychological Works of Sigmund Freud, Volume III (1893–1899): Early Psycho-Analytic Publications* (pp. 41–61).

Freud, S. (1895 [1950]). Project for a Scientific Psychology (1950 [1895]). In: *The Standard Edition of the Complete Psychological Works of Sigmund Freud, Volume I (1886–1899): Pre-Psycho-Analytic Publications and Unpublished Drafts* (pp. 281–391). *SE*, IV.

Freud, S. (1900). The Interpretation of Dreams. In: *The Standard Edition of the Complete Psychological Works of Sigmund Freud, Volume IV (1900): The Interpretation of Dreams (First Part)* (pp. 9–627).

Freud, S. (1905). Three Essays on the Theory of Sexuality (1905). In: *The Standard Edition of the Complete Psychological Works of Sigmund Freud, Volume VII (1901–1905): A Case of Hysteria, Three Essays on Sexuality and Other Works* (pp. 123–246).

Freud, S. (1912). The Dynamics of Transference. *SE*, XII.

Freud, S. (1914a). On Narcissism. In: *The Standard Edition of the Complete Psychological Works of Sigmund Freud, Volume XIV (1914–1916): On the History of the Psycho-Analytic Movement, Papers on Metapsychology and Other Works* (pp. 67–102).

Freud, S. (1914b). Remembering, Repeating and Working-Through (Further Recommendations on the Technique of Psycho-Analysis II). In: *The Standard Edition of the Complete Psychological Works of Sigmund Freud, Volume XII (1911–1913): The Case of Schreber, Papers on Technique and Other Works* (pp. 145–156).

Freud, S. (1915a). Instincts and Their Vicissitudes. In: *The Standard Edition of the Complete Psychological Works of Sigmund Freud, Volume XIV (1914–1916): On the History of the Psycho-Analytic Movement, Papers on Metapsychology and Other Works* (pp. 109–140).

Freud, S. (1915b). Repression. In: *The Standard Edition of the Complete Psychological Works of Sigmund Freud, Volume XIV (1914–1916): On the History of the Psycho-Analytic Movement, Papers on Metapsychology and Other Works* (pp. 141–158).

Freud, S. (1915c). The Unconscious. In: *The Standard Edition of the Complete Psychological Works of Sigmund Freud, Volume XIV (1914–1916): On the History of the Psycho-Analytic Movement, Papers on Metapsychology and Other Works* (pp. 159–215).

Freud, S. (1917a). A Metapsychological Supplement to the Theory of Dreams. In: *The Standard Edition of the Complete Psychological Works of Sigmund Freud, Volume XIV (1914–1916): On the History of the Psycho-Analytic Movement, Papers on Metapsychology and Other Works* (pp. 217–235).

Freud, S. (1917b). Mourning and Melancholia. In: *The Standard Edition of the Complete Psychological Works of Sigmund Freud, Volume XIV (1914–1916): On the History of the Psycho-Analytic Movement, Papers on Metapsychology and Other Works* (pp. 237–258).

Freud, S. (1918). *From the History of an Infantile Neurosis. SE*, XVII

Freud, S. (1920). Beyond the Pleasure Principle. In: *The Standard Edition of the Complete Psychological Works of Sigmund Freud, Volume XVIII (1920–1922): Beyond the Pleasure Principle, Group Psychology and Other Works* (pp. 1–64).

Freud, S. (1921). Group Psychology and the Analysis of the Ego. In: *The Standard Edition of the Complete Psychological Works of Sigmund Freud, Volume XVIII (1920–1922): Beyond the Pleasure Principle, Group Psychology and Other Works* (pp. 65–144).

Freud, S. (1923). The Ego and the Id. In: *The Standard Edition of the Complete Psychological Works of Sigmund Freud, Volume XIX (1923–1925): The Ego and the Id and Other Works* (pp. 1–66).

Freud, S. (1924). The Economic Problem of Masochism. In: *The Standard Edition of the Complete Psychological Works of Sigmund Freud, Volume XIX (1923–1925): The Ego and the Id and Other Works* (pp. 155–170).

Freud, S. (1926). The Question of Lay Analysis. In: *The Standard Edition of the Complete Psychological Works of Sigmund Freud, Volume XX (1925–1926): An Autobiographical Study, Inhibitions, Symptoms and Anxiety, The Question of Lay Analysis and Other Works* (pp. 177–258).

Freud, S. (1940 [1938]). An Outline of Psycho-Analysis. In: *The Standard Edition of the Complete Psychological Works of Sigmund Freud, Volume XXIII (1937–1939): Moses and Monotheism, An Outline of Psycho-Analysis and Other Works* (pp. 139–208).

Grotstein, J.S. (2007). *A Beam of Intense Darkness. Wilfred Bion's Legacy to Psychoanalysis*. London: Karnac.

Jones, E. (1927). Die Frage Der Laienanalyse: Unterredungen Mit Einem Unparteiischen. *International Journal of Psycho-Analysis*, 8: 86–92.

Kant, I. (1787). *Kritik der reinen Vernunft (The Critique of Pure Reason)* Frankfurt a.M: STW.

Langer, S.K. (1942). *Philosophy in a New Key*. Cambridge, MA: Harvard University Press.

Laplanche, J., and Pontalis, J.-B. (1972). *Das Vokabular der Psychoanalyse*. Frankfurt am Main: STW.

Meltzer, D. et al. (1975). *Explorations in Autism*. Perthshire: Clunie Press.

Nissen, B. (2014). Die Szene im psychoanalytischen Erstinterview. texte. *Psychoanalyse*. Ästhetik. Kulturkritik. 34, Heft 4. Wien, Passagen-Verlag.

Nissen, B. (2015). Faith (F) and Presence (O) in Analytic Processes: An Example of a Narcissistic Disorder. *International Journal of Psycho-Analysis*, 96.

Strachey, J. (1926). Editor's Note to "The Question of Lay Analysis". In: *The Standard Edition of the Complete Psychological Works of Sigmund Freud, Volume XX (1925–1926): An Autobiographical Study, Inhibitions, Symptoms and Anxiety, The Question of Lay Analysis and Other Works* (pp. 179–181). *SE*, XX.

Winnicott, D.W. (1971). *Playing and Reality*. London: Tavistock Publications.

Winnicott, D.W. (1974). Fear of Breakdown. *International Review of Psycho-Analysis*, 1: 103–107.

7

The analyst and his odyssey

Like Ulysses, we must not forget the return journey . . .

Monica Horovitz[1]

Ithaka gave you the marvelous journey.
Without her you would not have set out.
– C.P. Cavafy, Collected Poems, 1992, p. 35

Wisdom or oblivion – take your choice.
From that warfare there is no release.
– W.R. Bion, A Memoir of the Future, 1979, p. 136

"Why revisit the subject of lay analysis today?" Because, as J.-B. Pontalis (1985) writes, "the question of lay analysis lies at the heart of analysis itself" (p. 12).

> The status of psychoanalysis has always been uncertain and disputed when approached from a scientific view that demands evidence and is easily conflated with scientism. Today, part of the return of the medical model via the neurosciences reflects the anxieties inherent in the analytic endeavor and the undiminished yearning for some kind of unquestionable credibility. Re-reading Freud I find this theme weaving through all his work. In this context, the radical aspects of Freud's conceptualizations must be rediscovered by each new generation. Freud remains a guide for how to travel in the turbulent waters of psychoanalytical discovery.

> To speak of lay analysis is thus to speak of psychoanalysis in its specificity. This is exactly what Freud himself said when he stated that the essential difficulty of the task he was undertaking in 1926 lay in making his imaginary interlocutor understand that "Analysis is a procedure *sui generis*, something novel and special, which can only be understood with the help of *new* insights – or hypotheses".
>
> (Freud, 1926, pp. 189–190, Freud's emphasis)

And yet an attempt to take stock of the current relevance and validity of Freudian theory inevitably leads us to realize that our current philosophical, political and social developments constantly call into question, in every way possible, this singularity of psychoanalysis. At the same time, we are bound to make a parallel observation: the psychoanalytic community, whose passion for work and theoretical advances cannot be questioned, struggles to defend this specificity in any way other than resorting to the appeal of magic, to the point that we may ask ourselves if the so-called singularity, by dint of its apparent self-evidence, has not become a blind spot for psychoanalysts.

This specificity of psychoanalysis appears clearly, right from its beginnings, in what may be called, without blushing or shuddering, the Freudian *politics* of psychoanalysis which, like all politics, cannot do without such figures of castration as choices, separations, oppositions and distinctions. If we cast our minds back for a moment to the conflicts and ruptures with Jung, Rank and Ferenczi, among others, we will always find, whether a matter of theory or practice, the question of the singularity of psychoanalysis, the question of lay analysis.

But beyond this field of the politics of psychoanalysis, we need to identify in the literature of psychoanalytical theory, and in the various forms of its practical application, the nature of this lay quality, this specificity. In short, very modestly, it may be necessary, once again, to return to Freud, just as Ulysses returned to Ithaca, and "continue to work", as Freud himself invited Pfister to do in October 1923, adding: "You know that the truth often has to be said many times" (letter of Freud to Pfister, dated October 30, 1923, in Freud and Pfister, 1963, p. 90). Freud asserts, for example, that the question of medicine in its totality, with everything that it entails in terms of denying the transference (and even banalizing it) and excluding sexuality, is no longer at the heart of lay analysis.

This brutal and, as such, provocative formulation is only there to introduce what I would venture to call a thesis, namely, that the question of lay analysis remains centred on its relationship to medicine, not only throughout Freud's entire work, from *The Interpretation of Dreams* (1900) to *Moses and Monotheism* (1939), but still today, behind the deceptive masks of current developments, those of psychology in particular.

In the famous postscript to his essay on lay analysis, which he wrote in the wake of the debate that followed its first edition, Freud makes some important clarifications which have been taken up recently by various authors concerned with identifying certain aspects of the contemporary crisis in psychoanalysis, beginning with those who express themselves through a certain confusion in terms:

> For practical reasons we have been in the habit – and this is true, incidentally, of our publications as well – of distinguishing between medical and applied analysis. But that is not a logical distinction. The true line of division is between scientific analysis and its applications alike in medical and in non-medical fields.
>
> (Freud, 1926, p. 257)

Taking this "line of division" into consideration leads to a distinction between the related, but not identical, forms of concrete existence of lay analysis in three registers.

Medical and non-medical applications of psychoanalysis constitute, then, one of the aspects of this *line of division*, the other being the register that Freud calls *scientific analysis* – that of psychoanalytic theory proper. In this context, the specificity of psychoanalysis, lay analysis, is expressed primarily at the epistemological level, and the essential question alludes to the nature of the said scientificity of psychoanalysis.

It is the epistemological traces of this scientificity (of its construction and of the rejections it implies), insofar as it is constitutive of the specificity of psychoanalysis, that I want to identify briefly in Freud's writings, and show their enduring presence, from *The Interpretation of Dreams* to *Moses and Monotheism*, the last work in which two aspects of lay analysis, that of scientificity and that of its non-medical applications, are juxtaposed. What is involved here is the slow, painful process of gestation of psychoanalysis – in the nature of a transformation or mutation rather than a rupture, with what the latter implies in the way of rapidity and immediateness – which began very early on, at least as early as the *Project* (1950 [1895]) and the letters to Wilhelm Fliess, and continued up until *The Interpretation of Dreams* (1900), of which these texts are the prolegomena.

The process, as we know, was endless and consisted in delimiting, step by step, the space peculiar to psychoanalysis. The goal was to establish the foundations of its specificity while rejecting all other approaches (neurological, physiological, medical and psychological, as well as philosophical and later religious) which aimed to take its place by way of their empirical or spiritual objects. Or worse, they sought to argue that this domain did not exist at all, invariably striving to mask or invalidate the unconscious, the contours of which Freud was beginning to discern.

The abandonment, in 1897, of the theory of seduction already meant abandoning the reassuring shores of concrete facts that could be referred to very real acts, with what such a step implies in terms of linear causality. Isn't it possible to read here, already, one of the lines of fundamental tension that we will re-encounter, unchanged, forty years later in his *historical novel*? There he stated his fear that his "hypothesis that Moses was an Egyptian" was "based only on psychological probabilities" which "lacked any objective proof" (Freud, 1939, p. 17).

The imperious necessity of abandoning these comfortable shores of certainty, but also the risk inherent in negotiating the turbulence of the plausible, will thus be constantly underlined, right up to the end. Moreover, Freud will never fail to point to the illusion of definitively established knowledge as a form of resistance to which psychoanalysts are most vulnerable. This is indeed what he tells Pfister in January 1926 when, in informing him about the forthcoming publication of his essay *Inhibitions, Symptoms and Anxiety* (1926), he predicts that: "Analysts who above all want peace and certainty will be disconcerted at having to revise their ideas" (Freud & Pfister, p. 102).

Freud makes a departure of the same order concerning another piece of "objective proof" when he refutes the relationship that Fliess wants to establish between bisexuality as a theoretical, conceptual hypothesis, and the bilaterality invoked to serve as empirical foundation: "It seems to me that I object only to the permeation of bisexuality and bilaterality that you demand" (letter from Freud to Fliess dated January 4, 1898, in Masson, 1985, p. 292). And it is to Fliess, who already envisions the finished dream book in March 1898, that he swiftly replies, letting slip what may be understood both as a regret and as a satisfaction: "It seems to me that the theory of wish-fulfilment has brought only the psychological solution and not the biological, or rather, metapsychological one" (Masson, 1985, p. 301).

So, if one must leave behind the highly reassuring coordinates of biologists and physiologists (psychologists in Masson's translation) – the physiologists of whom he will say (when the book is almost finished) that they will "in any case find enough to rail against, but a thing like this turns out just as it will" (ibid., p. 368) – perhaps there is a chance of feeling less alone, of distinguishing other points of support, for example, in the border zone where philosophy and psychology rub shoulders. He thus finds in the writings of Lipps, a philosopher and psychologist who seems to him to have the "clearest mind" of anyone of his time, the exposition of his own principles, an exposition that is almost too perfect and, in any case, "perhaps rather more so than I would like" (ibid., p. 325). Only a few months will be needed for this point of support to be swept away, in turn, by the storm of *The Interpretation of Dreams*.

A book on dreams. A book devoted to objects with no empirical existence which only exist through the account that the dreamer can give of them – a partial, truncated and distorted account and, as such, highly unreliable in comparison with the foundations on which a scientific approach worthy of its name is supposed to be based. Of this object he will say as follows in "On Dreams" (1901a), a text whose publication followed the principal work:

> One day I discovered to my great astonishment that the view of dreams that came nearest to the truth was not the medical but the popular one, half involved though it still was in superstition.
> (Freud, 1901a, p. 635)

Of this object he reaffirms that "we have in fact no knowledge or, speaking more correctly, we have no guarantee that we know them as they actually occurred" (1900, p. 512). This idea, emphasized in the famous Chapter 7 of *The Interpretation of Dreams*, a chapter to which commentators have rightly attached great value, may already be found in "the scientific literature dealing with the problem of dreams", a devalued chapter if ever there was one, devalued even by the author himself. It is with the positivists he takes issue now, those who, like Tissié, want nothing to do with the psychic origin of dreams and affirm that *"les rêves d'origine absolument psychique n'existent pas"* ["dreams of purely psychic origin do not exist"] or *"les pensées de nos rêves nous viennent du dehors"* ["thoughts in our dreams reach us from outside"] (1900, p. 41).

This negation of the psychic essence of dreams and beyond, of the potential existence of what he has already called the *psychical apparatus* (a subject he will develop in Chapter 7), he emphasizes right away. He does so in a manner that serves to confirm, already, the presence, even in the terms employed, of the question of lay analysis, which is completely in line with "the prevailing trend of thought in psychiatry today" (p. 41). On this point he adds (and there can be no doubt that each of the terms used has been carefully weighed):

> It is true that the dominance of the brain over the organism is asserted with apparent confidence. Nevertheless, anything that might indicate that mental life is in any way independent of demonstrable organic changes or that its manifestations are in any way spontaneous alarms the modern psychiatrist, as if a recognition of such things would inevitably bring back the days of the Philosophy of Nature and of the metaphysical view of the mind. The suspicions of the psychiatrists have put the mind, as it were, under tutelage, and they now insist that none of its impulses shall be allowed to suggest that it has any means of its own.
>
> (Freud, 1900, p. 41)

In other words, the epistemological and theoretical space that Freud is creating, namely, that of the *independence of mental life*, dismisses the alternative that opposes brain science (and psychiatry played a part in this just as it is playing a part today, at the risk of hastening its own disappearance) to the metaphysics of the mind. This alternative, which Freud rejected in 1899, is precisely the one we face today. The respectability of a "cognitive science", the appendage and partially authorized spokesman of neuroscience, a "cognitive science" which, at the most, can admit the idea of an unconscious as long as it is cerebral, is being opposed to the darkness of obscurantism – the realm of superstition and popular beliefs, of religious and irrational approaches.

If, since 1900, the struggle for the autonomy of psychic life, for the independence of mental life has remained just as bitter, it is worth noting that in 1939, during the intermediate stage of our journey constituted by *Moses and Monotheism*, the question is approached in precisely the same terms. To justify the concordance between individual and group processes on the one hand, and to compensate for the failure of history and archaeology to give the history of Judaism a plausible explanation on the other, he has to draw attention to the most accomplished aspect of psychoanalytic theory: "I will add the further comment that the psychical topography that I have developed here has nothing to do with the anatomy of the brain" (1939, p. 97).

The more external forces resist the Freudian breakthrough, the more the creation of this space independent of a science of the mind involves the need for boldness, and the more it is necessary to be demanding and uncompromising with regard to ideas and to the way they are expressed. Once it has been shown (though history will confirm that the issue has never been resolved once and for all) that brain medicine, however respectable it may be when it remains on its own territory, is of no help when it goes beyond it, once this *psychical apparatus* – which Freud stresses is a theoretical object, "a psychical locality", thus avoiding the temptation to "determine psychical locality in any anatomical fashion" (1900, p. 536) – has been elaborated, it is necessary to turn towards closer neighbours who have gone beyond the superstition stage. To do so, one must know how far one can go in the company of this or that ally and when one must break off relations – differentiate, whatever the cost. That is why, once again, we come across Lipps, with whom, for a while, cordiality is still a requirement: "The problem of the unconscious in psychology is, in the forcible words of Lipps, less a psychological problem than the problem of psychology itself" (1900, p. 611).

A further step with this same Lipps makes the following assertion possible:

> It is essential to abandon the overvaluation of the property of being conscious before it becomes possible to form any correct view of the origin of what is mental. In Lipps's words, the unconscious must be assumed to be the general basis of psychical life. . . . The unconscious is the true psychical reality.
>
> (Freud, 1900, pp. 612–613)

Only a page later, and the separation is accomplished; it is based on the very simple affirmation of the specificity of the unconscious as psychoanalysis, henceforth definitively autonomous, conceives it:

> It is not without intention that I speak of "our" unconscious. For what I thus describe is not the same as the unconscious of the philosophers or even the unconscious of Lipps. . . . Thus there are two kinds of unconscious, which have not yet been distinguished by psychologists. Both of them are unconscious in the sense used by psychology; but in our sense one of them, which we term the *Ucs.*, is also *inadmissible to consciousness*.
>
> (Freud, 1900, pp. 614–615)

One could happily go on reading this text, which becomes more fascinating and astounding every time and attests to the emergence of a field of knowledge in which each advance implies the simultaneous reaffirmation of a specific scientificity. What should be stressed here, with regard to my research into the persistence of the concern for lay analysis, is that this masterpiece is the theatre of a double operation. The first, which took place notably at the time of the *Project* (1895) and whose active traces have been discerned in psychiatry, consists in taking note of the mutation that occurred in medicine at the end of the nineteenth century and increased in pace during the following century up to the present day.

Freud experienced this mutation without really being able to theorize it. It is Jacques Lacan (1966), much later on, who discerns it and names it as the advent of the *scientific function* of medicine to the detriment of what he calls its *sacral function*, which gave the doctor a place that was similar but not identical to that of the priest. This place, which involves listening to the symptom, is inscribed in the field of a demand-centred clinical practice that is capable of taking into account, alongside the biological body, the erogenous body enmeshed in it, that is, the body as a vehicle of the dimension of jouissance.

Scientific medicine and its prevalence, which marked the inception and implantation of the "medical age" (see Pontalis, 1988), could portend nothing positive with regard to a study of psychic life whose primary aim is to respect its autonomy. Yet, this does not mean that this medicine was uninterested in the psyche, quite the contrary. In an attempt to occupy the territory of the psyche, to make the psyche its object, scientific medicine dispatched a sort of expeditionary force whose essential element was psychology, a spearhead that was followed at a distance by the philosophical and religious battalions. Scientific medicine attentively watched this expeditionary force and supplied it with logistical support for its operations. This, in my view, is where the object of the second operation, for which *The Interpretation of Dreams* provides the framework, is situated – an operation that consists in nothing less than showing the impossible coexistence of psychology and the unconscious, which, we should recall, is less "a psychological problem than the problem of psychology" (1900, p. 611).

In the battle for psychoanalysis, everything shows that Freud saw psychology as a kind of Trojan horse, as a lure, a ruse, and it is as such, and only as such, that it can hold our attention. A lure it is, because it presents itself as the most authorized source to speak about the psyche, as the only mode of psychic expression. This "evident fact" can even, at least in the course of the difficult gestation of an autonomous and specific theorization of the psyche, produce curious paradoxes that are identifiable particularly in the *Studies on Hysteria* (1895).

From different horizons and in different times, many commentators have noted how, when Josef Breuer tried to free himself from the neurophysiological view by asserting that "psychical processes will be dealt with in the language of psychology" and adding, "it cannot possibly be otherwise" (1895, p. 185), he was actually neurologizing his text, whereas Freud, who was still trying to express himself in physiological terms, realized that he was presenting his clinical cases as if they were psychological fictions totally foreign to this psychology that was an appendage of physiology. A lax discourse of consciousness which, as Freud writes in his short text "On Dreams", is unaware of the origin of phobias and obsessions, a complacent chatter of the ego about itself, psychology collides with the obstacle of the unconscious; it can neither hear it (since it is based on the agency of the ego or, if you will, on the perception-consciousness system which repudiates its manifestations) nor survive it.

All too briefly, with the help of a few examples, I have tried to show the persistence of the modes of lay analysis and its defence in the register of scientific psychoanalysis up to and including Freud's final work, *Moses and Monotheism* (1939). Nevertheless, this last work (and this is what I suggested right at the beginning of this chapter) also provides a framework for expressing the same concern, this time in the register of the non-medical application of scientific psychoanalysis. About this register Freud said on many occasions, and from the very beginning of the psychoanalytic adventure, that it was called upon to occupy an equally specific, equally irreducible place in the field of the sciences of the mind which seek to explain (and more often to describe) the social and collective modes of functioning of humankind.

How are we to account for the production, development and transmission of certain ideas? How are we to analyse the function, be it positive or negative, of the sway of these ideas, religious ones in particular? Freud was obliged to recognize, which he did very early on, in "Thoughts for the Times on War and Death" (1915), that in this register, as in that of scientificity, nothing remains unaltered. Psychoanalysis would have to contend in this domain with every kind of rejection (and this is still the case today); it would have to protect itself against all attempts to assimilate and reduce it; it would have to find the courage to name the impasses of other approaches, take risks and have the boldness to move forwards, as he says himself in *Moses and Monotheism*, "like a dancer balancing on the tip of one toe" (p. 58).

You will recall that in his letter to Pfister he emphasized the equivalence between his text on lay analysis and that which followed it, *The Future of an Illusion* (1927). In one case it was a matter of protecting psychoanalysis from doctors, and in the other from priests. Once again he had his back to the wall: How is the essence of religion to be apprehended, how is it that humans have produced this view of the world and its history and submitted to it to such an extent? How is it that they believe in it so passionately? How can psychoanalysis, a science of the human mind, deal with this collective and universal obsession?

Does psychoanalysis have anything specific to say about this phenomenon? But, first of all, should it?

> From then on I have never doubted that religious phenomena are to be understood only on the pattern of the individual neurotic symptoms familiar to us – as the return of long since forgotten, important events in the primaeval history of the human family – and that they have to thank precisely this origin for their compulsive character and that, accordingly, they are effective on human beings by force of the historical truth of their content.
>
> (Freud, 1939, p. 58)

When summarizing the first version of *Moses and Monotheism* for Lou Andreas Salomé a few years before, he employed the following striking formula: "what makes religion powerful is not its *real*, but its *historical* truth" (Andréas-Salomé, 1966, p. 253). Tirelessly repeating, without getting discouraged (while knowing that he would never be reassured by what could constitute irrefutable *proof*), that only psychoanalysis, a theory of the human psyche, could assert something about the "real truth" of religion, was an ever-present way, in 1939 as well as today, of defending the analysis which, in this context, deserves even more to be called *lay* analysis.

Still, it seems to me that, years after its publication, the reading and rereading of Freud's final work suggests that he was tackling a domain other than that of religion alone, namely, the domain of politics. Furthermore, even if he was unable to explore the matter in any depth, he considered that psychoanalysis could apprehend, if not the real truth of politics in its entirety, then at least some of its most insistent and obscure dimensions. It is in particular in the second part of the third essay in this book that Freud discusses politics from a very specific angle, one that he admits might seem to be a regressive approach at a time when the dominant explanations (he does not name Marxism here or the common use that is made of it, but it is clear that this is what he has in mind) give priority to socio-economic causes, an angle which is revealed mainly through the figure of the *great man*.

About this figure, regarding which Freud admits that he cannot easily find "a connotation . . . that is unambiguously determined", for that "would lead us far away from our goal", he nonetheless notes, underlining in so doing his permanent vigilance concerning possible metaphysical and psychologizing slippages (which would not fail to occur in the form, for example, of psycho-history), that it is not his essence that should hold the attention of the psychoanalyst, but how "he influences his fellow-men". However limited they may be, and even if they have given rise to somewhat hasty interpretations (having, as such, an effect of closure) which have flourished even to the point of caricature – I am thinking here of the comparison of the great man to a father figure – the few arguments that nourish these last pages of *Moses* . . . seem to me to indicate a specific field of processes. We might call such field the *religiosity* of politics and of the successive stages of its *increasing tendency towards religious fervour*, whose *real truth* (as far as that part of philosophy is concerned which made politics its object and thus speaks of *totalitarianism*) also belongs, and perhaps even more, to the specificity of psychoanalytic theory.

To conclude, we should keep in mind that the Freudian odyssey gives shape to our destiny as analysts. Like Ulysses, we must not forget the distance that still has to be covered. As for the poet who composes by improvising poems that have already been sung, for anyone who speaks without the support of an already written text, forgetting is the most negative verb; forgetting the "return journey" means forgetting the poems called *nostoï*, his hobby horses. Memory really counts for individuals, communities and civilizations.

Whether it is a matter of the register of the non-medical applications of psychoanalysis, a register still largely unexplored which calls, at least as much as in 1933 (Freud, 1933), for new elaborations, or of the other two, namely, scientific analysis or medical applications, the struggle for the specificity of psychoanalysis, for the independence of mental life remains unchanged. It is only if we take account together of the traces of the past and of the project of the future that we are allowed to do what we want to do in the present. Becoming without ceasing to be and being without ceasing to become.

Note

1 Translated by Andrew Weller.

References

Andreas-Salomé, L. (1966). *Corréspondance avec Sigmund Freud*. Paris: Gallimard, 1970.

Bion, W.R. (1979). *A Memoir of the Future*. Book Three: The Dawn of Oblivion.

Cavafy, C.P. (1992). *Collected Poems*. Trans. Edmund Keely and Philip Sherrard. Ed. George Savidis. Revised Edition. Princeton: Princeton University Press.

The Complete Works. Volume XIV. Ed. Chris Mawson. London: Karnac, 2014.

Freud, S. (1900). The Interpretation of Dreams. *SE*, 4–5.

Freud, S. (1915). The Unconscious. *SE*, 14: 159–215.

Freud, S. (1926). The Question of Lay Analysis. *SE*, 20: 183–258.

Freud, S. (1927). The Future of an Illusion. *SE*, 21: 1–56.

Freud, S. (1933). New Introductory Lectures to Psychoanalysis. *SE*, 22: 1–182.

Freud, S. (1939). Moses and Monotheism. *SE*, 23: 1–137.

Freud, S. (1950 [1895]). Studies on Hysteria. *SE*, 2.

Freud, S., and Pfister, O. (1963). *Psychoanalysis and Faith: The Letters of Sigmund Freud and Oscar Pfister*. London: Hogarth.

Lacan, J. (1966). La place de la psychanalyse dans la medicine. In: *Le Bloc-Notes de la psychoanalyse* (pp. 9–38), 1987, 7, Geneva: Georgia.

Masson, J.M. (Ed.) (1985). *The Complete Letters of Sigmund Freud and Wilhelm Fliess, 1887–1904*. Cambridge, MA: Belknap.

Pontalis, J.-B. (1985). Preface to the new French translation of *La question de l'analyse profane*. Paris: Gallimard.

Pontalis, J.-B. (1988). Une idée incurable. In: *Perdre de vue*. Paris: Gallimard.

8

The problem of pluralism in psychoanalysis

Charles Hanly

Every analyst has first followed another profession. Freud was a biologist and a medical neurologist before he discovered the fundamental facts of human psychic nature that are the foundations of psychoanalysis as a body of knowledge and a therapy for neurosis. Institutes have admitted to training, for some time, applicants who are already medical doctors, clinical psychologists or social workers with few exceptions. Not a few of these few exceptions are academics. I am intrigued by the subject of this book because I happen to be one of these academic exceptions, and the only such analyst to be elected president of the IPA thus far.

My first control case was my first therapeutic experience other than as a patient. It is true that Wittgenstein, who was aware of Freud's ideas (Freud had treated one of Wittgenstein's sisters and other members of the Vienna Circle were interested in psychoanalysis), considered his own method of linguistic reflection to be a therapy for the "intellectual cramps" that made the meaningless statements of metaphysics appear to be meaningful answers to real problems according to the verification theory of meaning. But it was a lack of understanding of psychoanalysis and an exaggerated fantasy of the therapeutic worth of philosophical forms of thought, including his own, that allowed Wittgenstein to liken his reflections on language to a therapy (Hanly, 1971). Nothing that Wittgenstein had to offer and in general none of my studies in and teaching of philosophy provided me with any useful orienting experience or preparation for clinical work in psychoanalysis other than my own analysis. However, I shall argue that philosophical studies do provide candidates with intellectual skills and knowledge that can be useful for psychoanalysis.

Freud (1926) commented on the need for medically trained analysts to abandon the exclusiveness of the first premise of their medical training expressed in the guiding medical question "what is the organic or physical source of this malfunction" in order to consider the question "is there a psychic cause for this apparently physically caused malfunction?" I had no such need for this forgetfulness, although my mind was far from being a *tabula rasa* since I was already a philosophical naturalist, materialist or positivist by the time I began taking a serious interest in becoming a psychoanalyst. The first work of Freud I read was "The Future of an Illusion", which articulated some basic philosophical ideas toward which my studies of philosophy had already led me. I was especially impressed by the conceptual and logical acuity and the intellectual modesty that Freud (1927) brought to the task of understanding religion as evidenced by his argument that showing that religious beliefs are illusions does not, by itself, prove that they are false and his idea of our continuing helplessness in adulthood causing non-neurotic ontological anxiety eased by religious belief. But more importantly, despite this intellectual agreement with the premises and conclusions of Freud's work on religion, my preconscious resistances to self-knowledge opposed, no less vigorously than those of any physician analysand, my becoming a Socrates of my own psyche sufficiently to be an analyst. This psychological resistance to self-knowledge is the great equalizer of candidates for analytic training from diverse backgrounds.

In my opinion, one crucial factor in becoming an analyst can be defined as follows: it is not enough to intellectually acknowledge the universality of the Oedipus complex; it is important to be able to remember being Oedipal oneself and to be able to identify within oneself any current disguised derivatives of its powerful libidinal and aggressive wishes and anxieties, in order to be able to sufficiently understand the part played by Oedipal conflicts in the psychic lives of patients and to be able to identify and to therapeutically interpret their manifestations in their associations and transferences. Being able to recall the ecstasy and agony of being Oedipal allows one to be sceptical about the universality of the Oedipus complex while also being able to observe its potential derivatives in the lives of others without disregarding other factors. It is being able to remember what one does not want to remember that protects us against treating psychoanalysis as an ideology rather than as the science of human nature that it is (Hanly, 1993). Curiosity about psychic life is inhibited by abstract intellectual learning and, especially, by idealizing identificatory persuasions because the resistances to the self-knowledge that requires remembering will remain unresolved to play mischief with one's attitudes, observing and understanding. In this sense, psychoanalysis is also the great equalizer of its aspirants because of the self-understanding, which depends on the revival of Oedipal memories, which I cite here, but which are only one class of memories among others depending on constitutional inheritance, family experience and the life lived, that psychoanalysis requires of all of us to be able to remember or, at least, to calmly and equitably contemplate what is beyond our experience in order to practise well its healing art. I am of the view that the drift from psychoanalysis to relational psychotherapy among psychoanalysts, currently proceeding at a rapid pace, is caused more by this training failure than by financial hardship or the culture of haste.

I have suggested that being an academic offers no particular advantage in psychoanalytic training. And academics have some unlearning to do. An intellectual or scholarly solution to a problem is perfectly adequate for academic research and teaching purposes. But it is worse than useless for the practise of psychoanalysis. Neuroses cannot be cured by means of sound deductive and inductive reasoning and scholarly and scientific knowledge, even if they may help. Of course, thinking the unthinkable by remembering the repressed includes reasoning, but reasoning on its own does not bring about a curative instinctual motivational maturation nor an awareness in analysts and patients of the internal conflicts that cause their symptoms and inhibit their thinking about the motives that animate them, and the pleasures they seek to gratify or have to avoid. Intellectualism on the part of the analyst at best cooperates with symptom preserving resistances and at worst it strengthens them by adding yet another resistance. Different professional backgrounds offer various liabilities and advantages for psychoanalytic training. I had pursed literary as well as philosophical studies in preparation for my academic career the last twenty years of which were entirely devoted to teaching Freud to undergraduates and graduates. The study of character and motivation in literature and their interpretation obviously benefits psychoanalytic thinking (e.g. Hanly, 1986, 2009). The usefulness of philosophy is not obvious as a background for the acquisition of psychoanalytic knowledge and clinical skills. Freud, for example, had a legitimately ambivalent attitude toward philosophy (Hanly and Lazerowitz, 1970; Hanly, 1977). One of the useful things philosophy brings to psychoanalysis is not fundamental assumptions let alone substantive theories (for example, both the empiricist Locke and the rationalist Descartes assumed that consciousness is a defining property of any mental activity) but the ability to identify consistencies and inconsistencies and their implications among alternative, competing psychoanalytic theories.

I believe that psychoanalysis as a body of knowledge is in serious trouble on account of the complacency of analysts about theoretical pluralism. Cooper (2009) has concisely described the problem, "Psychoanalytic pluralism . . . has not unexpectedly, evolved into a multiplicity of opposing theoretical and technical dogmatisms. What we lack are the means to arrive at decisions concerning the superiority of one or another of these views" (p. 265). Mainstream psychoanalysis has overflown its banks and has become lost in a quagmire of schools that have abandoned enquiry for the absolutism of chronic quarrel or the relativity of personal invention. Psychoanalysis, generically defined as theories espoused by groups of analysts, is not a coherent body of knowledge; core propositions of the different schools of thought do not merely differ, they are often inconsistent, i.e. they are often contraries (both cannot be true) or contradictory (if one is true the others are false).

A current example of contrary theories is the Freudian and self-psychological theories of the Oedipus complex. The Freudian theory of the Oedipus complex traces its origin to a precocious instinctual libidinal development that is etiologically independent of, while being bound up in child-parent and parent-child relations. Kohut's theory of the Oedipus complex rejects Freud's idea of an instinctual origin and attributes the occurrence of the psychopathogenic Oedipus complex to parental empathic failures. Kohut's phenomenological description of the Oedipus complex once formed is identical with Freud's; the contradiction arises with its causation. Self-psychology explains any occurrence of the Oedipus complex as the result of unempathic parenting responses to the onset of romantic affection for the parent of the opposite sex (e.g. asexual fantasies of marrying) and unambivalent boisterous competitiveness toward the parent of the same sex as the child. The romantic affection is not sexual and, therefore, not incestuous. The aggressive competitiveness is neither parricidal nor matricidal (e.g. non-destructive fantasies of doing what the mother or father do appear to do). This position implies that the Oedipus complex involving incest wishes and hostile ambivalence do not occur in the presence of good enough empathic parenting; they are caused by parental unempathic responses to these developing feelings, which sexualizes them making them incestuous and which causes the aggressive trend to become destructive and ambivalent. The classical explanation is that incest wishes arise spontaneously in the drive life of all children, even those with ideally empathic parenting, bringing about the structural completion of the capacity for moral self-mastery as a consequence of the completion of the formation of the super-ego with its prohibitions and ideals sanctioned by guilt deriving from castration anxiety in boys and fears of infertility or deformed babies in girls. Freud's theory affirms that all occurrences of the Oedipus complex are instinctual; Kohut's theory affirms that no occurrences of the Oedipus complex, as described by Freud, are instinctual. These logically contrary theories cannot co-exist in a coherent body of knowledge. Their explanations of the genesis of the Oedipus complex are logical contraries; if either is true, the other is false. This same inconsistency with classical theory is to be found broadly, although sometimes without being explicitly formulated, in much of relational psychology. It is part and parcel of a tendency to play down the Oedipus complex, infantile sexuality and sibling rivalry and to repudiate the drives and psychic determinism. Relational psychoanalysis is continuing to add to the already existing inconsistent theories and part theories in psychoanalysis.

A more complex conceptual and logical difficulty of this sort is to be found in relation to Freud's death instinct theory. Freud

(1920) postulated that aggression is intrinsically masochistic in its structure and destructive in its dynamic. Klein adopted Freud's theory of aggression and drew from it the correct inference that, if this is so, then one of the infant's first experiences along with oral gratification from sucking on the breast or its substitute, there will also be an attack of annihilation anxiety caused by the infant's own spontaneous aggression (Klein, 1932, 1946). The infant is driven, according to Klein, to seek to reduce the danger to itself of its own destructive aggression by projecting it into the infant's experience of the primary object to which it is attached, the breast or its substitute. The breast or substitute is then experienced by the infant as both loving and nourishing and also persecutory, threatening and dangerous, giving rise, independently of any trauma of privation caused by the mother or substitute care givers, to what Klein named the paranoid-schizoid position. (The reader will notice that, contrary to Klein, I have treated this projection as projection, i.e. as a modification of the experience of the object only and not as a modification of the object.) Segel (1979) reaffirmed the essentially instinctual nature of this first annihilation anxiety. Independently of clinical observations and reconstructions, Klein was logically justified in postulating the occurrence of infantile annihilation anxiety given Freud's definition of aggression.

Then why did Freud not subscribe to Klein's valid and reasonable inferences from the masochism and destructiveness of his death instinct theory of aggression? Freud had not overlooked the potential in his new dualistic theory of a dangerous conflict between the ego instinct of self-preservation and the death instinct. To solve this problem, Freud added the qualifying postulate that the death instinct is, at least, aligned with or even takes over the functions of self-preservation depending on one's view of the ego instincts in Freud's late theory. (For the argument I am making here which alternative is correct is academic, although for other arguments it may well be consequential.) Freud (1920) thus postulated that the death instinct brings about the extinction of each of us according to our own genetic timetable inscribed in the cells that make up our bodies which then vigorously oppose any extrinsic causes that could bring death about in an "untimely" way. Weary of life as he was, Macbeth nevertheless defied the witches' prophecy and went into battle to defend himself. Hence, the death instinct does not threaten premature death unless the individual human genome is also genetically programmed with a fatal defect. And even an infant with a fatal heart defect would not suffer instinctual annihilation anxiety on Freud's understanding of it because the death instinct would oppose all threats that might shorten life including a genetic mutation that causes the development of a fatal heart failure in early adulthood such as arrhythmogenic right ventricle cardiomyopathy (ARVC), a genetic disorder that predisposes individuals to cardiac arrest. Infant primary "structural" narcissism (structural because the neonate has minimal capacities for subject-object differentiation), which Freud (1914) described as the libidinal complement of self-preservation, is not consistent with instinctually driven annihilation anxiety because of the consequent omnipotence that wards off anxiety. These considerations suggest that the annihilation of the self only begins to acquire fully realistic self-representation with the first indications of diminished biological and physical capacities toward the end of mid-life in men and with menopause in women (Hanly, 2013). If aggression is a death instinct, it could be argued that it is genetically programmed in concomitance with libido to experience instinctual annihilation anxiety much later with the occurrence of reduced, impaired or lost libidinal and motor capacities that anticipate the death that has always been irreversibly on its way. Of course, annihilation anxiety can result from externally caused trauma much earlier in life but these instances would not be caused by instinctual development according to Klein's development of Freud's death instinct theory. Certainly, people normally take whatever measures are available to them from surgery and medications to yoga to delay the inevitability of death as best they can. These efforts, which must eventually fail, are motivated by a death instinct acting according to Freud's (1920) postulated modification of the death instinct which makes it, at least, an ally of self-preservation.

These last reflections are not attributed to Freud, although they are intended to be Freudian; their purpose is to remind the reader of the internal, inferential difficulties of the assumption that aggression is intrinsically a masochistic, destructive instinct. Britton (2003) has questioned the idea that aggression is intrinsically masochistic; Fenichel (1945), Parens (1973) and Mitchell (1993) have questioned the idea that aggression is intrinsically destructive. Theoretically, if the death instinct takes the self as an object only in order to impose moral constraints on the ego (Freud, 1923) until later in life because of its fusion with narcissistic libido and its alliance with self-preservation, annihilation anxiety ceases to be an implication of its postulation. It is this logical state of affairs that allowed Hartmann (1948) and Hartmann et al. (1949) to subscribe to the death instinct together with its neutralization without subscribing to annihilation anxiety or the paranoid/schizoid position. My argument is that despite the obvious logical soundness of Klein's derivation of annihilation anxiety and the paranoid/schizoid position from Freud's death instinct theory, it turns out that this derivation is inconsistent with the weight that Freud seems to have assigned to self-preservation, to the beginnings of self-object differentiation and reality testing during the oral phase (Freud, 1895), to primary narcissism (Freud, 1914) and the neutralizing effect of the fusion of developing object love with aggression. These psychological factors could trump Klein's impeccable logic. Or Klein's derivation of annihilation anxiety and the paranoid and schizoid position could be sustained by other psychological factors identified by Klein and indicated by her clinical work with children. And although Hartmann (1948), Hartmann et al. (1949) as well as Eissler (1971) adopted Freud's theory of aggression as a death instinct, other Freudians have adopted a dual instinct theory of libido and aggression without the additional attributes of being intrinsically masochistic and destructive. Finally, a potential problem for Freud's account of the death instinct is, at least an apparent problem of accounting for aggressive destructive violence directed toward others. Since a death instinct depends upon fusion with libido to become directed toward objects, libido should, for the most part, inhibit the destructiveness of aggression. For the same reason, when libido is withdrawn from the object, the sadistic aggression invested in the object will revert to its masochistic form and attack the ego in some way, for example by a self-righteous inhibition of libido or a renewed libidinal investment in an unsuitable object. When libido is withdrawn from an object a vicissitude of libido also occurs, there is an increase of narcissistic libido. This narcissistic libido is the libidinal compliment of the ego instinct for self-preservation, which could have the effect of harnessing the augmented masochistic aggression in the tasks of protecting the ego by strengthening defences against instinctual demands, including aggressive ones, essentially by augmenting moral masochism. Thus, the philosophical conceptual, inferential and logical analysis of theories and arguments can be usefully applied in the search for more integrated and coherent theories in psychoanalysis.

Philosophy can also contribute more substantively to psychoanalytic theorizing. As we have seen, there is a basic disagreement between Freud and Klein concerning the awareness of death and, hence, of annihilation anxiety in infants and children (Blass, 2014). It is obvious that no conscious, let alone unconscious, verbal representations of death can occur in the infant psyche before the acquisition of language. However, empiricist philosophers (for example, Hobbes, 1651; Hume, 1748) have advanced the idea that images are used in thinking prior to and after the acquisition of language. This early use of images for thinking implies that meaning does not entirely depend on language. The earliest occurrence of symbolization, the use of one thing to represent another, hence of the beginning of intentional meaning, is the neonate's discovery of the pleasure of thumb sucking when the breast is not available. Inherent in this activity is a first intentionality or reference to the greater, because nutritive, pleasure of the breast for which the thumb becomes a substitute. Eventually words can substitute for things and can be used to describe them. Initially children treat words animistically as though they were connatural with the objects they name and believe that names are descriptive rather than conventional. This is also true of human intellectual history. The issue of the natural or conventional nature of words was still somewhat ambiguous even in Plato (1997, *Cratylus*). The question of prelinguistic thinking with images is important for a realistic appreciation of Klein's attribution of ego strengths to infants. As soon as infants are able to remember repeated sensory experiences they would be able to form integrated images of the object that gives rise to them. Freud (1895) located the first beginnings of subject-object differentiation during the first days of life as infants turn from the quasi-hallucinatory memory image that does not satisfy to the breast that does. This capacity for differentiation is also the first beginning of reality testing and a rudimentary capacity for philosophy and the basic theme of Plato's *Cratylus* dialogue! It also calls in question assumptions about myelinization (e.g. by Brenner, 2002), which begins before birth and continues into adolescence. I think that Klein has been unfairly criticized (e.g. by Brenner, 2002) for attributing a capacity for propositional thought, which depends on words, to neonates, because myelinization is not sufficiently advanced for language acquisition and propositional thinking to occur. There are two issues here: Is myelinization sufficiently advanced at birth for memory to occur? (e.g. Grunberger, 1971, 1989 attributed nirvana elational states in adults in part to prenatal memories of illusory umbilical self-sufficiency); and does thought depend on language and thus arise only after myelinization has sufficiently advanced to sustain language acquisition? Klein needed only to have postulated a capacity in infants to think by means of images before the acquisition of language drawing upon Freud's (1895) account of first subject-object differentiation and Freud's account of primary process thinking in dreams and symptoms in which thinking by means of images plays a predominant part. Primary process thinking persists in adult dreaming as described or implied by Freud (1900) in several contexts, including in "considerations of representability" in which logical connectives required by reasoning are provided by images of cross roads or double staircases to stand for alternation (either . . . or . . .) and succession to stand for hypothetical (if . . . then . . .) (p. 339ff.) and in formal regression in the formation of dreams and symptoms. Prior to the acquisition of language, logical relations between images can be represented by images of pre-logical spatial or temporal relations even though thinking with images is limited in a way that thinking with words is not; images of alternatives cannot differentiate between exclusive and inclusive alternation while thinking with words can, and succession falls woefully short of hypothetical or causal thinking with words. But all that Klein's hypothesis of an instinctual annihilation anxiety requires is that an image of the cessation of consciousness in sleep be invested with the instinctual energy of an aggression that is intrinsically masochistic in its organization and destructive in its dynamic. Thus, some philosophical ideas can make substantive contributions to psychoanalytic enquiry, in this illustration, by drawing on empiricist postulates concerning the cognitive role of thinking by means of images.

In addition, in Plato (*Republic*) we find the insight that dreams of incest, parricide and matricide reveal instinctually originated impulses in all humans, including "the most decent among us" (IX, 572). Aristotle (*Poetics*) offers evidence for the importance of the Oedipus complex in individual destiny when he cites Sophocles *Oedipus Rex* as a paradigm of the capacity of tragedy to articulate what is essential to the human condition whereas history has to occupy itself with what is accidental. And Spinoza (1677) had argued that the inner sense of free will is an illusion of consciousness that obscures psychic determinism, which opened the door to Freud's (1901) explanation of this illusion by repression and unconscious motivation. But philosophical premises and arguments cannot be simply taken at their face value. Both Descartes (1641), the father of European rationalism, and Locke (1690), the father of British empiricism, held, contrary to psychoanalysis, that the idea of unconscious thought activity is contradictory. Both held that consciousness is a defining property of all psychic activity. More recently, Sartre (1943) and Merleau-Ponty (1945) have paid homage to this erroneous illusion of consciousness. We are reminded that it is futile to seek in philosophy what can only be found by means of the observation of human nature made available to analysts in clinical observations of free associations and transference (Hanly, 1990). Freud made this mistake when he "found" confirming evidence for his dual instinct theory in the pre-Socratic cosmologist Empedocles' (*Fragments*) ideas of cosmic love and strife (Hanly, 1997).

The purpose of these reflections is not to prove or disprove any specific theory of aggression; it is to identify some of the contradictions or contrarieties and the uncertainties they cause among some current alternative psychoanalytic theories of drives, the Oedipus complex and aggression. There are many more to be found. I have examined inconsistencies, where one might assume there are only consistencies, in Freud's death instinct and Klein's adoption, extension and elaboration of it (see also Blass, 2014). Empiricism in science and philosophy teaches us that a conceptual and logical analysis of theories cannot establish the probability or improbability of a theory. Only facts can do that. But a conceptual analysis of theories can reveal to what extent within the generic idea of psychoanalysis as a body of knowledge the "mainstream of clinically most probable theories" has been lost. It could be argued that the Diaspora of theory in psychoanalysis is so far reaching that it has become meaningless to speak of a mainstream psychoanalytic theory. Clearly, if there is at least a remnant of "mainstream" psychoanalysis, it does not yet have a coherent theory of aggression. One utility of philosophy for psychoanalysis is its ability to identify consistencies and inconsistencies in proliferating alternative theories and work out their implications in a search for the grounds of coherence within compatible groups of theories. Since coherence is a necessary but not a sufficient criterion of truth, this analysis falls short of Cooper's reasonable wish to be able to arrive at "decisions concerning the superiority of one or another of these views". Only observation (primarily clinical, but also with the help of relevant non-clinical observation) can achieve that goal. In this connection it is worth recalling that Freud did not shrink from the task of making psychoanalytic theory consistent. When Freud (1920) introduced aggression as a death instinct, he realized that it was inconsistent with the primacy of the pleasure principle, with dreams as invariably wish fulfilling and with masochism being an internalization of sadism; he modified these earlier theories to make them consistent with a compulsion to repeat painful experiences and with the masochism of a death instinct. And even while having doubts about the clinical evidence Freud (1920) cited on behalf of the repetition compulsion, we can agree that clinical evidence must decide the question. It is because only reliable clinical evidence can enable us to discriminate between what is true or false in theory that I conclude with epistemology.

In recent decades Freud's epistemology of scientific realism, the tenants of which are to be found throughout his work and in particular and appropriately in the first paragraphs of "Instincts and Their Vicissitudes" (Freud, 1915), has been vigorously criticized on the basis of subjectivist epistemological ideas largely imported from postmodernist arguments but also because of concerns about the objectivity of clinical observations. These ideas have contributed to the idea that psychoanalytic theory is intrinsically and unavoidably pluralistic. But before proceeding further with the argument let us first briefly consider the nature of philosophical subjectivist epistemologies as represented by Protagoras who originated the idea of the subjectivity and relativity of knowledge and Kant who, during the enlightenment having been aroused, as he said, from his dogmatic slumbers by Hume, constructed what is probably the most ingenious, even if also misguided, form of such epistemologies.

Protagoras of Abdera, a 5th-century B.C. sophist, held that "Of all things the measure is man, of the things that are that they are, and of the things that are not that they are not" (Frag. 1), (Owens, 1959). Plato who was born in the last two decades of the 5th century understood that Protagoras was referring to individual persons in his use of "man". If so, Protagoras was affirming that things are as they are experienced to be by individuals so that truth becomes relative to individual subjective perspective and experience. Two paradoxical implications of this epistemological premise are: "it is just as true that the sun rotates around the earth as it is that the earth turns on its axis every day" and "it is as true that the human species is the result of a special act of creation of a designer god as it is that humans have evolved from inanimate chemical processes". The most recent philosophical advocate of the paradoxical view that there can be more than one true theory about the same thing is Putnam (1981). Plato (*Republic*), an idealistic realist, argued against Protagoras, "Does a bed really differ from itself when you look at it from the side or from straight in front or from any other point of view, or does it remain the same but appears different? And so with other things. The second alternative is right. . . . It appears, but is not different" (10: 598). Plato's argument brings out the radical perspectivism of the experiential relativity of a subjectivist epistemology.

The subjectivity of Kant's transcendental deduction of space, time and the categories of understanding is of the species rather than the individual. Kant (1781) argued that the human senses necessarily experience things and events in space and time, which he named "pure forms of intuition", and that our understanding necessarily imposes categories on our knowledge of others, society and nature the most prominent of which are causality and substance/attributes which he called pure categories of understanding. Kant conceived of these forms of intuition and categories of understanding conditions of perception and knowledge which are imposed *a priori* by the mind itself as conditions of any possible experience or thought. His fundamental point, contrary to empiricism, was that the forms of intuition and the categories of the understanding do not derive from our experience of things and events. As a result, the human mind is not able to experience or comprehend what things are like in themselves apart from these conditions imposed by the mind on knowledge. Knowledge is limited to the *phenomenal* world, which is the world as we experience it and understand it subject to the *a priori* conditions for experience and thought imposed by the mind; the mind can have no access to what Kant called the *noumenal* world of things in themselves except through the experience of moral duty. The reason for this profound limitation on human knowledge is that the forms of intuition (sensory experience) and the categories of the understanding (descriptions and explanations) owe their origin to the mind and not to experience. In opposition to Kant, philosophical and scientific empiricism is realist because it assumes that we acquire our ideas of space and time, causality and substance/attributes and other categories from our experience of things and events as they are. Thus, Kant's epistemology, for example, makes the nature of space out to be universally and necessarily Euclidean, i.e. rectilinear on the grounds that the human mind can only experience objects as existing in a rectilinear space in which the shortest distance between two point is a straight line and parallel lines retain their distance from each other indefinitely.

In opposition to Kant, scientific empiricism acknowledges that, while experience can be illusory, scientific enquiry is not bound by or to these illusions (we continue to experience the apparent rotation of the sun even though we now know that it is a perceptual illusion caused by the diurnal rotation of the earth) and can grasp the truth of what is actually happening in nature by means of abstract thought centuries before astronauts could actually observe the earth's diurnal rotation. Accordingly, by elevating the knowledge of space, to the exalted spiritual heights of the *a priori*, as Einstein (1921) put it, Kant put our knowledge of space out of the reach of experience and Einstein's discovery that, in the real world, space exerts an influence on the behaviour of material things because it is not at all always and necessarily rectilinear as it appears to be in our quotidian experience (except for intercontinental flight routes on the earth's curved surface) but can observationally be proven to curve in the vicinity of mass. Scientific empiricism, which from its beginning has espoused a critical realist epistemology, allows our knowledge of space to depart from our everyday sensory impressions of it when facts of nature – in this case, *inter alia*, the behaviour of light passing through the sun's gravitational field – agrees with Einstein's predictions based on Riemannian rather than with Newton's predictions based on Euclidean geometry. Philosophical scientific philosophy accepts that physics has disproven Kant's version of subjectivist epistemology (Reichenbach, 1951). With this background let us turn to a consideration of subjectivist epistemologies in psychoanalysis. In doing so, a critical question should be kept in mind: What if psychoanalytic knowledge is *sui generis* because its object is human psychic life the structure and dynamics of which differentiates it from other objects of knowledge? If psychoanalysis is not a natural science, then critical realism may not apply.

Goldberg (1976) asserted that

> When two individuals with roughly similar neurophysiological equipment view the same thing or event and each sees it differently, it is not necessarily true that one is incompetent or even wrong; rather, it may be that they each observe with a different theory. In science, theories are guides or tools to direct our observations. No one can make an observation that is devoid of a guiding theory and no theory can stand without the empirical evidence to substantiate it.
>
> (p. 67)

This statement was made in defence of self-psychology when criticisms were made based on the classical analysis of patients. There is an ambiguity in Goldberg's assertion that "no theory can stand without the empirical evidence to substantiate it". On the face of it, the statement implies the realist idea that the truth of a theory depends upon the observational evidence that supports it or falsifies it. But we have just been told by the sentences that precede it that what we observe clinically depends upon the theories that "direct our observations". In order to observe, one must have a theory and the theory with which one observes will necessarily condition what one observes such that a Freudian will find evidence of an instinctually caused Oedipus complex and a self-psychologist will find evidence for an Oedipus complex caused by parental empathic failure. Neither clinical observer will be "incompetent or even wrong". What an analyst will observe will be decided by the theory he brings to the task. Thus both the Freudians and the self-psychologists are, on this account, true to their observations of the aetiology of the Oedipus complex even though what they claim they observe logically cannot both be true; for, as we have seen earlier, they are contraries and, therefore, are logically incompatible. The clinical observations of Freudian analysts cannot provide evidence for the Freudian theory of the Oedipus complex without falsifying the self-psychological theory of the Oedipus complex and conversely.

The purpose of the argument is to avoid this logical dilemma by safeguarding the self-psychological theory from refutation by clinical evidence that appears to falsify it. But the argument is a two-edged sword. It protects self-psychology from falsifying clinical evidence from classical analysis but it equally, and for the same reason, protects classical theory from falsifying self-psychology clinical evidence. The effect of the argument is to conceptually and logically isolate Freudian clinical evidence from Kohut's theory and conversely. The epistemological subjectivism of Goldberg's argument which makes clinical evidence relative to the theory that guides its observation lies between the subjectivity of each individual of Protagoras and Kant's subjectivity of the species.

It is this epistemic and logical isolation that contributes to the dogmatism of pluralism referred to by Cooper (2008, 2009). Goldberg's argument, if sound, would provide an explanation of why psychoanalytic theory is irremediably pluralistic. Whether or not Goldberg's argument is sound ultimately depends on whether or not being guided by a psychoanalytic theory alters clinical observation in such a way that disconfirming evidence cannot appear. Any theory imposes blinkers. The underlying assumption of his argument is that because the Freudian analyst is guided by drive theory he/she is rendered pure blind to clinical evidence of the self-psychological object relational theory. The problem is that making truth relative to theory in this way makes it impossible to observationally test the theory by coming upon negative instances. The clinical observations that could test these contrary theories guide observations so rigidly that they become constitutive of the observations made under its guidance. In this argument, theory is made to be the incarnation of a limited form of Descartes' Malignant Deceiver.

It is not difficult to find philosophical epistemologies that are in agreement with Goldberg's position. Representative of them is Putnam's (1981) view that "the very (experiential) inputs upon which our knowledge is based are conceptually contaminated" (p. 54) from which assumption Putnam (1981) correctly infers that there may be more than one true theory about the same thing. What could be a better vindication of Goldberg's thesis and for theoretical pluralism in psychoanalysis than this philosophical confirmation? A Protagorean analyst has gone beyond Putnam or Goldberg by affirming that "there is no such thing as a clinical fact". But the problem remains that philosophical and scientific empiricism can be cited to vindicate the opposite view. Philosophy as such does not offer an authoritative solution to which an appeal can be made because of its own pluralism. The only alternative is to consider the arguments for and against each view the nub of which, in this context, is whether or not our ideas govern our observations in a way that prevents them from being factually tested. Philosophical empiricism can accept that we need ideas and methods to make observations. But empiricism rejects the assumption that being guided by ideas necessarily so alters our observing that we become unable to make observations of any facts that falsify them.

Philosophical epistemologies have taught philosophers to differentiate the knowing subject from the object to be known including the difficulties that may stand in the way of objectivity. This differentiation poses the question of intersubjectivity. The term "intersubjective" in ordinary language and science denotes an observation of something about which qualified observers agree. Intersubjectivity is lost in the subjectivism of Protagoras' epistemology since each individual has his/her own perspective. Plato opposed this loss in his affirmation that objects remain the same and only appear to be different when they are seen from different perspectives. As suggested previously, a qualified form of Protagorean subjectivism is implicit in Goldberg's argument. It is qualified because it allows Freudian analysts to agree or disagree with each other and self-psychology analysts to agree or disagree with each other while insulating them logically and epistemologically from each other. This insulation offers a rationalization of dogmatic pluralism; if this epistemological assumption is true, then psychoanalytic theories cannot be dogmatic.

Schafer's (1976) argument primarily concerns the nature of the object to be known. The implication of his general epistemological assertion is that human psychic reality is not sufficiently "definite" to be known other than by means of multiple perspectives. Faced with this difficulty the knowing subject must rest content with more than one way of understanding psychic reality each of which is as true as any other. Schafer (1976) makes two further assertions that support Goldberg's (1976) argument, "there are more ways than one to understand reality" and further "reality is not, as Freud usually assumed, a definite thing to be arrived at or a fixed and known criterion of objectivity" (p. 66). This statement about reality, if true of psychic reality, would add to the explanation of why it is that ideas guiding observation can so influence our experience of the psyche (Goldberg, 1976; see also Stolorow and Atwood, 1992).

Schafer's epistemological statements appear to generalize the quantum mechanical uncertainty principle from the physics of subatomic particles to all objects of knowledge. One hears the popular postmodern generalization "we now know that the observer always changes the object observed". Schafer (1983) employed a narratological argument to claim that what a patient says to a particular analyst is inadvertently and inevitably influenced by the analyst to whom he speaks (Hanly, M.A.F. 1996). Schafer's view draws our attention to the fact that knowledge of a given object can often be improved by considering it from more than one perspective, although it is also true that the intersubjectivity of the observations of expert and experienced observers constitutes evidence that the observations are reliable.

Schafer's hypothesis about the knowability of objects has a number of difficulties. The hypothesis fails in so far as it is based on an inference from the uncertainty principle in physics. The uncertainty principle applies to the microscopic world of subatomic particles but not to the macroscopic world of terrestrial mineral, plants and animals and suns, planets and galaxies which permit simultaneous observations of location and velocity along with other quantities and qualities (Coyne, 2009; Weinberg, 1996; Hawking, 2001). The analogical stretch from subatomic physics to the neurons that make up the central nervous system and the impulses, motives, perceptual experience and thought activities they sustain that are the objects of psychoanalytical enquiry strains one's credulity. Freud as well as Klein and many other analysts have assumed that unconscious psychic processes and contents are sufficiently definite to be known objectively and described as they are or have been as well as their influence of psychic functioning and character. But it is could be argued that unconscious psychic processes unlike the symptoms they cause are evasive when we seek to know them. Perhaps their nature alters depending on the analyst to whom they are told. After all, are not patients, who are perfectly familiar with their obsessional or hysterical symptoms and can describe them convincingly, not only mystified about what causes them but are also resistant to finding out? Perhaps this inevitable resistance involves an evasiveness on the part of unconscious psychic processes that is somewhat analogous to the inability of knowing the location and velocity of subatomic particles. An exploration of this issue, which is specific to psychoanalysis, can be found below.

There are further logical and conceptual problems to be considered. First, Schafer's epistemological assertions about the knowability of unconscious processes and contents could be thought to imply that the proliferation of points of view is essential to the growth of psychoanalytic knowledge by eventually preparing the way for theory integration. The integration of different perspectives needs to be pursued as far as possible because of the complexity of the interactive processes of the human psyche. Two or more different points of view may generate apparently inconsistent theories because of their use of different terms when in fact they are describing two real aspects of a complex totality. Although little work has been or is being done in this direction, multiple perspectives, while essential, will only take us part way toward but not as far as an integrated mainstream theory composed of consistent elements of current alternative theories. The reason for this is that many of the alternative theories we now have are contradictory or contrary, in which case, both cannot be true. They cannot be integrated. These theories do not describe aspects of one and the same complex totality; they claim that the object is not at all as another theory claims it to be as, for example, the alternative theories (above) of Freud's and Kohut's theories of the origins of the Oedipus complex. Rangel's (2006) admirably optimistic metaphor of the Freudian tree trunk with alternative theory branches fails to take into account this logical obstacle.

Second, Schafer's fundamental epistemological premise is self-contradictory. If the hypothesis is true that unconscious psychic processes and contents are not "a definite thing to be arrived at" then it is false because the premise itself claims to have arrived at a definitively objective epistemic description of all unconscious processes and contents. It is true that patients will often enough be vague and indefinite about the causes of their difficulties and they may persist in this for some time. But this vague, amorphous indefiniteness is a resistance to the pain of remembering and we routinely find that it does not result from the indefiniteness of the unconscious sources of the egoistical self-image demanding the protection of repression or of the unconscious repudiated libidinal and aggressive wishes; it results precisely from specific, identifiable, intrinsically simple wishes whose ownership patients find it hard to bear. Topographically, the vagueness and indefiniteness are conscious ego states. These qualities need not be shared by the ideas we form of them nor by the instinctual repressions nor the idealized self-images that defensively contrive them. Instinctual repressions and repressed object relational traumas are of the macroscopic order of things and share their epistemological characteristics. Psychoanalysis illuminates them by enabling the unconscious memories, fantasies and affects to become conscious. Unconscious psychic processes and contents do not have the observational problem of subatomic particles with the impact of light necessary for locating them or measuring their velocity. This epistemic issue in psychoanalysis will be considered further below. But if we are able to save the epistemic worth of unconscious psychic processes and objects we still have to contend with the question of the disturbing influence of the analyst on what the analyst observes to which we now turn.

Renik (1993) advanced the epistemological premise that the analyst's clinical observation of conscious and unconscious psychic processes and contents is always subject to the "irreducible subjectivity" of the analyst. It is important to appreciate that Renik (1999) does not question the objectivity of scientific knowledge generally, nor does he question the possible objectivity of psychoanalytic knowledge. On the contrary, Renik (1998, 2004) argues that this definition of "irreducible subjectivity" is not inconsistent with objectivity. The first premise of his argument is that objective scientific knowledge depends upon being able to predict what will be observed, if a given hypothesis is true. This premise is classically exemplified in the observations made of the passage of light particles through the sun's gravitational field which were much more accurately predicted by Einstein's theory than Newtonian predictions. Renik's (1998) second premise is that psychoanalysis is able to predict as well as retrodict the structure and dynamics of psychic functioning and its changes in the lives of people. While the argument is sound for other kinds of knowledge, it would not apply to psychoanalysis, if the clinical observations of the analyst actually are irreducibly subjective. For, if so, would not the observations and their explanation, on which any predictions are based, be "irreducibly subjective" in the case of psychoanalytic knowledge (i.e. more about the knower than the object to be known) and would not the truth testing observations to verify the prediction also be irreducibly subjective? Would not the implication of Goldberg's thesis apply; would not the analyst's theory govern the observations? Would not the predictions and their confirmation be governed by the subjectivity (personality) of the analyst, if not by the conscious or unconscious theory favoured by the analyst? Would not everything unfold as though Schafer's thesis of the indeterminate multifaceted nature of the object were sound? Would not the likelihood of this epistemologically subjective state of affairs be further increased by Sandler's (1996) idea of private and public theories (Hanly, 2012)? Is there not an implication that analysts would, of psychological necessity, always seek confirmations of their own favoured conscious and unconscious ideas and fail to consider what observations of change in the patient(s) would falsify them, if the analyst's observing is always and necessarily governed by irreducible subjectivity? There is no disputing that just this misguided complacently ideological treatment of clinical experience all too frequently occurs as analysts seek confirmation for their consciously and unconsciously preferred ideas with an ideological zeal that causes them to overlook falsifying evidence in the transference and associations. It is to oppose just this theoretical and observational complacency that Renik proposes his epistemological idea of irreducible subjectivity. The purpose is right but is the assertion that all analysts are irreducibly subjective the best means? Everything turns on the meaning of "irreducible subjectivity".

According to a standard dictionary, "subjectivity" means "the quality or condition of viewing things exclusively through the medium of one's own mind or individuality" (*OED*, p. 2058);

"irreducible" means "that [which] cannot be reduced to a desired form, state, condition etc." (*OED*, p. 1046). But is it not reasonably expected that the analyst be able to respond with appropriate affect and understanding that tallies with what is going on in the patient? For Renik, the purpose of his epistemological assertion is to facilitate this response in analysts to patients. But does not the idea of the "irreducible subjectivity of the analyst" provide an epistemological justification for a fundamental relativity of analytic truth to individual analysts? Has not psychoanalysis been rendered Protagorean? Individual analysts because of psychological factors at work in their observing and thinking cannot do better than find themselves in their patients. Does not this view of psychoanalytic knowledge go beyond Kantian epistemological subjectivity which is limited to the species *homo sapiens* in the direction of Protagorean individual relativism.

There is a fundamental subjectivity characteristic of human experience that *is* irreducible and which has elsewhere been named ontological or psychological subjectivity because of its nature and its difference from epistemological subjectivity (Hanly and Hanly, 2001). Each individual's experience is his or her own. This subjectivity derives from the fact that the brain is the organ that sustains psychic activity. The wonderful inner-world of each person is in each person's head; it is theirs and is private to them. In the same way and for the same reason, each person's experience of others, society and nature belongs to the person whose experience it is. But this subjectivity, while it is irreducible, is not epistemological even though it brings it about that each individual's experience is perspectival. The basic flaw of Protagorean-like epistemology is that it assumes that perspectives are all that there is and that they are incorrigible. The tricky part is that they remain experientially incorrigible even after they have been corrected cognitively.

However, we are not always fooling ourselves and others when we can share our perspectives and their influence on our experience and our evaluation of objects; we can learn by doing so; we can become better at seeing things as they are or we can disagree and explore further by articulating the reasons for disagreeing with other perspectives. The important truth in Schafer's view of unconscious psychic reality is that knowledge of it can often be gained by considering different perspectives on it because of its complexity and also because of our fear and dislike of it. The fundamental reason that we can do so, despite our inevitable perspectivism is because, contrary to Schafer, self, others and objects have determinate natures and characteristics along with complexity that provide grounds for consensus when we hit upon appropriate and effective means of knowing them. Paradoxically, radical epistemological subjectivism of the Pythagorean kind is a form of naive realism because of its basic assumption that each individual can only know things as they appear to him/her. It is because Schafer denies that objects have stable natures that can be known that he takes sides with Protagoras' individual perspectivism in opposition to Plato's realism.

The need for epistemological reflection arises naturally and elementally within our experience when we realize that even consensus among observers about what they are experiencing may not yield knowledge of what is real. For example, very small children learn without being taught that the perceived convergence of railroad tracks at a distance is a perceptual illusion that does not convey the real continuity of their size, location and stasis (how they will appear close up) even though children and adults must always perceive the illusory convergence. In general, the apparent diminution of objects with distance in the visual field is recognized and "corrected" without alteration of the individual fields of each individual by considerations of how things would appear close up. In general, we are accustomed to reducing the subjectivity (perspectivism) of our sense experience of things. It was, in part, for this reason that Locke (1690) introduced the idea that our perceptions are "representations" of things.

This distinction between appearance and reality is fundamental to epistemology. In cognitive development, this elementary distinction first arises (Freud, 1895, 1917) early in the oral stage when the infant differentiates the hallucinated fantasy breast that does not satisfy from the real breast that does and continues to wail until the real breast comes to remedy the discomfort of hunger. Telling the difference between how things appear and how they are is evidence (one could cite much more) that our ontological subjectivity does not make us irremediably cognitively subjective. To be sure, only fairly recently, since Copernicus, Kepler, Galileo, Descartes and Newton and only after bitter struggles waged against their discoveries from the perspectives of Ptolemy, Aristotle and the evidence of everyday experience, have the many been able to realize that the perception of the diurnal movement of the sun, planets and heavens is caused by the rotation of the earth, etc. This knowledge does not alter our subjective perspectival experience of the sun's state of relative motion or rest or our use of it to organize our daily lives on the equally illusory experience of the flat earth on which we live them and which also makes Euclidean geometry seem self-evident. But this utility has no bearing on the truths of a globular earth defining a day by its diurnal rotation and bringing in the seasons and the years by an annual tilting motion as it rotates. Despite the utility for daily life of the astronomical beliefs these perceptual illusions engender, these beliefs are unequivocally false because they fail to correspond with the reality of the earth's geometrical structure and motion relative to its location in the solar system to the sun and other planets. It is a mistake to assume that truth is necessarily relative to perspective or that perceptual illusions cannot be corrected cognitively even though the perceptual illusions continue to be subjective and uncorrected. But even if inorganic and organic objects and the cosmos are knowable, what about unconscious psychic processes and contents? Are they also knowable as they are and not only as they appear to be in their observable derivatives?

Analysts scarcely need reminding of the loss of reality testing in neurotic symptom formation (Freud, 1924). It is important to be clear about its logical bearing on the question of the irreducibility of epistemological subjectivity of the analyst and the psychic unconscious. Consider the following much abbreviated but telling clinical material from the analysis of an obsessional neurosis. A talented, highly educated and cultured young business executive, Jacob, had proven his mettle at work in making decisions about investments in merchandizing projects in the face of unavoidable market uncertainty. Nevertheless, he found himself overwhelmed by anxiety about causing an accident while driving his car despite its improbability. The symptom developed in the aftermath of an accident in which he, when riding a bicycle, had collided with a motorcycle causing body injuries to himself and the motorcyclist. Jacob felt entirely responsible for the accident even though the police report had found the cyclist and the motorcyclist equally responsible. He was wracked by a conscious fantasy that his career and his life would be ruined by a court proceeding that would find him guilty of deception and criminal negligence and would punish him with humiliating and life devastating imprisonment. This anxiety quickly spread to causing a serious car accident, being deprived of immigration rights (he had applied for Canadian citizenship) and being dismissed by his corporate employer. It also quickly infected all contacts with insurance brokers and forms relating to insurance coverage for the cycling accident, to customs officials at borders, immigration officials and any papers required by his citizenship application and the police. He was terrified that some official would find out about some negligence on his part which, when known, would result in his being found guilty and ruinously punished. He was aware that none of this was true, that the punishment he anticipated was out of all proportion to anything he had done or was likely to do, but he also believed it not only to be true that he had caused an accident and that he was at risk of it's becoming known. He gave updriving his car and travelled to his appointments by public transit only to be seized by the anxiety that he would cause an accident by walking across the quiet street he had to take to get to his analysis. Thus, although he knew that his anxiety was unrealistic, this knowledge based on sound reasoning and self-encouragement and the same from family and friends could not release him from his bondage to the idea that he was at grave risk of causing an accident that would be his ruination. It is obvious that Jacob's experience of these things was epistemologically subjective and caused by displaced unconscious memories and fantasies. This displacement had not destroyed his reality testing which he continued to exercise very well in his work; but it had suspended its credibility in this sphere of his experience along with its demands for evasive precautions and inhibitions. The ontological (psychological) subjectivity of his experience is evidenced by the fact that despite his intense suffering the people he worked with had no idea that he was struggling with such a difficulty in his life. Jacob's epistemic subjectivity had its origin in his own genetic psychological endowment and life experience. But was it reducible? Could Jacob's reality testing about causing accidents be restored?

Early in his analysis, Jacob's distance from, hatred for and fear of his father became evident in his complaints that his father had allowed and even seemed to condone his being bullied, teased, tricked and derogated as the baby of the family by his three much older siblings. His hatred for his father was matched by his love and admiration for his father's strengths and his capacity for stoicism, for controlling his feelings, his athletic prowess, professional success, wealth and social status. Occasionally into this history of his family and adult life and his symptoms, but affectively isolated from them, came Jacob's memory from his fifth year, that his father had nearly drowned in a sailboard accident when he had been swept by wind and currents far out from the beach. Jacob remembered seeing his father struggling for breath, vomiting and exhausted on the beach after being rescued. He remembered being on the beach and that he had been a detached observer without any feelings about it then or now. In due course, I interpreted this experience as having aroused in him a wish, of which he had not been aware, that his father had drowned. I added that this wish to get rid of his father had so deeply frightened him, because he also needed his father to protect him, that he had not been aware of his fear or the wish that aroused it. Jacob denied any awareness of any such destructive wish. But the interpretation was followed by a series of dreams over subsequent months in which an older man was killed not by him but in his presence. His associations to this murdered man went from his analyst to older, male, authority figures by a variety of pathways to his father until he was not only observing the killing but was doing the killing himself in his manifest dreams. As this process of dreams and interpretations proceeded, Jacob's anxiety about causing an accident began to give way until they ceased when he was confidently driving his car again without neurotic anxiety. His unconscious fantasy of having killed his father lost its efficacy and his conscious anxieties about police, customs officers, government forms about citizenship, etc., had steadily melted away. His experience of them had become realistic. The subjectivity with which Jacob's experience of these objects had been deeply stained by having become symptoms of an unconscious parricidal crime and punishment had returned to objectivity about what and how they actually were rather than what he feared them to be.

This bit of clinical history refutes the premise of irreducible epistemic subjectivity. Refutation of a generalization requires only one counter instance. Inductive proof is more difficult. For proof it is but one instance of the many required while ruling out other causal factors. However, I could cite many more as can other psychoanalysts including Schafer and Renik. While highly individual in its details, the essentials of this analytic process are ordinary and expectable in the return to realism from the displacements and compulsions of neurotic anxiety. In this respect, its logic is the same as Aristotle's (Poetics) argument that tragedy reveals more of the reality of the human condition than history. It shows that the interference in our grasp of reality caused by neurotic symptoms is not irreducible. As for the analyst, if at various points in the work the analyst drew blanks, failed to be empathic, became impatient as a result of becoming anxious about some severe bouts of regression and the rapidly increasing spread of the patient's anxiety despite the driving inhibition and, especially, the anxiety about crossing the street to get to his appointments, these subjectively caused failures of the analyst were sufficiently contained that they did not interfere with the basic interpretive work or its efficacy. It is to facilitate the development of this capacity for containment that psychoanalytic training requires a personal analysis at a high frequency. This capacity for containment contradicts the epistemological premise that analysts must always suffer from irreducible epistemological subjectivity.

Similarly, Schafer's theses of multifaceted indeterminacy and the absence of criteria for the objectivity of objects and, especially, for unconscious contents and processes are not borne out by these observations. It is the awful simplicity and forceful demands for satisfaction of a parricidal wish that requires the obfuscations and compulsion of displacements and condensations that cause symptoms, the loss of reality testing and resistance to remembering despite the suffering that the symptoms also bring. The disguises, obfuscations and resistances certainly give the appearance of multifaceted and shifting obscurity and the impression of indeterminacy. But the wish that the father had drowned and the guilty unconscious fantasy that the patient had caused him to drown are neither complex nor indeterminate. And the analytic recovery of the causes reveals that the choice of symptom is determined in its details by antecedent developments and events. Contrary to Schafer's claim, unconscious contents and processes provide a criterion of objectivity when they undergo beneficial change caused by interpretation in the analytic relation.

To this psychoanalytic argument a philosophical argument can be added. Subjectivist epistemological premises of this kind are paradoxical or self-contradictory. Some analysts are so enthusiastic about paradoxes that they neglect their possibly being self-contradictory by focusing exclusively on the possibility that they only *seem* to be "absurd though [they are] . . . really well founded statements" (*Shorter OED*). The philosophical argument is, "If Schafer's premise is true that unconscious psychic processes and contents are not 'a definite thing to be arrived at' then it is false because the premise itself claims to have arrived at a definitively objective epistemic description of all unconscious processes and contents". The assertion of the irreducible subjectivity of the analyst has the same logical problem: "If the statement that analyst's interpretations are irreducibly subjective is true, then it must be itself irreducibly subjective and, therefore, false". Empiricist realism does not have this problem. For empiricism, whether or not our knowledge of an object is only perspectival irreducibly subjective is always an open question the answer to which depends upon how well our knowledge corresponds to the object, how coherent the knowledge is and whether or not it can be used to bring about changes in it. Epistemological affirmations are generalizations like any other and their soundness and utility, their objectivity, depends on the evidence for and against them. For psychoanalysis this evidence concerning the nature of psychoanalytic knowledge of unconscious processes and contents will be derived from factual descriptions of what happens in analysis. The advantage of this approach is that it allows for the possibility that psychoanalytic knowledge is, contrary to assumptions guiding this paper, *sui generis*. This argument concludes that subjectivist epistemological premises are not "well founded statements" but neither are they "absurd", despite appearances. They are well-founded precepts to guide us in the search for psychoanalytic objectivity.

A self-contradiction arises in another way that is primarily psychoanalytic and only secondarily philosophical. Goldberg, Schafer and Renik have written clear and convincing clinical accounts of unconscious processes and contents at work in their patients on the implicit assumption that they are to be taken as being objective and not merely an expression of the analyst's theoretical point of view (Goldberg), or merely a perspective among several (Schafer) or of the analyst's life and personality. Subjectivist epistemological theories of this kind provide rationalizations for pluralism in psychoanalysis even while remaining inconsistently committed to realism. This logical inconsistency is evident in Renik's (1998) prediction argument but also in his view that "it is precisely at those moments when we believe that we are able to be objective-as-opposed-to-subjective that we are in the greatest danger of self-deception and departure from sound methodology" (p. 562). It is as though two things had happened. First, the inevitable ontological (psychological) subjectivity of the mind is transferred to perceptual and cognitive activities. Second, empirical epistemological ideas are treated as *a priori* principles with the result that things that certainly can go wrong resulting in epistemological subjectivity, such as following theory when it ceases to apply (Goldberg), transferring the evasiveness of resistances to unconscious contents (Schafer) and assuming that the patient is more like the analyst than he/she is, are treated as though this is what must inevitably happen. The results are statements that have the conceptual and logical character of radical epistemologies that seem to imply Protagorean solipsism when they are actually methodological exhortations disguised as epistemologies. In the case of Goldberg, "Take care not to become so committed to a theory that you are unable to make clinical observations that could falsify it". In the case of Schafer, "Be careful not to assume that you have fully grasped theoretically and clinically the structures and dynamics of psychic reality when you may have only grasped an aspect of it that is, perhaps, correct but, even so, it can turn out to be incomplete!" And in the case of Renik (1998), "be careful lest your conviction that you are following a sound (objective) methodology is a denial because your observations of your patient are being shaped by your own unconscious processes rather than by the transferences and associations of your patient!" The contradictions disappear when these insights into real epistemic and methodological difficulties inherent in psychoanalytic observation and theorizing are treated as heuristic precepts rather than as substantive epistemological theories. These ideas also cease to serve as incentives and rationalizations for an isolating, dogmatic pluralism. Instead, they become gadflies for self-critical enquiry into psychoanalytic therapy and theory needed by psychoanalysis to find its way beyond dogmatic pluralism to critical enquiry. The problem with these subjectivist affirmations is not that they do not express truths about the difficulties in the way of objectivity in clinical psychoanalysis but that they are stated as though they were *a priori* epistemological principles when they are empirical generalizations about the special problems of psychoanalytic clinical observation and reasoning (Hanly, 2014). They are precepts that underline the great importance of the "critical" in critical realism.

Philosophy is able to contribute in three ways to psychoanalysis. First, philosophy can assist in the identification and conceptual study of consistencies and inconsistencies in alternative psychoanalytic theories. In this way, philosophical analysis can make a contribution to the important task of integrating psychoanalytic knowledge. Second, philosophy can sporadically and intuitively contribute substantively to psychoanalytic knowledge. But what counts as an intuitive contribution to psychoanalysis and its place in psychoanalytic knowledge needs to be decided by psychoanalytic judgement. Third, philosophy can contribute to the study of the implicit basic epistemological assumptions required by psychoanalysis, a subject to which this chapter seeks to contribute. However, because philosophical epistemology is itself pluralistic it cannot, as a humanistic discipline, provide authoritative epistemological assumptions to which psychoanalysts can appeal for the adjudication of their own differences about the nature of psychoanalytic knowledge. The burden of proof is on the shoulders of psychoanalysis.

References

Aristotle. (1958). (*Poetics*). Trans. G.M.A. Grube. Library of Liberal Arts. Indianapolis, New York: Bobbs-Merrill.

Blass, R. (2014). On "the Fear of Death" as the Primary Anxiety: How and Why Klein Differs from Freud. *International Journal of Psychoanalysis*, 95: 613–617.

Brenner, C. (2002). Reflections on Psychoanalysis. *Journal of Clinical Psychoanalysis*, 11(1): 7–37.

Britton, R. (2003). *Sex, Death, and the Superego*. London: Karnac.

Cooper, A.M. (2008). American Psychoanalysis Today: A Plurality of Orthodoxies. *The Journal of the American Academy of Psychoanalysis*, 36: 235–253.

Cooper, A.M. (2009). *Psychoanalytic Disagreements in Context. By Dale Boesky*. Lanham, MD: Jason Aronson, 2008, *Psychoanalytic Quarterly*, 78: 265–274.

Coyne, J. (2009). *Why Evolution Is True*. New York: Viking Press.

Descartes, R. (1641). Meditation on First Philosophy. In: *Philosophical Works of Descartes* (pp. 133–199), Vol. 1. Trans. E.S. Haldane and G.R.T. Ross. New York: Dover Press, 1955.

Eissler, K.R. (1971). Death Drive, Ambivalence, and Narcissism. *Psychoanalysis of Study Child*, 26: 25–78.

Empedocles. (Fragments). The Cosmic Cycle. In: *The Presocratic Philosophers* (pp. 326–331). Trans. G.S. Kirk and J.E. Raven. Cambridge: Cambridge University Press, 1962.

Einstein, A. (1921). *The Meaning of Relativity: Four Lectures Delivered at Princeton University*. Trans. P. Adams. London: Methuen, 1922.

Fenichel, O. (1945). *The Psychoanalytic Theory of Neurosis*. New York: W. W. Norton and Company.

Freud, S. (1895). Project for a Scientific Psychology. *SE*, 1: 295–359 (1950).

Freud, S. (1897). Letter 69. *SE*, 1: 259–260

Freud, S. (1900). The Interpretation of Dreams. *SE*, 4–5.

Freud, S. (1901). The Psychopathology of Everyday Life. *SE*, 6: 1–291.

Freud, S. (1914). On Narcissism: An Introduction. *SE*, 14: 73–102.

Freud, S. (1915). Instincts and Their Vicissitudes. *SE*, 14: 117–140.

Freud, S. (1917). Mourning and Melancholia. *SE*, 14: 237–259.

Freud, S. (1920). Beyond the Pleasure Principle. *SE*, 18: 3–64.

Freud, S. (1923). The Ego and the Id. *SE*, 19: 3–66.

Freud, S. (1924). Loss of Reality in Neurosis and Psychosis. *SE*, 19: 183–190.

Freud, S. (1926). The Question of Lay Analysis. *SE*, 20: 183–238.

Freud, S. (1927). The future of an illusion. *SE*, 21: 5–56.

Freud, S. (1929). The Future of an Illusion. *SE*, 21: 1–56.

Goldberg, A. (1976). A Discussion of the Paper by C. Hanly and J. Masson on "A Critical Examination of the New Narcissism". *International Journal of Psychoanalysis*, 57: 67–70.

Grunberger, B. (1971). *Le Narcissisme: Essais de psychanalyse*. Paris: Payot.

Grunberger, B. (1989). *New Essays on Narcissism*. London: Free Association Books.

Hanly, C. (1971). Wittgenstein on Psychoanalysis. In: A. Ambrose and M. Lazerowitz (Eds.), *Ludwig Wittgenstein: Philosophy and Language*. London: George Allen & Unwin.

Hanly, C. (1977). An Unconscious Irony in Plato's *Republic*. In: *The Problem of Truth in Applied Psychoanalysis*. New York: Guilford, 1992.

Hanly, C. (1986). Lear and his Daughters. *The International Review of Psychoanalysis*, 13: 211–220.

Hanly, C. (1990). The Concept of Truth in Psychoanalysis. *International Journal of Psychoanalysis*, 71: 375–383 or *The Problem of Truth in Applied Psychoanalysis*, Ch. 1. New York: Guilford, 1992.

Hanly, C. (1993). Ideology and Psychoanalysis. *Canadian Journal of Psychoanalysis*, 1(2): 1–17.

Hanly, C. (1997). Psychoanalysis and the Uses of Philosophy. In: Arnold Richards et al. (Eds.), *The Perverse Transference and Other Matters* (pp. 269–284). London: Jason Aronson.

Hanly, C. (2012). Theoretical and Clinical Reflections on Public and Private Theories. In: Jorge Canestri (Ed.), *Putting Theory to Work*. London: Karnac.

Hanly, C. (2013). Interview with Charles M.T. Hanly (Canada). In: Guillermo Julio Montero, Alicia Mirta Ciancio de Monteero, and Liliana Singman de Vogelfanger (Eds.), *Updating Midlife: Psychoanalytic Perspectives* (pp. 103–112). London: Karnac.

Hanly, C. (2014). Skeptical Reflections on Subjectivist Epistemologies. *Psychoanalytic Quarterly*, 83: 949–968.

Hanly, C., and Hanly, M.A.F. (2001). Critical Realism: Distinguishing the Psychological Subjectivity of the Analyst from Epistemological Subjectivism. *Journal of the American Psychoanalytic Association*, 49(2): 515–532.

Hanly, C., and Lazerowitz, M. (1970). Editors Introduction. In: *Psychoanalysis and Philosophy* (pp. 1–3). New York: International Universities Press.

Hanly, M.A. (1996). "Narrative" Now and Then: A Critical Realist Approach. *International Journal of Psychoanalysis*, 77: 445–457.

Hanly, M.A. (2009). Sibling Jealousy and Aesthetic Ambiguity in Austen's *Pride and Prejudice*. *Psychoanalytic Quarterly*, 78(2): 445–468.

Hartmann, H. (1948). Comments on the Psychoanalytic Theory of Instinctual Drives. *Psychoanalytic Quarterly*, 17: 368–388.

Hartmann, H., Kris, E., and Loewenstein, R.M. (1949). Notes on the Theory of Aggression. *Psychoanalytic Study of the Child*, 2–3: 9–36.

Hawking, S. (2001). *The Universe in a Nutshell*. London: Bantam Spectra.

Hobbes, T. (1651). *The Leviathan*. Ed. M. Oakeshott. Oxford: Blackwell.

Hume, D. (1748). An Enquiry Concerning Human Understanding. In: E.A. Burtt (Ed.), *The English Philosophers from Bacon to Mill* (pp. 585–689). New York: Random House, 1939.

Kant, I. (1781). *Immanuel Kant's Critique of Pure Reason*. Trans. N.K. Smith. London: Macmillan, 1950.

Klein, M. (1932). *The Psychoanalysis of Children*. Seymour Lawrence: Delacourt Press, 1975.

Klein, M. (1946). Notes on Some Schizoid Mechanisms. *International Journal of Psychoanalysis*, 27(3).

Locke, J. (1690). An Essay Concerning Human Understanding. In: *The English Philosophers from Bacon to Mill* (pp. 238–402). New York: Modern Library, 1939.

Merleau-Ponty, M. (1945). *Phenomenology of Perception*. Trans. C. Smith. London: Routledge & Kegan Paul, 1962.

Mitchell, S. (1993). Aggression and the Endangered Self. *Psychoanalytic Quarterly*, 62: 351–382.

Owens, J. (1959). *A History of Ancient Western Philosophy*. New York: Appleton Century Croft.

Parens, H. (1973). Aggression: A Reconsideration. *Journal of the American Psychoanalytic Association*, 21: 34–60.

Plato. (1948). *Republic*. Trans. B. Jowett. New York: Liberal Arts Press.

Plato. (1972). *Phaedo*. Ed. R. Hackforth, New York: Cambridge University Press.

Plato. (1972). Phaedo. Translated and edited, R. Hackforth, Bobbs Merrill: Indianapolis, New York. The dialogue was originally published by Cambridge University Press which gave to Bobbs Merrill the right to republish. This last is the publication from which I actually worked.

Plato. (1997). *Cratylus*. Trans. C.D.C. Reeve. Indianapolis and Cambridge: Hackett; reprinted in J.M. Cooper. Ed. *Plato. Complete Works*. Indianapolis and Cambridge: Hackett.

Putnam, H. (1981). *Reason, Truth and History*. Cambridge: Cambridge University Press.

Rangell, L. (2006). *The Road to Unity in Psychoanalytic Theory*. Lanham, MD: Jason Aranson.

Reichenbach, H. (1951). *The Rise of Scientific Philosophy*. Berkeley, Los Angeles: University of California Press.

Renik, O. (1993). Analytic Interaction: Conceptualizing Technique in Light of the Analyst's Irreducible Subjectivity. *Psychoanalytic Quarterly*, 62: 553–571.

Renik, O. (1998). The Analyst's Subjectivity and the Analyst's Objectivity. *International Journal of Psychoanalysis*, 79: 487–497.

Renik, O. (1999). Discussion of Roy Schafer's (1999) Article. *Psychoanalytic Psychology*, 16(4): 514–521.

Renik, O. (2004). Intersubjectivity in Psychoanalysis. *International Journal of Psychoanalysis*, 85: 1053–1056.

Sandler, J. (1996). Comments on the Psychodynamics of Interaction. *Psychoanalytic Inquiry*, 16(1): 88–95.

Sartre, J.-P. (1943). *Being and Nothingness*. Trans. H.E. Barnes. New York: Philosophical Library, 1956.

Schafer, R. (1976). *A New Language for Psychoanalysis*. New Haven: Yale University Press.

Schafer, R. (1983). *The Analytic Attitude*. New York: Basic Books.

Segal, H. (1979). *Klein*. Glasgow: Fontana Collins.

Spinoza, B. (1677). Ethics. In: J. Wild (Ed.), *Spinoza Selections*. New York: Scribner, 1930.

Stolorow, R., and Atwood, G. (1992). *Contexts of Being: The Intersubjective Roots of Psychological Life*. Hillsdale, NJ: Analytic Press.

Weinberg, S. (1996). Sokal's Hoax. *New York Review of Books*, August, pp. 11–15.

9

On "The question of lay analysis" by Sigmund Freud

Abel Fainstein

I am grateful for the possibility to reread the 1926 Freudian text in light of our own experience in the practice and transmission of psychoanalysis, which I work to develop in Buenos Aires and occasionally in visits to other countries in the region.

Our "Porteña" and "Rioplatense" culture is the required setting of my reflections, and is surely very different from the Vienna of Freud or the Northern Hemisphere of today. Our Latin American region has quite distinct cultures and legislation and this necessarily shapes the views of those who think and practice psychoanalysis and who train psychoanalysts. In this regard, Freud warns us:

> it does not arise in all countries with equal significance.
> (Freud, 1926, p. 183)

The article before us refers to the possibility of lay people practicing psychoanalysis, and was prompted by an accusation brought against Theodore Reik for practicing it illegally. Freud had a completely favorable position regarding its practice by lay people, and gives his arguments. Lay people, at that time, were not medical doctors.

However, after more than 100 years, we must ask ourselves: Who are lay people today? In general, the practice of psychoanalysis exclusively by doctors has been placed to the wayside, though not without lawsuits in the midst.

There is considerable consensus regarding the training tripod necessary to becoming a psychoanalyst that includes analysis of the analyst, supervisions and clinical theoretical studies beyond having an undergraduate degree. However, different analytical groups and theoretical perspectives often claim exclusivity of its practice, leading, in some cases, to others being denied their condition as analysts. The lack of academic and professional accreditation by a competent authority further complicates this matter.

In this context, I think that we are required to agree on what being an analyst implies and what is the necessary training to become one. This consensus, however, should be based on the premise that there is no longer a single psychoanalysis nor is there only one notion of the unconscious that supports it. The plurality of theories and practices that have greatly enriched psychoanalysis during these last 100 years translates to this.

It was Angel Garma, one of the founders of the Argentine Psychoanalytic Association and analysand of Theodore Reik, whose clear position in favor of the practice of psychoanalysis by non-medical analysts, marked the initial structure of our society and the spirit that sustains it, beyond compliance with current laws regarding professional practice.

The Freudian text adds a very clear explanation in its account to the "impartial person" as to why psychoanalysis has nothing to do with medicine. The text places emphasis on the usefulness of the diagnosis, the evaluation of the conditions of the patient's ego, and the part thereof that will always be for the doctors. These are points I will try to highlight in my reflections.

In his Editor's Note to this Freud's text, Strachey considers

> what was perhaps his most successful non-technical account of the theory and practice of psychoanalysis, written in his liveliest and lightest style" and underlines that "The theoretical part in particular has the advantage over his earlier expository works of having been composed after the great clarification of his views on the structure of the mind in The Ego and the Id.
>
> (Freud, 1926, p. 181)

Although it refers us to the beginnings of our discipline, it is of great topical importance because, in addition to the theory, it touches on the practice, including the practice of child psychoanalysis, the necessary training and way to for it, giving priority to the initial diagnosis. I will try to comment on my perspectives with regards to each of these points.

Buenos Aires is the site of three IPA psychoanalytic societies, that since 1942, 1977 and 1996 have developed intense scientific, cultural and training activities. In addition, there are societies in Mendoza, Cordoba and Rosario, other important cities in Argentina. As a whole, however, they constitute only a small proportion, approximately 10 percent, of the local psychoanalytic map. It is assumed that there are more than 100 groups and small institutions that offer psychoanalytic training, and it is estimated that there are more than 20,000 professionals working in and with psychoanalysis, of which only a small percentage are medical doctors; the majority are psychologists.

The Argentine Psychoanalytic Association (APA), founded in 1942 by Celes Cáramo, Guillermo Ferrari Hardoy, Angel Garma, Marie Langer, Arnaldo Rascovsky and Enrique Pichon Riviere, was, in this regard, a pioneer in the region and in much of the world, and included, since its beginning, non-medical analysts. I have already made reference to the importance of Garma, analysand of Theodore Reik, for this. However, this initial willingness that had permitted the training of prestigious colleagues, such as Arminda Aberastury, Madeleine and Willy Baranger, Betty Garma, to name only a few, was affected by a law, passed in the early 1950s, that prohibited the practice of psychotherapy, including psychoanalysis, by non-medical doctors. This law, in effect for more than 30 years, stipulated that psychologists were only allowed to practice analysis under the supervision and responsibility of a physician. This limited analytical training in the APA to medical doctors. However, analysts who were already members of the association continued to practice and teach without much difficulty.

This situation encouraged many professionals from other disciplines to train individually in numerous non-IPA institutions which, in general and over time, ascribed to Lacanian movements. Many of these professionals came to hold university faculty teaching positions, replacing APA members such as Joseph Bleger or David Liberman, who, upon retreating to the psychoanalytic societies, left their teaching posts vacant. The implications of this change will be evaluated further on.

It was not until the return of democracy in 1983, following a period of military dictatorship that had begun in 1976, that the law regarding the professional practice of psychology was passed. It authorized the practice of psychotherapy, including psychoanalysis, by psychologists. This resulted in the acceptance of psychologists for analytical training in IPA societies, but that continues to prohibit the training of those who are neither medical doctors nor psychologists.

Among us, however, there is considerable acceptance toward not requiring that an analyst be a doctor or psychologist. Many non-IPA institutions train writers, philosophers, educators, etc. for the practice of psychoanalysis. In fact, many analysts of the IPA seek to reanalyze with some lay analysts of prestige, thereby erasing limits imposed by the different societies and their training proposals.

Having described the state of the professional practice of psychoanalysis, I will now turn to the central themes of Freud's text.

The practice of psychoanalysis by non-medical analysts

As I have said, there is a fair amount of consensus among us regarding the practice of psychoanalysis by non-medical analysts, even though IPA societies continue to train only medical doctors and psychologists in order to avoid violating the laws governing professional practice.

Freud made it clear that psychoanalysis had little to do with medicine and that in general it had hindered its development.

> Doctors have no historical claim to the sole possession of analysis. On the contrary, until recently they have met it with everything possible that could damage it, from the shallowest ridicule to the gravest calumny. You will justly reply that that belongs to the past and need not affect the future. I agree, but I fear the future will be different from what you have foretold.
> (Freud, 1926, p. 229)

We agree with him that the practice of psychoanalysis requires specific training that the IPA institutes offer today, though not exclusively. I will refer to them in the next section. Lay people today then are those who have not been trained as psychoanalysts, regardless of their university degree.

However, difficulties posed in some cases by the diagnosis and the importance of having medical knowledge is of interest to Freud. In his opinion, once organic pathology has been ruled out, one can only be entrusted to an adequately trained analyst who may well be a physician, but need not be. During treatment and in cases of disease of an organic nature or the presumption thereof, a doctor will need to be consulted. Among us, however, the psychologization of the medical practice, while beneficial in many ways, has nevertheless generated frequent diagnostic problems that in some cases have been serious.

We are aware that this becomes more complex when a psychoanalyst, trained as such but with no medical or even psychological knowledge, is the patient's first contact with the field of mental health. This occurs frequently in our context and in private practice, but can be resolved by entrusting the diagnostic stage to an interdisciplinary team that includes a physician. Despite advances in biological psychiatry, this structure is the most commonly used in mental health services in hospitals, especially in the large urban centers of our country. The pioneering experience of psychiatrists such as Enrique Pichon Riviere introduced psychoanalysts to hospital practice. They were first introduced to psychiatric hospitals (Jorge García Badaracco among others) and then to general hospitals (Mauricio Goldenberg).

The insistence on discarding organic pathology should be taken into account when training analysts, especially non-medical analysts. For those who work with children, the intervention of developmental specialists, speech therapists, pediatricians or child neurologists, as well as physicians and psychologists, is often required.

Returning now to the aforementioned, in the following sections I will try to update my perspectives on analytical training, the societal structure and its role in the exchange between colleagues that is the basis of ongoing training processes.

Finally, I will address the importance I assign to the study of the structuring of the psyche and to diagnosis, especially of the ego conditions of the patient, following the ideas Freud expounds in The Question of Lay Analysis.

The training of a psychoanalyst

The principal aim of training analysts is to continue to have people who have the desire to train as analysts.

Jacques Alain Miller in dialogue with Daniel Widlocher – (2003, p. 1066)

This remains a central theme after more than 100 years of psychoanalysis. As we have said, only good training separates psychoanalysts from those for whom there is consensus in considering lay people in psychoanalysis.

Garma (1959) proposed greater freedom for individuals and groups within a unit: making only a few courses mandatory; allowing for curricular freedom and choice of professors; favoring scientific and educational liberty; avoiding excessive work; remunerating professors; developing knowledge of the initial stage and origins; achieving gratitude and disseminating psychoanalysis.

After almost 60 years, I think his ideas remain valid. They have guided much of the developments of the Argentine Psychoanalytic Association and the institute that bears his name. Although currently subject to revision, it includes an open educational system with curricular and academic freedom. Although, in general, it is restricted to professors of the same institution, the large number of seminars offered, many of which include guest professors from outside the APA, allow for this openness.

What lies ahead is the implementation of individualized theoretical and clinical training courses and the carrying out of needed debates for their preparation.

Beyond the state of affairs in our association, there is significant consensus worldwide regarding the importance of the tripod that makes up personal psychoanalysis, supervisions of its clinical tasks and clinical theoretical studies in the training of a psychoanalyst. The importance of dialogue and debate among colleagues has recently been added.

Encouraging exchanges regarding clinical practice and theories should be the essential goal of psychoanalytic societies and their continuing educational programs. This requires societal structures and training programs that serve as environments enabling their achievement.

As Goldstein, Moise and others, I think of the institution of psychoanalysis not as a noun that refers to something already completed and is sometimes crystallized, but rather as a permanent action that forces us to agree on what defines our work, and how to sustain it, despite our differences.

Although Freud speaks more of the value of people's inclinations than of arguments, he proposes an authority that determines what analysis is and the training required to become an analyst. My understanding is that this ambiguity should be maintained in order to keep our work from becoming bound by regulations. We need institutions and institutions require regulations. They should, however, be conducive to generating an enabling environment for the transmission of the experience of the unconscious and the teaching of psychoanalysis in its different variants.

In my Master's thesis on the psychoanalytic institution I wrote:

> Considering that the transmission of the experience of the unconscious cannot be guaranteed and that it is strictly personal, neither the institutions nor their institutes are able to ensure achievement. They can, however, offer favorable conditions toward making it so. This means not only not interfering with it, but also favoring it. It is, as Szpilka (2002) puts it, the peculiar nature of the unconscious needs to be protected in institutions that shelter it and conversely, paradoxically, institutional structures need to subsist, tame, appease and soothe the object whose transmission they sustain.
>
> This tension is inevitable and its management depends on the effectiveness of the institutions in the transmission of psychoanalysis.
>
> In order to fulfill this task, institutions also require integration to the scientific, academic, social and community settings in which they work.

In the IPA, the psychoanalytic societies have institutes that are responsible for training analysts. The first one was in Berlin.

> At these Institutes the candidates themselves are taken into analysis, receive theoretical instruction by lectures on all the subjects that are important for them, and enjoy the supervision of older and more experienced analysts when they are allowed

> to make their first trials with comparative slight cases. A period of some two years is calculated for this training. Even after this period, of course, the candidate is only a beginner and not yet a master. What is still needed must be acquired by practice and by an exchange of ideas in the psycho-analytical societies in which young and old members meet together. Preparation for analytic activity is by no means so easy and simple. The work is hard, the responsibility great.
>
> (Freud, 1926, p. 228)

As we see, Freud thought of two years of training, followed by required practice and exchange with more experienced analysts from a psychoanalytic society. This has changed: today, in some institutes, training takes six or more years, the majority of which are on-site. In some cases, students are required to be in analysis throughout the duration of their training. It goes without saying that no other post-graduate, masters or doctorate degree demands these requirements. And, as is in our case, this training is carried out and completed without receiving official academic credit. This latter encourages those who are interested, many of whom have a strong transference with psychoanalysis, to seek training options elsewhere.

In addition to this, there is, in general, a poor systematization of institutional scientific activities that had constituted for Freud the complement to the basic two years of training.

> And the same will happen in the case of psycho-analysts: anyone who decides in favour of this new specialized branch of medicine will, when his studies are completed, take on the two years training you spoke of in a training institute, if it really requires so much time. He will realize afterwards, too, that it is to his advantage to keep up his contact with his colleagues in a psycho-analytical society, and everything will go along swimmingly. I cannot see where there is a place in this for the question of lay analysis.
>
> (Freud, 1926, p. 229)

Despite Freudian indication, psychoanalytic societies in general and including the IPA, lack ongoing training programs, an issue that was discussed with Eduardo Agejas in 2000.

I recently suggested that IPA be more of a scientific institution, orienting its ongoing training rather than dedicating itself to controlling "standards" of analysis based on session frequency, a task which, alone, has little to do with psychoanalysis and is little operative. Taking into consideration that there is more than one psychoanalysis, its definition based on the number of weekly sessions is debated by many today, yet it guides much of our institutional efforts. It has taken more than 20 years of discussions to move from one standard to three training models, and today it is still taking time to accept regulations of three to five sessions of analysis per week plus the monitoring of patients, instead of the four that is part of the classical Eitingon model. This is occurring simultaneously to the acceptance of three weekly sessions in the French or Uruguayan models.

This same duality happens in relation to the use of electronic devices for analysis or supervisions, which are accepted in the Psychoanalytic Institute Eastern Europe (PIEE) or Instituto Latinoamericano de Psicoanálisis (ILAP) centers, even in the Far East. The use of devices, however, is not accepted in far-reaching places such as Argentina or Brazil, or in very large cities such as Mexico City or Buenos Aires, in which movement is both difficult and chaotic.

In 2004, Kirsner addressed the risks of basing psychoanalytic policy on standards that are difficult to implement rather than on policies of cultural, community and academic integration. I think we are facing this challenge.

Equally, there is little information and, in general, there is no consensus regarding the theoretical and clinical contents that should be taught to a future analyst, nor the best way to carry it out.

I agree with Otto Kernberg, who identifies an institute as being between a science and arts faculty, and who places special value on knowledge and enthusiasm of those who teach. He suggests that candidates be included in curriculum design and evaluations of professors.

I agree with him in the desirability of avoiding singular discourse, and adding contemporary contributions and seminars from related sciences and disciplines such as philosophy, neuroscience, anthropology, literature sociologies, etc. to the Freudian texts. I also agree, in order to favor this process, with stimulating the study of different methods of investigation beyond content. Unlike this author, I think of psychoanalysis as psychotherapy, more or less centered on the typical cure, so that the teaching of psychoanalytic psychotherapy that it proposes is implicit in a broad perspective of our work that should be taught to analysts in training.

Leticia Glocer Fiorini (2007) introduced amongst us the concept of "limit", proposed by Trias. For this author, the confrontation of the work of contemporary pluralism demands confrontation, and this cannot go hand in hand with the search for an improved synthesis but rather of the epistemologies of complexity. This, in turn, can only occur within the limit of each theory. Unlike the center, which is a reassuring place of imparted knowledge, it works on delimiting omnipotence and all-encompassing ambition. I think it is an appropriate framework for the interdisciplinary work required for psychoanalytic training.

On the other hand, the lack of academic recognition of the training we impart impedes teaching in universities, and lends to the absence of IPA analysts there, particularly in psychology and in medicine. This movement, which accentuated among us in the 1960s, favors the occurrence of the first transferences with teachers who have generally trained outside our institutions and who belong to Lacanian groups.

Aware of what isolation from the university implies, I am in favor of encouraging academic integration of our graduates through specializations, master and doctorate programs that meet the requirements of each country.

This has been carried out in different societies through distinct organizational formats. Becoming university institutes, for example, or, as in the case of the APA, associating with local prestigious universities. I defend, in particular, this latter variant and have strongly promoted its development in our society. This format respects the discourse and unique modality of each of the institutions involved and does not compromise the institution as a whole nor the training it imparts.

I agree with Madeleine Baranger that an institution should have a structure consistent with the discipline it develops. State regulations, as well as academic and graduation requirements and university discourse, do not, in my experience, constitute the most appropriate environment for the development of psychoanalysis or the training of analysts.

In relation to the societal structure, we part from the premise that institutions are based on identification with common ideals, and we need them. Therefore, we should be aware of the weight that imaginary identifications have in their functioning, and to quote Horenstein: "Their emotional ups and downs, betting on symbolic identifications as founding support".

What Fernando Ulloa has described among us, the "virtual institution", which groups the three components of the tripod, although not within the same walls but rather in the mind of the analyst, is a model that many analysts currently use. It is worth exploring, as it respects the essentials of training and makes it more open and flexible.

I think that within the IPA we are facing difficult competition with the other options if we want to continue forming analysts. That wager requires clearly established policies and institutions to carry them forward. If we do not carry out this work, there will be analysts but trained by others.

Regarding the selection of candidates, I agree with Kernberg in favoring a variety of health related professions. As I have said, I lean towards the French training model of the IPA: it evaluates the results of prior analysis in terms of the relationship with the unconscious rather than requiring analysis during the training.

Considering analysis as the axis of training, I will expand further on this topic here, leaving supervisions and clinical and theoretical studies for another opportunity.

Analysis of the analyst

Freud emphasized that this experience was essential in anyone who wanted to practice psychoanalysis. In favor of the objective he sought to ensure, which was the conviction in the existence of unconscious dynamisms, we should add having had a satisfactory experience in terms of alleviation from suffering, therefore being able to rely on its results.

However, Freud recommended six months to a year of analysis, which he practiced with daily sessions, six times a week.

Today, although in some societies it is limited to 300 hours, training in IPA institutes generally requires three to five weekly sessions for at least four and sometimes up to six and eight years. In addition to these years of analysis, generally carried out in person, there are also supervisions of at least two cases of high-frequency session for two or more years.

Each of these experiences, over time, has become increasingly difficult to carry out. In addition, there are theoretical developments that support the effectiveness of other ways of practicing psychoanalysis.

In our milieu, therapeutic psychoanalysis is frequently practiced in one to two sessions per week, to which family, multi-family, groups, couple, and parent-child relational approaches have been added. In addition to cultural changes, with regards to the significance of high-frequency analysis of four or five weekly sessions, which was standard practice until the 1980s or 1990s, are added distances and travel times in large cities. This latter makes it difficult to hold a high number of weekly sessions. Patients and analysts have discovered the benefits of one or two weekly sessions, and even treatments on demand. That makes that even those of us who value more sessions per week, value these practices and develop theories to better support them.

Theoretical clinical pluralism of contemporary psychoanalysis offers these alternatives. Today, it is difficult to think of there being only one psychoanalysis. The so-called typical cure is only a small portion of our work.

Returning to the issue of training, in many institutions outside the IPA, analysts are trained for the diversity of practices. In general, younger colleagues with 10, 15 or more years of analysis, attending one or two sessions a week, practice psychoanalysis in the same way, in their private practices as well as in hospitals. Those who value a deep psychoanalytic experience of frequent weekly sessions are unable to ignore this reality, a product of different psychoanalysis.

Let us remember again that Otto Kernberg considered the possibility of adding a total of 600 sessions regardless of frequency, and that we are always able to evaluate the results of that analysis in terms of subjective change, psychic growth, etc.

Times have changed dramatically toward acceleration, after more than 100 years. We fly from one continent to another in a few short hours, words have been replaced, in large part, by instant images or video clips. Virtual exchanges are increasingly possible and are of higher quality due to technology, and communication through the Internet is used more frequently in academic settings. We continue, however, thinking about analytic training centered on a model that is more than 100 years old. Madeleine Baranger referred to this as something "outrageous".

I believe that the in-person analytic experience is very useful and is recommended. However, online or telephone analysis can also be beneficial. These processes can be studied longitudinally for use in the training of analysts. If we follow Freud, and the aim of training analysis is to achieve conviction in the existence of unconscious dynamisms, perhaps it is worth studying in order to determine if this is not possible with more extensive use of these new technologies. As I have said, in our country, there are many who are interested in training to become psychoanalysts, but they are anywhere from 250 to 3,000 kilometers away from any training institutions. They would benefit from not having to travel frequently for training. This would be very similar to the way that the IPA accepts colleagues from countries in which there are no analysts.

The training requirements of institutions in our context, some of which are not very psychoanalytic, make it difficult for new generations of analysts to train in IPA societies. Dozens of existing institutions, many of which offer official titles, as well as some hospitals, train psychoanalysts. In the latter, analysts train while also carrying out work in the hospitals. All of these training programs require analysis of the analyst although without specifying length or frequency of weekly sessions. At the same time, case supervisions, theoretical and clinical studies and, in some cases, internships in psychoanalytic practice are required.

Let us recall that Freud was skeptical regarding the intervention of the authorities in psychoanalytic practice:

> I come now to a question the discussion of which seems to me more important. Is the practice of psycho-analysis a matter which should in general be subject to official interference, or would it be more expedient to leave it to follow its natural development? I shall certainly not come to any decision on this point here and now, but I shall take the liberty of putting the problem before you for your consideration.
>
> At all events, I shall not spare you my unauthoritative thoughts on the subject. In my opinion, a superabundance of regulations and prohibitions injures the authority of the law. It

> can be observed that where only a few prohibitions exist, they are carefully observed, but where one is accompanied by prohibitions at every step, one feels definitely tempted to disregard them. Moreover, it does not mean one is quite an anarchist if one is prepared to realize that laws and regulations cannot from the origin claim to possess the attribute of being sacred and untransgressable that they are often inadequately framed and offend our sense of justice, or will do so after a time, and that, in view of the sluggishness of the authorities, there is often no other means of correcting such inexpedient laws than by boldly violating them.
>
> (Freud, 1926, p. 235)

Although he was referring to those who enforce the law, I understand his reflections, in general, apply to the practice of psychoanalysis. Its regulation is very difficult apart from strictly adhering to psychoanalytic method. This is why, and because experience indicates that more weekly sessions are not necessarily associated with effects, I consider it more consequential to evaluate if there were effects from that experience than to regulate its development.

Although three models exist within the IPA, the majority of the societies follow the Eitingon model, requiring four to five weekly sessions of analysis with a teaching analyst of the same institution. The French and Uruguayan models accept three weekly sessions, and in the French model, analysis although required, do not have to be simultaneous with the rest of the tripod.

Personally, I think that a high frequency of weekly sessions is desirable when undergoing training analysis. This is what I have done for years. In any case, the need for a particular number of sessions will be linked to the analyst's referential scheme and, in particular, to their perspective on regression. However, in my opinion, flexibility should be exercised, over all evaluating the results and avoiding that the organizations take on a policing role over these devices. I have already pointed out the coexistence of very different criteria within the IPA regarding what is accepted as psychoanalysis suitable for training.

Regulations do not only cover the frequency of weekly sessions, they also stipulate that they take place with an analyst of the same institution. In my Master's thesis on the psychoanalytic institution, I described the problems that accompany closed training systems that require analysts of the same institution. The institutions favor imaginary identifications, psychology of the masses, family and power groups. These are questions that undermine, the objectives, in psychoanalytic terms, of freeing individual subjectivity as a premise for creative training. Having a structure and institutional leadership that transcend these identifications should be the premise if we seek to train psychoanalysts.

In 1958, Clara Thompson advocated toward openness in psychoanalytic education:

> So institutes do not have to be homes from which there is no escape. Their graduates should be encouraged to think and act for themselves. On the other hand, teachers from outside should be brought in, in order to stimulate constructive appraisal of the institute's theories. Psychoanalysts need to see themselves as part of a developing science to which they have a specific contribution to make, rather than as members of some isolated group, fantastically loyal. There are too many family groups in psychoanalysis, and if they continue, they may well make impossible its contribution to the science of human nature.
>
> (Thompson, 1958, p. 51)

More recently Patrick Guyomard, following Antigone, described the consequences of this imprisonment in incestuous terms.

I am in favor of leaving the choice of an analyst in the hands of the candidate, whether the analyst be of the same institution or not, and evaluating the effects of the analysis to determine admission to the institute. Although in my teaching functions I respect the Eitingon model with its variants adopted by my society, as I said before, I am drawn more to the French system among those accepted by the IPA.

About the mental apparatus and its structure

> What do you mean by the "mental apparatus"? and what, may I ask, is it constructed of?

> For we picture the unknown apparatus which serves the activities of the mind as being really like an instrument constructed

> of several parts (which we speak of as "agencies"), each of which performs a particular function and which have a fixed spatial relation to one another: it being understood that by spatial relation – "in front of" and "behind", "superficial" and "deep"- we merely mean in the first instances a representation of the regular succession of the function.
>
> (Freud, 1926, p. 194)

Following *On Narcissism: An Introduction* and especially *The Ego and the Id*, the structure of the ego was of interest to Freud. Freud emphasizes the importance of the relative strength of the ego organization and the indomitable strength of the instincts in this article:

> Only let us hold fast to this: the nodal point and pivot of the whole situation is the relative strength of the ego organization. We shall then find it easy to complete our aetiological survey. As what may be called the normal cause of neurotic illness we already know the feebleness of the childhood ego, the task of dealing with the early sexual impulses and the effects of the more or less chance experiences of childhood. Is it not child's life? For instance, an innate strength and unruliness of the instinctual life in the id, which from the outset, sets the ego tasks too hard for it? O, a special developmental feebleness of the ego due to unknown reasons? Such factors must of course acquire an aetiological importance, in some cases a transcendent one. We have invariably to reckon with the instinctual strength of the id; if it has developed to excess, the prospects of our therapy are poor. We still know too little of the causes of a developmental inhibition of the ego. These then would be the cases of neurosis with an essentially constitutional basis. Without some such constitutional, congenital favouring factors, a neurosis can, no doubt, scarcely come about.
>
> (Freud, 1926, p. 242)

The work of representation, identifications, constructs the ego and the superego and in some cases fails. The clinic varies greatly depending on the level of symbolization, the thickness of the preconscious, the strength and flexibility of the ego in each case, and therefore the importance in its evaluation a priori and in some moments of the treatment.

Carlos Mario Aslan highlighted the importance of considering instances as functions that Freud introduces following *The Ego and the Id*. In this sense, we speak of "the unconscious" instead of the unconscious, or of identifications with ego or superego functions emphasizing its function rather than its geography. Localization models are nevertheless interesting in the dialogue with the neurosciences. Mark Solms has recently described interesting perspectives on the conscious id.

The evaluation of the psychic instances and especially the ego is approached by Freud in his article that then poses the psychopathological conditions and the therapeutic goals within this context:

> You are right. So long as the ego and its relations to the Id fulfill these ideal conditions, there will be no neurotic disturbance.
>
> (Freud, 1926, p. 202)

> It is easy now to describe our therapeutic aim. We try to restore the Ego, to free it from its restrictions, and to give it back the command over the Id which it has lost owing to its early repressions. It is for this one purpose that we carry out analysis; our whole technique is directed to this aim. We have to seek out the repressions which have been set up and to urge the Ego to correct them with our help and to deal with conflicts better than by an attempt at flight. Since these repressions belong to the very early years of childhood, the work of analysis leads us, too, back to that period.
>
> (Freud, 1926, p. 205)

Anna Freud has described the diagnoses of normality and pathology based on the evaluation of psychic instances. I think it is a very useful resource when thinking about a possible course of normal or pathological development. The extension of psychoanalysis to border states, psychosomatic symptoms, narcissistic disorders, depressions, make this evaluation indispensable, particularly in the case of ego functions in order to determine the type of approach required.

The traumatic, for its part, is a broad area for contemporary psychoanalysis, and Benyakar described "the disruptive" to define its scope to the processes that affect representational ligature. The stimuli that do not achieve this effect are only "disruptive" for the ego and this differentiation extends to the clinical approach.

The ego alteration characterizes these cases that exceed the framework that Freud imagined for his technique.

This also applies to psychoanalysis with children. These have their ego in structuring and therefore are without sufficient strength in relation to the adult. In this article, Freud strongly supports his practice.

> What? You have had small children in analysis? Children of less than six years? Can that be done? And is it not most risky for the children?
>
> It can be done very well. It is hardly to be believed what goes on in a child of four or five years old. Children are very active-minded at that age; their early sexual period is also a period of intellectual flowering. I have an impression that with the onset of the latency period they become mentally inhibited as well, stupider. From that time on, too, many children lose their physical charm. And, as regards the damage done by early analysis, I may inform you that the first child on whom the experiment was first ventured, nearly twenty years ago, has since then grown into a healthy and capable young man, who has passed through puberty irreproachably, in spite of some severe psychical traumas. It may be hoped that things will turn out no worse for the other "victims" of early analysis.
>
> (Freud, 1926, p. 214)

The more than 100 years since little Hans and the experiences of Anna Freud, Melanie Klein, Winnicott, Dolto, Aberastury and many others have consolidated the analytic practice with children beyond their differences. Today the IPA proposes a model of integrated training for adults and for children and adolescents which, in some societies, is in addition to their university accreditation. For the benefit of the clinic, psychoanalysis is deeply related to development, pediatrics and education.

Finally, the study of the structure of psychic or mental apparatus has become particularly important with the contributions of psychoanalysis. Unlike evolutionary psychology that proposes a conventionally linear model of development, psychoanalysis proposes a time in torsion that includes the a posteriori.

Although psychoanalysis includes the genetic model, where what happens before determines what happens next, for example in the description of the libidinal phases or in the processes of mourning, it introduces the historical model where what is next determines what is before in an original way. The history is described later and we know that it not only reconstructs facts, but also builds them. It is the basis of much of the contemporary psychoanalytic clinic that Hornstein described as "symbolizing historicity", which we apply when there are flaws in the processes of symbolization. In this manner he develops the Freudian "construction", classically articulated to interpretation among the resources of the analyst.

Finally, there is a consideration of what is called the "personal influence" of the analyst. In analysis we do not use the suggestive factor to suppress symptoms as in hypnosis.

> What you say about the special influence of the analyst certainly deserves great attention. An influence of the kind exists and plays a large part in analysis – but not the same part as in hypnotism. It ought to be possible to convince you that the situations in the two cases are quite different. It may be enough to point out that we do not use this personal influence, the factor of "suggestion", to suppress the symptoms of the illness, as happens with hypnotic suggestion. Further, it would be a mistake to believe that this factor is the vehicle and promoter of the treatment throughout its length. At its beginning, no doubt. But later on it opposes our analytic intentions and forces us to adopt the most far-reaching counter-measures. And I should like to show by an example how far diverting a patient's thoughts and talking him out of things are from the technique of analysis.
>
> (Freud, 1926, p. 190)

He acknowledges however that this personal influence exists and that it plays a large role in analysis. We can locate it in relation to different contemporary developments:

1. the results of the intersubjective encounter
2. the capacity of empathy of the analyst
3. the drive of the analyst

I think that each of these, described by authors such as Renik, Bolognini, Marucco and many others, plays an important role in analysis and models the influence of the analyst in each process.

In summary

I have tried to update and clarify some points of view on the central themes from the article at hand: conditions for the practice of psychoanalysis and its practice by non-physicians; what is expected from the training of analysts and the evaluation of psychic instances of the mental apparatus in order to understand normality and conditions of pathology.

References

Aberastury, F. (2002). El futuro del psicoanálisis y las instituciones psicoanalíticas. In: A. Varios (Ed.), *60 Años de Psicoanálisis en la Argentina: Pasado. Presente. Futuro* (pp. 287–293). Buenos Aires: Comisión de Publicaciones de la APA y Editorial Lumen.

Agejas, E. (2001). Razón de ser del pluralismo (inédito). *Presentación en Asamblea Científica de la APA*, de diciembre 18.

Aulagnier, P. (2005). *Un intérprete en busca de sentido*. 2nd ed. Buenos Aires: Siglo XXI Editores.

Aryan, A. (2005). *Symposium: Las instituciones psicoanalíticas frente a la clínica y práctica actuales*. Buenos Aires: APdeBA.

Azouri, C. (1995). *He triunfado donde el paranoico fracasa*. Buenos Aires: De la Flor.

Baranger, W. (1987). Mesa Redonda del Claustro de Candidatos de la APA del 25/6/85. In: *Vicisitudes del análisis didáctico*. Buenos Aires: Nueva Librería.

Baranger, M. (2003). Formación psicoanalítica. La reforma del '74, treinta años después. *Revista de Psicoanálisis*, LX(4).

Bernard, M., and Bianchi, H. (1995). Entrevista con René Kaës. *Revista de Psicoanálisis*, LII(2): 470.

Bernfeld, S. (1962). On Pychoanalytic Training. *Psychoanalytic Quarterly*, XXXI(4): 453–482.

Bleger, J. (1972). *Simbiosis y ambigüedad*. Buenos Aires: Paidós.

Bolognini, S. (2013). *La empatía psicoanalítica*. Buenos Aires: Editorial Lumen.

Borgogno, F., and Casullo, G. (2010). Who, Where, What, in Which Way and to Whom: Upon and About the Results of a Questionanaire on the Present State of the Relation between Psychoanalysis and the University in Europe. *International Forum of Psychoanalysis*, 19(4).

Cabral, A. (2002). El Manifiesto de 1974 y la polaridad Enseñanza-Transmisión en la institución psicoanalítica. In: A. Varios (Ed.), *60 Años de Psicoanálisis en la Argentina. Pasado. Presente. Futuro* (pp. 433–442). Buenos Aires: Comisión de Publicaciones de la APA y Editorial Lumen.

Comisión Nacional de Evaluación y Acreditación Universitaria (CONEAU). Ministerio de Educación, Ciencia y Tecnología. (2004). *RESOLUCION N° 526/04. Instituto Universitario de Salud Mental de ApdeBA*, 14-octubre. Retrieved 2012, 19-agosto from www.coneau.edu.ar/archivos/818.pdf

Campalans Pereda, L. (2012). *Transmisión del psicoanálisis. Formación de analistas*. Buenos Aires: Psicolibro.

Cohen, P. (2007). Freud Is Widely Taught at Universities, Except in the Psychology Department, November 25, 2007. *The New York Times*, www.nytimes.com/2007/11/25/weekinreview/25cohen.html

Czander, W. (1993). *The Psychodynamics of Work and Organizations: Theory and Application*. New York: Guilford.

Emory University. (n.d.). *History & Tradition*. Retrieved 2012, 20-agosto from www.emory.edu/home/about/history/index.html.

Escuela Freudiana de Buenos Aires. (1977). Primeras y Segundas Jornadas sobre Institución Psicoanalítica (1976–1977). In: *Cuaderno Sigmund Freud*. Buenos Aires: Escuela Freudiana de Buenos Aires.

Fainstein, A.M. (2002). La APA hoy, algunas reflexiones. In: A. Varios (Ed.), *60 Años de Psicoanálisis en la Argentina: Pasado. Presente. Futuro*. Buenos Aires: Comisión de Publicaciones de la APA y Editorial Lumen.

Fainstein, A.M. *"Institución Psicoanalítica" Tesis de Maestría en Psicoanálisis*, Universidad del Salvador- Asociación Psicoanalítica Argentina. Unpublished.

Francese, G., Weissmann, F., Canovi, R., and Weissmann, J. (2005). *La crisis del psicoanálisis (inédito)*. Proyecto subsidiado por IPA, bajo el programa Development Psychoanalytic Practice and Training.

Freud, S. (1926). The Standard Edition of the Complete Psychological Works of Sigmund Freud. Volume XX. *The Question of Lay Analysis*. London: The Hogarth Press.

Freud, S. (1910/1979). *Sobre el psicoanálisis silvestre*. 1st ed., Vol. XI: Obras Completas. Buenos Aires: Amorrortu Editores.

Freud, S. (1919/1979). *¿Debe enseñarse el psicoanálisis en la universidad?* 1st ed., Vol. XVII. Obras Completas. Buenos Aires: Amorrortu editores.

Freud, S. (1921/1979). *Psicología de las Masas y análisis del yo* 1st ed., Vol. XVIII. Obras Completas. Buenos Aires: Amorrortu editores.

Freud, S. (1926/1979). *¿Pueden los legos ejercer el análisis? Diálogos con un juez imparcial*. 1° ed., Vol. XX Obras Completas. Buenos Aires: Amorrortu editores.

Freud, S. (1927/1979). *El porvenir de una ilusión*. 1st ed., Vol. XXI: Obras Completas. Buenos Aires: Amorrortu editores.

Freud, S. (1937/1979). *Análisis terminable e interminable* 1st ed., Vol. XXIII. Obras Completas. Buenos Aires: Amorrortu editores.

García, J. (2011). Comentario al trabajo "La nostalgia del absoluto en la institución psicoanalítica" de Mirta Goldstein. *Asamblea Científica de la APA.*

Garma, A. (1959). Las relaciones entre analistas. *Revista de Psicoanálisis,* XVI.

Glocer Fiorini, L. (2007). Pluralidad de teorías y prácticas clínicas. *Revista de Psicoanálisis,* LXIV(4): 809–819.

Goldstein, M. (2001). La práctica científica institucional. *Asamblea Científica de la APA,* 18 de diciembre.

Goldstein, N. (2002). El futuro de la transmisión del Psicoanálisis y las relaciones entre analistas. In: A. Varios (Ed.), *60 Años de Psicoanálisis en la Argentina. Pasado. Presente: Futuro* (pp. 457–468). Buenos Aires: Comisión de Publicaciones de la APA y Editorial Lumen.

Goldstein, M. (2011). *La nostalgia del absoluto en la institución psicoanalítica,* 18 de setiembre.

Goldstein, M., and Moise, C. (comp.). (2001). *Pensando la institución psicoanalítica.* Buenos Aires: El Escriba.

Gomberoff, M. (1991). Consideraciones sobre la institución psicoanalítica. In: J. Coloma and J. Jordan (Eds.), *Cuarenta años de psicoanálisis en Chile.* Santiago de Chile: Casaula Editores.

Gomberoff, M. (2005). *Symposium: Las instituciones psicoanalíticas frente a la clínica y práctica actuales.* Buenos Aires: APdeBA.

Gramajo Gallimany, N., and Siguel de Turjansky, D. (2002). Imaginar un futuro. In: A. Varios (Ed.), *60 Años de Psicoanálisis en la Argentina: Pasado. Presente. Futuro* (pp. 469–478). Buenos Aires: Comisión de Publicaciones de la APA y Editorial Lumen.

Horenstein, M. (2011). Personal Communication. Córdoba. Argentina.

Jacques, E. (1951). *The Changing Culture of a Factory.* Londres: Tavistock Publ. Ltd.

Jacques, E. (1965). Los sistemas sociales como defensas a las ansiedades persecutorias y depresivas. In: M. Klein (Ed.), *Nuevas Direcciones en Psicoanálisis.* Buenos Aires: Paidós.

Kernberg, O. (1984). Cambios en la naturaleza de la formación psicoanalítica, en la estructura y en las normas de formación. In: R. Wallerstein (Ed.), *Colección de Monografías.* Volume 4. Cambios en los analistas y en su formación (pp. 59–66). London: International Psychoanalytical Association.

Kernberg, O. (1996). Thirty Methods to Destroy the Creativity of Psychoanalytical Candidates. *International Journal of Psychoanalysis,* 77: 1031–1034.

Kirsner, D. (2004). Psychoanalysis and Its Discontents. *Psychoanalytical Psychology,* XXI: 339–352.

Lacan, J. (1981). Situación del psicoanálisis y formación del psicoanalista en 1956. In: *Escritos* 2. Buenos Aires: Siglo XXI.

Leibovich de Duarte, A. (2007). Psychoanalysis and the University: Contributions, Strategies and Dilemmas. Psychoanalysis and the University in Latin-America. In: *Congreso de la IPA*, Berlín.

Leibovich de Duarte, A., and Duhalde, C. (2007). Participation of Psychoanalysts in the University in Latin America. Presented in *Berlin International Psychoanalytical Congress*, 2009.

Loewenberg, P., and Thompson, N. (Eds.) (2010). *100 Years of IPA: The Centenary History of the International Psychoanalytical Association 1910–2010: Evolution and Change*. IPA & Karnac, London.

Lourau, R. (1975). *El análisis institucional*. Buenos Aires: Amorrortu Editores.

Marucco, N. (1998). *Cura analítica y transferencia*. Buenos Aires: Amorrortu Editores.

Morin, E. (2000). *La mente bien ordenada: Repensar la Reforma. Reformar el pensamiento*. Barcelona: Seix Barral. Los Tres Mundos.

Morin, E. (2006). *Articular los saberes ¿Qué saberes enseñar en las escuelas?* 1st ed. Monterrey, México: Instituto Internacional para el Pensamiento Complejo, bajo el auspicio de UANL, ENS.

Muller, F. (2008). Psychotherapy in Argentina: Theoretical Orientation and Clinical Practice. *Journal of Psyhcotherapy Integration*, XVIII(4): 410–420.

Peskin, L. (2002). Mesa redonda: 60 años de APA. In: A. varios (Ed.), *60 Años de Psicoanálisis en la Argentina. Pasado. Presente. Futuro* (pp. 42–46). Buenos Aires: Comisión de Publicaciones de la APA y Editorial Lumen.

Reider, N. (1953). A Type of Transference to Institutions. *Bulletin of Menninger Clinic*, XVII: 58–63.

Renik, O. (2002). Los riesgos de la neutralidad. *Aperturas Psicoanalíticas*, (10), 2002.

Rocha Barros, E. (2001). *10° Conferencia de Analistas Didactas*. Buenos Aires: APA.

Safouan, M., Julien, S., and Hoffman, C. (1997). *Malestar en el Psicoanálisis. El tercero en la institución y el análisis de control*. Buenos Aires: Nueva Visión.

Schroeder, D. (2006). Subjetividad y psicoanálisis. La implicación del psicoanalista. *Revista Uruguaya de Psicoanálisis*, (103).

Sociedad Psicoanalítica del Sur. (n.d.). *Home Page*. August 25, 2012, www.sps.org.ar/

Steiner, G. (2001). *La nostalgia del absoluto*. Madrid: Siruela.

Subsecretaría de Educación Superior de México. (n.d.). *Reconocimiento de Validez Oficial de Estudios Superiores Federales y Estatales*. August 29, 2012, www.sirvoes.sep.gob.mx

Szpilka, J. (2002). Sobre los cambios en APA en 1974. In: A. Varios (Ed.), *60 Años de Psicoanálisis en la Argentina. Pasado. Presente. Futuro* (pp. 170–179). Buenos Aires: Comisión de Publicaciones de la APA y Editorial Lumen.

Thompson, C. (1958). A Study of the Emotional Climate of Psychoanalytic Institutes. *Psychiatry* 21, 45–51.

Uriarte, C., and Costanzo, P. (2003). Maestría en Psicoanálisis de la Asociación Psicoanalítica del Uruguay. *Revista Uruguaya de Psicoanálisis*, (98): 9–17.

Weissmann, F. (2002). El análisis didáctico y la formación. Una contribución al 60° Aniversario de la fundación de la APA. In: A. Varios (Ed.), *60 Años de Psicoanálisis en la Argentina. Pasado. Presente. Futuro* (pp. 295–306). Buenos Aires: Comisión de Publicaciones de la APA y Editorial Lumen.

Widlocher, D., Miller, J.A., and Granger, B. (coord.). (2003). El porvenir del psicoanálisis. *Revista de Psicoanálisis*, LX(4).

Zak de Goldstein, R. (1994). ¿Caos, petrificación . . . o qué? *Revista Latinoamericana de Psicoanálisis*, I(1): 251–257.

10

Psychoanalysis is lay in its essence

Cláudia Aparecida Carneiro

I would like to begin this essay about *The Question of Lay Analysis* (Freud, 1926) by asking a question: Is there a psychoanalysis that is not lay? If this new way of thinking about the human condition that began with the Freudian discovery requires dismissing previous knowledge derived from theoretical and scientific models, to allow the knowledge of the unconscious, we will be dealing with knowledge arisen from the emotional experience, which is by nature lay. Psychoanalysis began with the discovery of the unconscious and was structured by the rules that govern it. This has been the starting point for the psychoanalytic function; therefore, psychoanalysis has been lay since its birth.

Before proceeding along this main road, which I imagine to be crucial in the discussion of 'lay analysis', it is important to go back a few steps and to focus on the term 'lay', which can lead to misunderstandings and semantic confusion.

Freud, in his book, states that 'lay' means 'not practiced by doctors'. At the time of the publication, there was a practical reason for the question as to whether non-doctors were allowed to treat people through psychoanalysis, or not – avoiding damage to patients. This is one of the reasons alleged by the medical profession that persists among psychoanalytic groups in countries where the State has not yet produced instruments to regulate the psychoanalytic practice. The specificity of the analytic treatment and the analyst's training led Freud to directly object to this way of control and to pose this statement for consideration; "It may perhaps turn out that in this instance the patients are not like other patients, that the laymen are not really laymen, and that the doctors have not exactly the qualities which one has a right to expect of doctors and on which their claims should be based" (Freud, 1926, p. 184).

It is opportune to explain the term 'layman' etymologically, which is used to designate a person who does not have deep knowledge of a certain area or subject. Originally, the word, which derives from the Greek *laikós*, referred to the people who did not have the necessary knowledge to participate in certain functions within the religious organization, being hierarchically submitted to an ecclesiastical elite. In classical Greek, it means 'people of lower class', and in Latin, it also means 'idiot', 'illiterate', 'secular'. It contrasts with *klerikós*, a reference to the prior knowledge of the literate, official member of the church (Nascentes, 1955).

Although the term 'lay' is used today in all human areas, its use in the psychoanalytic community suggests the existence of castes, or 'religious elites' who persist in underestimating the ability of non-doctor and non-psychologist professionals to become psychoanalysts and to efficiently attend the peculiar conditions demanded by this practice.

Who determines whether someone is a layman or not? Who has the legitimacy to decide if the analyst, who is called lay, is less capable to practice psychoanalysis, to be with his patient and to think with him, than medical professionals or psychologists? The issue seems to be related to the problem of truth and lies, as proposed by Bion (1974).

In a lecture occurred in São Paulo in 1970s, Bion addressed this topic, commenting on a participant's question about the problem of the liar and the practice of psychoanalysis by lay people. He emphasized that a person can be labeled as 'capable' or not, according to the vertex from which one is considered. He quoted Plato saying that the philosopher suggested that artists should be forbidden in his republic, because poets and painters *would be liars to corrupt society and the nation*. Bion invites us to think about the vertex with which we judge a situation and its ideological character. Here is his consideration, well suited to our theme: "It all depends on thinking the artist is teaching us something about the truth, about how a brick wall is, or that he is really fooling us. Consequently, it is important to determine *who* says a person is a liar and *why* he says it" (Bion, 1974, p. 66).

The question highlighted by Bion, regarding analysis, is the difficulty for the psychoanalyst to conform to the idea that the patient is either trying to deceive him/her or telling him/her one of many sides of truth. Bion teaches us that a psychoanalyst can investigate a misunderstanding in a way that is not accessible to a philosopher, since the philosophers are concerned with understanding and misunderstanding, but the analyst can observe and listen to a person *while* this person is immerse in his/her understanding or misunderstanding.

This debate also makes us think about the series of misunderstandings that the spread of the idea of a 'lay analysis' and a 'non-lay analysis' raises. Let us begin with Freud's position, strictly defended in his 1926 text, which can be summarized as follows: one who has undergone analysis with another and acquired a knowledge about his unconscious is no longer a layman for psychoanalysis. With this, Freud leads us to the *princeps* condition that is required by someone who wishes to become an analyst – the psychoanalyst is trained from his own experience as a patient.

The understanding of this Freudian postulate may be vague for those who have not gone through a deep, unique and intimate experience of analysis. How can we speak of a single emotional experience that can only be lived by two, in which there is no third person? How can we talk about it to someone who has not been through the experience of being analyzed?

These considerations led Freud to create a revolutionary text, written in just one month, to make a stand in favor of the freedom of psychoanalysis in relation to dogmatic models. He did that by placing this entirely new method of treating psychic suffering, which affects one's body and their relation with themselves and with the world. In a brilliant way, Freud prepared his 'impartial interlocutor', summoned in the text, to the nature of the psychic processes, the disorders of the soul that affect the person, and what is the work through analysis and the conditions for this to occur. The dialogue created by Freud helps the reader gradually to assimilate what is original and subjective in this *new kind of human knowledge*, which is distinct from scientific and philosophical models, although it maintains a relation of respect and cooperation with the others.

We know that this *new kind of knowledge*, meaning the understanding of the unconscious processes and the access to another knowledge that emerges in the analytic situation, implies a specific training of the future analyst. Freud details to his interlocutor what involves the training of a psychoanalyst, having as pillars the theoretical instruction, the clinical practice with supervision and, in particular, the personal analysis called training analysis. The learning is a non-stop process that continuous in the clinical practice, through several authors' thinking and in the exchange of ideas among colleagues of psychoanalytic institutions. Every analyst knows how long and arduous this course is. We will come back to that point later.

What we see while reading Freud's book is his indisputable position on the indispensability of the analyst's analysis. Thereby, the inventor of psychoanalysis has distanced the prior knowledge, preconized by the scientific field of that which can only arise in analytic experience. Knowledge governed by the laws of the unconscious, that is to say, the presence of resistances that operate to prevent access to the repressed, but which tend to subside as analysis proceeds. It is in the field of transference, which functions as the motor of the analytic process, that this knowledge is obtained, free from the illusion that we can have prior knowledge of the one who seeks us. It is what makes analytic experience different from other therapeutic forms.

Recalling the words of Freud addressed to his impartial interlocutor, at the point where he details the model of training that existed in the three European institutes of psychoanalysis at that time. Anyone who has passed through such a course of instruction, who has been analyzed himself, who has mastered the psychology of the unconscious and has learnt the technique of psychoanalysis, the art of interpretation, of fighting resistances and of handling the transference, *is no longer a layperson in the field of psychoanalysis*. For the meanings of the term 'lay' not to be confused, we must understand that Freud uses the term *layman* to describe the 'non-doctor' and, as he defends his position, he deconstructs the idea of 'not knowledgeable' and 'unqualified' attributed to non-doctors who practiced psychoanalysis.

The lay tradition in psychoanalysis

In the 1927 *The Question of Lay Analysis* post-essay, Freud clarified that he wrote the book in defense of his friend and disciple Theodor

Reik, a non-doctor member of the Vienna Psychoanalytic Society, accused in 1926, of illegally practicing psychoanalytic treatments. Reik was denounced by one of his patients. In a letter to the Viennese newspaper *Neue Freie Presse*, shortly after finishing the book, Freud acknowledges Reik's competence in the treatment of *particularly difficult cases*. In the postscript, he closed the debate with a criticism and his usually sharp tone. He addressed his colleagues who kept resistance to lay analysis – their practical and local actions "cannot affect any of the factors which govern the situation" and amount to "an attempt at repress" (Freud, 1926, p. 258). To my mind, the actions that today turn against the lay nature of psychoanalysis represent a transferential attack on Freud's own discovery.

The history of psychoanalysis has several examples of non-doctor and non-psychologist analysts who contributed (and contribute) remarkably to the expansion of the psychoanalytic movement and the development of this discipline. To name some of the well-known analysts of the international community, let us begin with the pioneers of psychoanalysis; among them there were the non-doctors Otto Rank, Hans Sachs, Leopold Bernfeld, as well as Theodor Reik. In 1926, when Freud discussed lay analysis, the International Psychoanalytic Association had 60 non-doctors, among its 344 members (Chasseguet-Smirgel et al., 1969).

Among the members of the Freudian circle, it is worth mentioning the importance of two laywomen, Lou Andreas-Salomé and Marie Bonaparte, both also presented with the famous rings reserved for members of the Secret Committee (Roudinesco and Plon, 1998). The contribution of Princess Marie for the preservation of the Freudian legacy was valuable. Anna Freud created a school in the field of child psychoanalysis, but surely the best example of a lay analyst's contribution to psychoanalytic theory and technique lies in the innovative ideas of Melanie Klein and her work as a whole. From her school names of great relevance came to psychoanalysis, among them Joan Rivière, Susan Isaacs, Money-Kyrle and Betty Joseph, all of them non-doctors.

Because of its importance in the international psychoanalytic movement, it is interesting to highlight the participation of the British Psychoanalytical Society in the defense of lay analysis. Historically, it has maintained among its members a significant number of non-doctor analysts, who collaborated and collaborate today with an original thinking and fertile theoretical production, such as Frank Philips and Christopher Bollas.

In France, we can point as examples of non-doctor analysts Jean-Bertrand Pontalis, Didier Anzieu, Janine Chasseguet-Smirgel, Monique Schneider, Julia Kristeva, Elizabeth Roudinesco and the couple Octave Mannoni and Maud Mannoni. Prior to their work with psychoanalysis, all of them came from different areas – philosophers, historians, writers, literary critics and political scientists.

In Brazil, the history of psychoanalysis cannot be told without pointing out the pioneering and achievements of Virgínia Leone Bicudo, a lay analyst who has paved the way for the diffusion of psychoanalysis and the training of many generations of analysts, who inherited her innovative actions. Virgínia Bicudo was the first woman and first non-doctor professional to become a psychoanalyst and a training analyst in Latin America (Abrão, 2010; Castro, 2010). She helped in the creation of the Sociedade Brasileira de Psicanálise de São Paulo and established the pillars of psychoanalytic training for that institution. There, Virgínia was the one who introduced the ideas of Melanie Klein, with whom she had supervision during the years of her training at the British Psychoanalytical Society.

The pioneering spirit of Virgínia promoted the spread of psychoanalysis in other regions of Brazil and contributed to the widespread dissemination of Freudian doctrine in this country in the 1950s and 1960s. Certainly, one of her greatest achievements was the introduction of psychoanalysis in Brasilia, the newly inaugurated capital of Brazil at that time. Virgínia's project was bringing psychoanalysis to the center of the political power. She believed that the political leaders, if analyzed, would have better conditions to govern with responsibility and social commitment (Abrão, 2010).

Virgínia's daring project was accomplished with her weekly trips from São Paulo to Brasília with some fellow analysts who supported her to train the first group of psychoanalysts in the capital. That was a pioneering experience in the international history of the institutes of psychoanalysis (Castro, 2010). Her perseverance resulted in the foundation of the Sociedade de Psicanálise de Brasília. Her legacy prevails; traditionally, we are the society that receives more laypersons for psychoanalytic training in Brazil. Among current members of our training Institute – that bears her name – 20% are doctors, 46% are psychologists and 34% are professionals from other areas.

The lay knowledge of the unconscious

The very large theoretical and clinical production of these psychoanalysts who I mentioned corroborates what Freud strongly stated – the psychoanalytic knowledge and practice are not learned in books or at any university, therefore they are not part of either the technical-scientific field of medicine (or psychology), or the academic theoretical field – because the analyst training is lay. Freud was a man of science, but he was essentially loyal to the truth of his discoveries and fought bravely to defend psychoanalysis from pre-established parameters. The Freudian experience showed that there is a knowledge in the unconscious, which is incompatible with the prevailing norms of scientific knowledge, and the former defines a person's uniqueness. This truth has led him to break with the medical scientific discourse, causing a strong reaction among his colleagues, including some of his followers.

Those professionals attributed to themselves the prerogative of the treatment of neurotics, supported by the idea of denouncing charlatanism and protecting people who sought the help of psychoanalysis. After the clinical development, the collaboration of new authors and the improvement of the psychoanalytical technique, psychoanalysis advanced in the field of psychoses, narcissistic structures and other severe pathologies. Curiously, this expansion of the psychoanalytic domain also serves as an argument for the movement against the access of non-doctors and non-psychologists.

What does, in methodological terms, such a break with classical scientific discourse mean? Psychoanalytic method proposes a differentiated listening of one's psychic suffering. However, how does the analyst listen to his/her patient? How does the analyst return to him/her something that might be useful for a pain that is *without smell, without taste* – using Bion's metaphor – and can neither be treated with drugs, directive methods nor ready-made recipes? What is the benefit that the patient could obtain from an analysis?

I think about a moment of the analysis of a young patient of mine, who was really worried about her role of a *good girl,* whose relationships with partners followed the trail of a roller coaster. In the first stages of her analysis, she frequently experienced her Cinderella fairy tale followed by the tragic outcome of her relationships that controlled her life. Her dream castle could collapse from one session to the next; this oscillatory movement, predominantly paranoid-schizoid, was frequent. She attributed all responsibility for her personal tragedies and despair to her partner.

This is how her analysis worked in the beginning; she could not understand these disintegration states as something that referred mainly to her. She did not recognize her participation in the misunderstandings that characterized her relationships. Every time she argued with her partner, she would come to me in tears and say, "How could he '*do this to*' me?" I saw a child facing me – a child who could not '*do anything for*' herself; her despair touched me.

My interpretations aimed at informing her that she was always waiting for other people, including me, to '*do that for*' her. Driven by her fear of abandonment, she allowed other people to '*do that to*' her, something she could not bear. I wanted to help her approach a forgotten truth, which was about a child rejected by her father – this fact was present in my mind and 'denied' by her. This fact was overshadowed by the presence of her loving stepfather.

When she was able to recognize the pain which seemed hidden – *without smell, without taste* – her attention turned to her symptom. She came to realize her tendency to be in 'roller coaster' relationships and the inability to tolerate the rejection and absence of the object. After that, her cry for help communicated a new state of anguish, "I ruin everything and I do not know how to '*do it*' differently, without going crazy". This perception gradually gave way to another one, "I see myself as an abandoned child, so I cannot be an adult".

However, an analytic work also concerns the analysis of the own analyst. Without experience, technique is empty and the transferential relationship with this patient enabled the analyst to construct a knowledge – *a posteriori* – of which she already knew in her unconscious. In the relation of this analytic pair, '*do with*' was being replaced by '*be with*'. New narratives have emerged from the experience shared by the pair; an opening for the analysand to leave a passive position and take responsibility for her life and her choices.

I chose to bring this clinical illustration to think about the logic of psychoanalysis, which, I believe, establishes itself by the affects and the unconscious experience. I will turn to the ideas and concepts developed by Antonio Muniz de Rezende, which are presented in the book *The 'Current' Psychoanalysis at the Interface of the 'New' Sciences* (Rezende and Gerber, 2001). If the analyst makes himself/herself in his/her own experience of analysis, Rezende says that the logic of psychoanalysis is "learned in psychoanalytic experience" (p. 10).

From this proposition, we can draw a line between formal scientific thought and psychoanalytic thought. The logic of psychoanalysis has an affective condition, which is based on uncertainties, possibilities and constructions of narratives, unlike classical logic, based on the certainty of ideas, reason and determination of facts. We can follow Rezende in his reflection by employing this poetic expression from Bion's reading – the psychoanalytic thought is a movement *from inside out*, since it starts from the experience, whereas other sciences and modes of thought make a movement from the outside in, guided by a ready-made logic.

Other therapeutic practices seek to obtain a nosological view of disorders, eliminate symptoms, reduce damage, cure diseases and change behaviors (Alves and Saad, 2009; Balbi et al., 2009). Psychoanalysis does not have the same goals. In this sense, we work with a clearly distinct object, which cannot be reproduced or refuted: the unconscious emerges in the patient's narrative; it is a movement *from inside out*, referred by Muniz Rezende.

This unicity of psychoanalysis in relation to other fields of knowledge does not take away from it its scientific character, defended by Freud. Through his scientific training and his rigorous commitment to research, Freud followed the tracks of the unconscious, which revealed itself in the speech and symptoms of Freud's hysteric patients. He kept his respect to scientific precepts throughout his life always being faithful to the truth of his own experience.

As psychoanalysis does not aim at a therapeutic objective, it maintains its scientific quality precisely in this coherence of the unconscious investigation. If we are humble enough to 'let go' of our eagerness to heal and if we dare to detach ourselves from the memory of narrated and known facts, from the desire to obtain answers and to understand the person's internal reality from a predetermined way, we may be working with the logic of psychoanalysis.

Bion (1970) tells us that the analyst should abstain from *memory, desire and understanding* to be willing to think psychoanalytically with his patient and let himself be 'carried away' by that experience; guided only by love for the truth, the way suggested by Freud and emphasized by Bion. They teach us that what heals is the truth and our reception of this truth.

Once, a young man came to me saying that he needed to be treated because he was suffering from anxiety, which prevented him from pursuing his career and moving out of his parents' house. However, he saw no reason for such fear. He had an urgent need for analysis in order to heal himself. Some years later, after he had overcome past difficulties, he told me: "The reason I looked for analysis no longer makes me sick, I cannot remember, I just feel the need to continue, without reaching any proper objective; I need myself more".

This piece suggests to me something new to psychic reality, in which the patient talks about an acquired knowledge about himself, from the emotional experience, which is possible in the analytic relationship. To my mind, those are moments of change and openness in which unconscious knowledge manifests itself, while one becomes aware of something in themselves. I feel the urge to bring a debate about healing and the end of analysis, reported by Rezende. It is about a patient who had been analysing for several years, and with a new analyst, he thought he would need an hour and a half in each session. A participant of the debate commented that this fact had led other people to believe that it was the proof that psychoanalysis had neither effect, nor could it heal.

Rezende highlights that analysis time or lifetime under analysis should be considered according to Freud's thinking when he refers to *endless analysis*. From this point of view, the concept of healing must be criticized; "It is not a question of reaching an exhausting end, where the analysis is closed. Healing does not mean putting an end, but checking if we are on the right path" (Rezende and Gerber, 2001, p. 155). Healing consists in continuing to seek – the author proceeds, in tune with Bion's thinking.

While searching for the truth with his/her analysand – which is a movement *from inside out*, the psychoanalyst abandons, on principle, the search for healing according to scientific precepts. He uses the logic of psychoanalysis, which is based on the logic of the unconscious. From the reading and re-reading of patient's and his own narratives, the analyst follows the careful and slow work of considering what comes to mind and dealing with the uncertainties and possibilities that open up to construct new narratives, new senses which create the analysis tissue.

My associations bring me back to Freud and his rigor in defending the legitimacy of the unconscious knowledge, which comes from narratives woven in the loom of the analytic relationship – *the lay knowledge*. That is not a work based on goals, but made on the day-to-day of the analytical experience and one's life. So, it is a work of renouncement and patience that consists of the (artisanal) management of removing from the raw material (the analysand's speech) what was hidden (the unconscious), just as the sculptor removes from the stone block the statue contained within.

In the dialogue maintained with his impartial interlocutor, Freud (1926) uses a similar metaphor to clarify that patient communications, forgotten experiences, and repressed instincts come in the form of raw material. The analyst will have to make up his/her mind to look at the material that the patient provides him/her in a quite especial way. Thereby, having to "extract the precious metal content from the raw ore" and to "be prepared to work over many tons of ore" (p. 219). As Freud points out, when we really practice analysis, we learn a lot of things.

We can relate Freud's metaphor – extract the precious metal content from the raw ore – to Bion's proposal – the analyst works *from inside out* – seeking to discover in his analytical practice the instruments that may be useful for him to think along with the analysand. Asserting that the logic of psychoanalysis is learned in experience (of one's own analysis) does not in any way reduce the scientific quality of psychoanalysis. Its model does not fit to the other sciences, and it is clear that other models cannot be applied to psychoanalysis without distorting its essence. We have our research instrument (the psychic) and we also have the fundamental rule of free association and evenly suspended attention. Analytic work, through transference, produces the knowledge that comes from the unconscious.

This model is foreign to medicine, even to psychology. Of course, psychoanalysis is not medicine, physics, nor psychology. Therefore, it does not reduce itself to the model of other sciences and has its own method. When it comes to the difference between fields and that of logic, Rezende clearly formulates the relation between psychoanalysis and other sciences:

> The presence of the unconscious is a new fact that the other sciences have no way of knowing, except with the help of psychoanalysis. In this sense, I would say that the relationship is reversed: concerning the unconscious, if the sciences have anything to say to psychoanalysis, psychoanalysis has a lot to say to the scientists. For this reason, the sciences cannot provide us with an epistemological model *from the outside in*. Psychoanalysis must discover its own model, in a characteristic experience that allows it to make its own norms clear, from inside out or even from *inside to within*.
>
> (Rezende and Gerber, 2001, p. 13)

In my opinion, what Rezende says strengthens the ideas brought before, not only in the sense of the specificity of psychoanalysis, which makes it different from other knowledge, but also in the sense of reconciling it with other sciences and vice versa (as the author expresses, in a dialogue with scientists, we need to listen, but also to be listened). Again, since psychoanalysis does not reduce itself to the model of other sciences, and seeks its own norms from inside out, from experience, in the meeting between conscious and unconscious, once again the *lay* quality of psychoanalysis becomes evident.

Concerning the theme proposed by Muniz Rezende and Ignácio Gerber – an interface between current psychoanalysis and the new sciences – I will make a brief digression, based on other readings, to talk about what these authors suggest as *a new way of being and thinking about our presence in the world*. This current moment of sciences is characterized by complexity, relativity and the uncertainty principle, according to these authors. Historian Yuval Noah Harari (2014), a doctoral fellow at the University of Oxford and a professor at the Hebrew University of Jerusalem, defined in his bestseller *Sapiens – A Brief History of Humankind*, this time as *the discovery of ignorance* – recalling Voltaire's expression.

Harari states in his book that the scientific revolution has not been a revolution of knowledge but a revolution of ignorance, because the great discovery was that humans do not know the answers to their most important questions. The historian points out the willingness to admit ignorance as a crucial aspect that differentiates modern science from all previous traditional models of knowledge. "We don't know everything [. . .] and the things we think we know could be proven wrong as we gain more knowledge" (Harari, 2014, p. 215).

This strong willingness to accept ignorance opens a path to a dialogue between new sciences and psychoanalysis. We cannot dismiss (in any way) what the sciences and philosophy have to tell us about the human condition, at the risk of psychoanalytic thought becoming old. However, anticipated knowledge can contribute nothing to an analyst training and psychoanalysis practice if truth is on the outside. Psychoanalysis can favor people insofar as it considers themselves in their singularity and recognizes that human experience is conflicted, and so it will be, as long as the individual has id, ego and superego! The analytic experience does not change this condition; it provides the person with the possibility of knowing himself/herself and gives him/her back the responsibility for himself/herself. This is an act of love and freedom, which can only take place from inside out. Learning from one's own experience, says Bion (1962).

From this point, *speaking about* psychoanalysis is not the same as *practicing* psychoanalysis. Bion discusses this aphorism in a fascinating and sincere way in the introduction of *Attention and Interpretation* (1970): "I doubt if anyone but a practising psycho-analyst can understand this book although I have done my best to make it simple" (p. 17). This means that, unlike those who learn psychoanalytic theories, only one who is practicing psychoanalysis can grasp Bion's meaning, because the analyst can experience for himself what Bion can only represent by words from his experience. Theories are useful and necessary, but they do not replace experience.

The analyst depends on non-sensuous experience

Another Bion's contribution, developed by Rezende in his work – and I want to emphasize here – concerns the binocular logic of psychoanalysis. Bion draws attention to the fact that the psychoanalyst cannot dispense with analysis of the conscious. What this tells me is that there is an opening suggested to the analyst to consider both the conscious and the unconscious, as we have several levels of reality. A person can have an idea about himself/herself, which is merged (in the affective experience) with the idea that others say about him/her. This confusion may persist and prevent a person from examining his/her life on another level of reality.

The clinical situation I will reproduce in the next lines suggests to me that we should be alert to talk to the patient in an effort to join the conscious and the unconscious. I think it would be something like putting reason and emotion together. A patient who had had episodes of depression and panic attacks in her youth felt guilty for giving up a bad marriage. For some sessions, she brought back the memories of things she had always heard her parents say about her – that she 'was no good', and now she heard the same from her husband. Her speech had sounded dissonant to me. Although she was a responsible and successful professional, a loving and dedicated mother, and very solicitous with her family and friends, she was convinced that she was not a good person, because she heard this from those she loved and cared for.

At some point, I said that she really seemed to believe everything people told her and if she had already thought about asking herself whether she 'was good' or not. The patient was surprised by the effect her parents' sentence, which was reproduced by her husband, had in her perception throughout her life and how much that conviction kept her imprisoned in a bad marriage.

How do these considerations become a part of the theme of lay analysis, as I understand it? An analyst can only advance in the investigation of the unconscious if he remains in the position of *not knowing*, if he takes into account that the knowledge that interests the analysis is constructed in a temporality and is revealed in the *after*, from experience, creating then a *before* which is already gone. This is the same as saying: one learns from what was already known in one's unconscious.

This perspective allows us to address the divergence between the physician's task and that of the psychoanalyst, according to Bion. In *Attention and Interpretation*, Bion (1970) devotes a chapter to reflect on the model of medicine. The author notes that, although the psychoanalyst, like the physician, also needs to recognize the disease, the physician considers the pain less important than its cure. The clearest point of this divergence, in Bion's words, is that "the physician's *realization* depends on sensuous experience; in contrast with the psychoanalyst who depends on experience that is not sensuous". While the physician "can see and touch and smell", the psychoanalyst "deals with realizations which cannot be seen or touched", because "anxiety has no shape or color, smell or sound" (p. 24).

It is worth recalling Freud's observation in the 1926 text about the training that the doctor receives at the university, "somehow the opposite" of what he would need if he were being prepared for psychoanalysis. "His attention has been directed to objectively ascertainable facts of anatomy, physics and chemistry; on the correct appreciation and suitable influencing of which the success of medical treatment depends" (Freud, 1926, p. 230). As we can see in Freud's observations, medical interest does not turn to psychic phenomena; although the psychiatrist deals with the disorders resulting from these phenomena, he also seeks the physical determinants and the treatment of the symptoms.

In a non-identical but similar way, psychotherapies distance themselves from psychoanalysis when they work to eliminate symptoms, resorting to prior knowledge for the prescription of conduct and technical procedures. The patient receives the 'suggestion medicine' to free himself/herself from conflicts. Of course, I do not question the therapeutic value and effectiveness of the several modalities of the psychological clinic to resolve problems and emotional disorders here. What we question here is the distinction between the field of psychoanalysis and that of psychology. Moreover, the notion that a psychologist, like a doctor, is not prepared to be an analyst, except through a specific training for it.

In the same way, as Freud cautions, there is no reason for an aspiring psychoanalyst to take a detour through medicine or, I add, through psychology. Medical training can alienate a person from the understanding of psychic phenomena – as Freud pointed out, speaking from his own experience as a physician. But the psychologist's training could also stifle the creative potential of the future analyst by establishing epistemological boundaries that permeate him/her with previous knowledge, in detriment of a logic of the unconscious.

On the other hand, the so-called layman (one without a prior medical or psychological training) may not correspond to what is expected of an analytical work. I only want to insist on Freud's position that the analyst should have the personal attributes that make him/her trustworthy to work with the logic of psychoanalysis, and that he/she has acquired the knowledge and experience (in his/her analysis) that enable him/her for the job. The analysis that all psychoanalyst candidates have to undertake when they start training continues to be, in Freud's view, the best means of forming an opinion of their personal aptitude for performing this activity (Freud, 1926).

Is a lay psychoanalyst prepared to deal with severe psychic disorders? In this regard, let us recall Freud's position about diagnosis in the 1926 text. He notes that in the case of some serious mental disorders, only a physician can take responsibility for deciding whether an analytical treatment is feasible or not. To the astonishment of many readers, I suppose, Freud insists that "in every case which is under consideration for analysis, the diagnosis shall be established first by a doctor" who may entrust the treatment to a lay analyst if there is no doubt about the psychogenic nature of the patient's disorder (Freud, 1926, p. 243).

What we see in clinical practice is that a non-doctor psychoanalyst would highly unlikely start the analysis of a severely compromised patient without psychiatric backup. The decision is even recommended for doctor analysts, since the place occupied by the psychoanalyst should not be confused with positions taken by the physician, even if they are the same people. A doctor psychoanalyst should not medicate his/her patient. It is an ethical position that requires the neutrality of the analyst. While he/she answers to the demand for healing, he/she is identified with the 'knowing position' where he/she is placed by the patient, and is conformed to another ethics, one that seeks the triumph over the symptoms or the psychosocial rehabilitation of madness (Balbi et al., 2009).

Deviations committed by lay people in psychoanalytic practice – yes, they also occur! – should not serve, by themselves, as a justification against the independence of psychoanalysis in relation to medicine and psychology; doctor and psychologist analysts are not free to distance themselves from the analytical position expected from these professionals.

The preparation of the analyst

One can understand why the training of the analyst has always occupied a prominent position in the work of several authors and in the internal debates of psychoanalytic institutions. Established almost a century ago and based on the tripod of personal analysis, theoretical and technical teaching and supervised clinical practice, the training model of the International Psychoanalytical Association (IPA) persists. However, the duration of the training has increased since the first recommendations made by the IPA. At that time, they advised two years of theoretical studies and training analysis, besides supervised practice. More precise training criteria had been discussed successively at the IPA congresses. In most affiliated institutions, regulations that have been in place remain valid for more than 50 years.

Since the beginning of the IPA training committees, they have decided that the rules for the selection of lay candidates would be the responsibility of each committee. Among the deliberations around the Eitingon model, they already stipulated that lay analysts ought to go through studies and experience inside psychiatric clinic. This criterion has been maintained since then by institutions that accept non-doctors and non-psychologists for training.

In this sense, the experience of the Sociedade de Psicanálise de Brasilia has been successful: for about 20 years, our training institute has had an agreement with a mental health clinic to train professionals from other areas selected for psychoanalytic training. In the first year of the training, candidates undergo a rich experience of learning and interaction with psychiatric patients in therapeutic activities, as well as participation in multidisciplinary clinical team meetings, supervisions and study groups on psychopathology topics. Having started my psychoanalytic training as a layperson, I am grateful to have been a pioneer in this local experience, which has given me daily contact with the mental functioning of severely disturbed patients. I have been able to accomplish what Bion names *learning from experience*.

More than the acquisition of certain knowledge and the familiarity with clinical states of psychiatry, the analyst's preparation depends on a certain sensitivity to what is unconscious and repressed (Freud, 1910, 1926). Moreover, the aspiring analyst is expected to have an aesthetic experience before undertaking the analytic training, as Bion (1974) recommends. Almost half a century later, his observation remains valid: our methods of mental investigation do not fit precisely to any discipline known to date.

He asserts; "It may be argued that this method is subjective, not scientific, but I know no better" (p. 94).

In order to enhance our discussion, it is worth mentioning Freud's proposal in the 1926 text for an educational program for the psychoanalyst, which is *yet to be created*: it should include the humanities, psychology, history of civilization, mythology, sociology, psychology of religion, literature, anatomy, biology and the history of evolution. Of course, this is an ideal proposition, Freud said; psychoanalytical faculties do not exist. Adding to the Freudian proposition, Bion (1974) suggests that the analyst should be, in his/her private practice, like a poet, an artist, a person of science or a theologian. Thereby he/she would be able to make an interpretation or a construction.

The State regulation as a thorn in the flesh of psychoanalysts

Psychoanalysis is not tuned to any model of teaching proposed by the university, in spite of the rich dialogue maintained between both. In 1918, at the V International Psychoanalytic Congress in Budapest, Freud (1919) defended the teaching of his doctrine in medical school, so that future physicians could learn about the relations between the mental world and the physical world.

In the academic context, the teaching of psychoanalysis can only be taught through theoretical lessons, which is valid for the scientific knowledge, but it does not add to the construction of the analyst who depends on his/her own experience of analysis. How is it possible to delegate to the university the personal analysis of the student, with high frequency of analytical sessions and their long duration? How do we guarantee a supervised clinical experience in the university context, years on end? The university cannot afford the instruments required for this.

Since psychoanalysis cannot be taught, it can only be transmitted, what makes the analyst and what authorizes him/her to practice in a clinic is not an academic curriculum but the contact with the unconscious, provided by the work of the transference in relation to the other who transmits psychoanalysis. Therefore, let us remember, there is no justification for the future analyst to be first submitted to the study of medicine or psychology. Freud had defended that psychoanalysis should remain lay, free of medical power and independent from the university. If the analyst has to deprive himself/herself of a position of power to maintain his/her freedom, this means that his/her logic is distinct from that logic of a field of power constituted of rules and prohibitions – like parallel lines which intersect in infinity.

This conflict of interests refers to the problem of the regulation of psychoanalysis by the State. I often say that the State regulation is a thorn in the flesh of the Brazilian psychoanalysts (Carneiro, 2012, 2013). In the last 50 years, not fewer than ten bills have mobilized Brazilian psychoanalytic community to react in order to prevent the State regulation of the psychoanalytic practice. These legislative actions have been encouraged by groups that had no commitment to the Freudian legacy and have been defended the interests of religious organizations or even corporations of psychotherapists.

One of the proposals that have been insinuated is the inclusion of psychoanalysis in the field of psychotherapies. These attempts led representatives of 65 psychoanalytic institutions to subscribe in 2001 to the 'Manifesto of Brazilian Entities of Psychoanalysis', with the support of ten non-psychoanalytic institutions, in the defense of the historical position of the international psychoanalytic movement (Amendoeira, 2009).

Self-regulation, intended by some groups of psychotherapists, is also inopportune because it seeks to include psychoanalysis in the wide list of the 'psy' universe. In her book *The Patient, the Therapist and the State*, Roudinesco (2005) reminds us that more than 700 psychotherapy schools have emerged in the world since 1950 in response to society's overwhelming demand for psychic care. Nothing more harmful to psychoanalysis and its survival than to include it in the same list of therapeutic practices, which have no relation to the psychoanalytic ethics.

The submission to the rules established by the State and the institutional control are incompatible with the essence of psychoanalysis. As an activity, it does not contain a registered specialist title in a professional council, which authorizes the psychoanalyst to practice it. The father of psychoanalysis wanted to protect it from State, religious, medical and academic domains. Because psychoanalysis is excluded from universities and sheltered in specific institutions, it has been maintaining its lay organization (Freud, 1919, 1928).

The debate in favor of the 'lay analysis' has divided the international psychoanalytic movement throughout its history. The clashes within psychoanalytic institutions, notably among Americans who reacted vigorously against lay analysis, aimed at the figure of the 'impostor'. Since Theodor Reik, several were accused of charlatanism for representing the heterogeneous, the strange, the *other* of the science and the reason, who escapes from the norms fixed by a power that is claimed to be hegemonic (Mijolla, 2005; Roudinesco, 2005).

In the middle of a clash between Brazilian psychiatry and psychoanalysis in the 1950s, Virgínia Bicudo was accused of charlatanism – and suffered severe attacks by medical professionals – for challenging a group who did not want to lose its hegemony, at a moment when the psychoanalytic movement in São Paulo had been gaining autonomy and independence from medicine (Abrão, 2010). Certainly, Virginia's leadership, her fearless and stubborn personality as well as her prominent position in the media made her a timely but not fragile target for the attacks. Virgínia never surrendered to criticism and obtained the respect of the scientific community in Brazil, as Abrão recalls in the biography dedicated to that psychoanalyst.

The analyst emerges from the *opening* to the unconscious

By including professionals from other areas, the psychoanalytic institution grows because of the diversity of knowledge. Without the preconceptions of the knowledge produced in courses of medicine and psychology, which can affect the analytical work, the 'lay' analyst brings with him/her the freedom to think based on his/her vertices. Perhaps, also a greater possibility of openness to the logic of the unconscious. Not wanting to generalize, what we notice in a psychologist's training is some rationalization of emotions, a kind of shield for the therapist's emotional experience, to the point of disqualifying the unconscious.

I resort to our best example of freedom in the psychoanalytic thinking and practice. Virgínia had an open mind. She was firm, sustained by the faith in the openness of psychoanalysis and in what this practice could offer to the person and to the community. A revolutionary mind which turned back on dogmas and the institutional superego, which usually restricts the candidate with theorizations, endangering the creativity and the freedom of the future analyst.

The following testimonies of two training and supervising analysts of the Sociedade de Psicanálise de Brasília add to our conviction that there is no analysis that is not lay. When he decided to 'give up' his job as a physician in the 1970s, the psychoanalyst Carlos de Almeida Vieira told his analyst Virgínia Bicudo, on her coach, that the analysis was giving him a chance to 'take off his white coat' and give up medicine. He remembers that this 'transgression' gave him a labyrinthitis for four months. From the confusion and the anguish of being non-institutionalized, the analyst inserts himself/herself in the exercise of psychoanalysis. Another testimony given to the author of this text revives our proposition: before starting the analytic training, the psychoanalyst Fátima Rebouças Malva had been feeling dissatisfied with her psychology course. Her outlook changed when she read Freud's first book. In an interview given to this author, Malva said that it was like a telescope that opened her vision to contemplate the universe; a path had been opened towards infinity.

In his book with Antonio Muniz de Rezende, the psychoanalyst Ignácio Gerber, of the Sociedade de Psicanálise de São Paulo, tells us how he began his psychoanalytic training. As an engineer, he believed that his earlier profession could get into the way of his training in psychoanalysis. Thus, he reports: "I soon realized that my previous engineering practice had everything to do with my current practice of psychoanalysis. In both, there is the search for an integrative sense from dispersed stimuli: a solution, a selected fact. There is also the music, something that I have always had present throughout my life" (Rezende and Gerber, 2001, p. 253).

Gerber discusses in this book the relation between Bion's ideas and the psychoanalytic formulations from mathematical concepts by the Chilean Matte-Blanco. Gerber developed an in-depth study of Matte-Blanco's work and his papers are recognized in Brazil and abroad. For that, he used his experience with engineering and music. He claims that the practice of engineering has brought him a comprehensive thinking, and he has drawn from physics and mathematics the ability to transcend rational understanding and develop psychoanalytic thinking, feeling and working.

My psychoanalytic training was preceded by 15 years of a journalistic career, most of this period devoted to political coverage. This experience has given me growing interest in issues such as power, ethics and personal motivations, truth and lies, and the politicians' internal relations with the public and the private. These questions lead a journalist to an undesirable and inevitable coexistence with the perverse face of the political world.

I left journalism and started my training as a psychoanalyst, during which I decided to study psychology, even though I was advised against it by some psychoanalysts from my Institute. Although I had already known that psychology should not help me to become a psychoanalyst, I graduated in that course. What I was looking for in psychology was the same I could seek in philosophy – an investigation about the human experience and the different approaches of the psychological thinking. Psychology has been useful for me to understand what psychoanalysis is not.

References

Abrão, J.L.F. (2010). *Virgínia Bicudo: a trajetória de uma psicanalista brasileira* [Virgínia Bicudo: The trajectory of a Brazilian psychoanalyst]. São Paulo: Ed. Arte & Ciência.

Alves, A.L., and Saad, L.A.-C. (2009). A psicanálise é leiga [The psychoanalysis is lay]. In: S. Alberti, W. Amendoeira, E. Lannes, A. Lopes, and E. Rocha (Orgs.), *Ofício do psicanalista: formação versus regulamentação*. São Paulo: Casa do Psicólogo.

Amendoeira, W. (2009). A articulação das entidades psicanalíticas brasileiras [The articulation of Brazilian psychoanalytical entities]. In: S. Alberti, W. Amendoeira, E. Lannes, A. Lopes, and E. Rocha (Orgs.), *Ofício do psicanalista: formação versus regulamentação*. São Paulo: Casa do Psicólogo.

Balbi, L., Lessa, M., and Becker, P. (2009). A psicanálise é leiga: da formação do psicanalista [The psychoanalysis is lay: about the psychoanalyst's training]. In: S. Alberti, W. Amendoeira, E. Lannes, A. Lopes and E. Rocha (Orgs.), *Ofício do psicanalista: formação versus regulamentação*. São Paulo: Casa do Psicólogo.

Bion, W. (1962). *Aprendiendo de la experiencia* [Learning from experience]. Trad. H.B. Fernández. Buenos Aires: Paidós, 1980.

Bion, W. (1970). *Atenção e Interpretação* [Attention and interpretation]. Trad. P.C. Sandler. Rio de Janeiro: Imago, 2006.

Bion, W. (1974). *Seminários de Psicoanálisis* [Bion's Brazilian lectures]. Trad. S.B. Abreu. Buenos Aires: Paidós, 1978.

Carneiro, C.A. (2012). A psicanálise e seus espinhos [Psychoanalysis and its thorns]. *Correio Braziliense*, May 28, Brasília: Opinião, p. 11.

Carneiro, C.A. (2013). A prática da psicanálise [The Practice of the Psychoanalysis]. *Psique Ciência & Vida*, March, 7(87): 72–78.

Castro, R.M.O. (2010). Virgínia Leone Bicudo: Pioneirismo e criatividade [Virgínia Leone Bicudo: pioneering and creativity]. *Alter Revista de Estudos Psicanalíticos*, 28(1): 29–34.

Chasseguet-Smirgel, J., Letarde, P., and Bourgeron, J.P. (1969). Notas sobre a questão dos psicanalistas não-médicos [Notes about the question of non-doctor psychoanalysts]. *Arq. Bras. Psic. Apl*, 21(4): 9–100.

Freud, S. (1910). Sobre psicanálise "selvagem" ['Wild' Psychoanalysis]. In: S. Freud (Ed.), *Obras completas, Volume 9* (pp. 324–333). Trad. P.C. Souza. São Paulo: Companhia das Letras, 2013.

Freud, S. (1919). Deve-se ensinar a psicanálise nas universidades? [On the teaching of psychoanalysis in universities]. In: S. Freud (Ed.), *Obras completas, Volume 14* (pp. 377–381). Trad. P C. Souza. São Paulo: Companhia das Letras, 2010.

Freud, S. (1926). The Question of Lay Analysis. *SE*, 20: 179–258. London: Hogarth Press, 1959.

Freud, S. (1928). *Correspondance de Sigmund Freud avec le pasteur Pfister (1909–39)* [Correspondence of Sigmund Freud with pastor Pfister (1909–39)]. Paris: Gallimard, 1966.

Harari, Y.N. (2014). *Sapiens: A Brief History of Humankind*. Canada: Signal Books, Penguin Random House.

Mijolla, A. de (Org.). (2005). *Dicionário internacional de psicanálise: conceitos, noções, biografias, obras, eventos, instituições* [International dictionary of psychoanalysis: concepts, notions, biographies, works, events, institutions]. Trad. A. Cabral. Rio de Janeiro: Imago.

Nascentes, A. (1955). *Dicionário etimológico da língua portuguesa* [Etymology dictionary of the Portuguese language]. Rio de Janeiro: Livraria Acadêmica, Livraria São José, Livraria Francisco Alves, Livros de Portugal.

Rezende, A.M., and Gerber, I. (2001). *A psicanálise "atual" na interface das "novas" ciências. O método psicanalítico e suas* aplicações [The 'current' psychoanalysis at the interface of the 'new' sciences]. São Paulo: Via Lettera.

Roudinesco, E. (2005). *O paciente, o terapeuta e o Estado* [The patient, the therapist and the State]. Trad. A. Telles. Rio de Janeiro: Jorge Zahar.

Roudinesco, E., and Plon, M. (1998). *Dicionário de psicanálise* [Dictionary of psychoanalysis]. Trads. V. Ribeiro, L. Magalhães. Rio de Janeiro: Jorge Zahar.

11

From the obvious to the unbridgeable

Avner Bergstein

Bion (1970) writes:

> Most people think of psycho-analysis, as Freud did, as a method of treatment for a complaint. The complaint was regarded as similar to a physical ailment which, when you know what it is, has to be treated in accordance with the rules of medicine. The parallel with medicine was, and still is, useful. But as psycho-analysis has grown so it has been seen to differ from physical medicine until the gap between them has passed *from the obvious to the unbridgeable.*
>
> (p. 6, italics added)

However, this gap seems to have already been discerned by Freud, whose passionate campaign in support of lay analysis was in fact a struggle for the very crux of psychoanalysis. Freud's struggle was in fact a decisive statement on the distinct essence of psychoanalysis encountering, alongside material reality, a non-sensuous, immaterial psychic realm and an ineffable truth. It was an implicit claim to relinquish the supremacy of the realm of the positive, knowable reality in favour of the unknown and unknowable. Hence, it is of no wonder that it aroused such tenacious resistance which is in fact resistance to psychoanalysis itself, even though its strongest opposition was from his fellow psychoanalysts. As Bion writes: "Any formulation felt to approximate to illumination of O is certain to produce an institutionalizing reaction" (1970, p. 81), with O denoting unknowable, ultimate reality threatening to disrupt psychic equilibrium and evoke change felt as catastrophic.

This institutionalizing reaction seems to have been a further repercussion to Freud's intervention into the society, which as Bion (1967a) said, created a serious upset. Freud must have felt he was in a position where either society was going to squeeze the life out of psychoanalysis, or else psychoanalysis was going to disrupt the conventions of society.

Many of Freud's arguments did in fact revolve more around practical issues than essential, intrinsic ones. Many of them referred to the study of medicine being unnecessary in becoming a psychoanalyst, a "roundabout road" (1926, p. 247), "an arduous and circuitous way" (1927, p. 252) or due to the prospective analyst's "impoverished material circumstances" (1927, p. 254). Freud was more cautious in asserting that medical studies were considerably inappropriate for the practice of psychoanalysis, or a possible handicap endorsing an unfit mode of observation which will have to be unlearnt in the course of becoming an analyst.

Even so, Freud does write that "the doctors [practicing psychoanalysis] have not exactly the qualities which one has a right to expect of doctors" (1926, p. 184). Further on he indicates that

> in his medical school a doctor receives a training which is more or less the opposite of what he would need as a preparation for psycho-analysis. His attention has been directed to objectively ascertainable facts of anatomy, physics and chemistry, on the correct appreciation and suitable influencing of which the success of medical treatment depends. The problem of life is brought into his field of vision so far as it has hitherto been explained to us by the play of forces which can also be observed in inanimate nature. His interest is not aroused in the mental side of vital phenomena.
>
> (1926, p. 230)

Bion (1970) elaborates on this:

> In physical medicine the patient may have a pain in his chest for which he can go to his doctor. To him he can explain its

> nature and its history and from him he can receive instructions to undergo further examination, say, by X-rays or microscopy, or certain forms of treatment. . . . [L]ater we may have reason to question this account. For the present it will serve to point the divergence of physical medicine and psycho-analysis. Suppose the patient complained not of physical but of mental pain; no one doubts the existence of anxiety or sees any incongruity in seeking help to cure it. We find it necessary to differentiate between the pain of a broken leg and the pain, say, of bereavement; sometimes we prefer not to, but exchange mental for physical pain and vice versa. . . . *The point that demonstrates the divergence most clearly is that the physician is dependent on realization of sensuous experience in contrast with the psycho-analyst whose dependence is on experience that is not sensuous*. The physician can see and touch and smell. The realizations with which a psycho-analyst deals cannot be seen or touched; anxiety has no shape or colour, smell or sound. For convenience, I propose to use the term 'intuit' as a parallel in the psychoanalyst's domain to the physician's use of 'see', 'touch', 'smell', and 'hear'.
>
> (pp. 6–7, italics added)

I would like to focus on Bion's radical writings beginning at the end of the 1950s and reaching their climax in the late 1960s and 1970s, where he seems to state more clearly and openly Freud's intuitive apprehensions concerning the 'over-positivation' of psychoanalysis. It was only when psychoanalysis had found its respected place in Western culture, institutionalized one might say, that these radical ideas could, and needed to, be revived and further elaborated. In fact, Bion's writings may reflect a developmental stage in the evolution of psychoanalysis. It is when the establishment begins to calcify and its borders begin to solidify, that a need arises for new propositions corresponding to the new clinical experiences. Exploration of Bion's thinking, deriving from these clinical experiences with patients whose thinking and dreaming capacities are defected, may shed light on psychic realms which Freud may have intuited but did not pursue. However, it was his foreknowledge of these dimensions that aroused him to react so vehemently in regard to the possibility of leaving analysis solely in the hands of medicine.

A non-sensuous realm

Freud described two forms of the same existence of reality – psychic reality and material reality (Sandler, 2005). Bion elaborated the notion of these two aspects of reality and wrote of 'reality sensuous *and* psychic'. It is not one or the other, and one is not superior to the other. Bion stresses the need for *binocular* vision on the part of the analyst. I would stress the need for a *'multi-ocular'* vision, since the psychic reality of a session has an *infinite* number of facets, which can be 'observed' from an infinite number of vertices. Psychic reality can thus be approached through the constant movement between the various vertices, for example, that which is perceived through the familiar senses and that which is intuited, even though they may be contradictory. This is illustrated by Bion (1979) with Segal's clinical description of the man who says he cannot play the violin because he won't masturbate in public. Could it be, Bion asks, that this man was 'seeing' something that most of us are prevented from seeing because we are too tied up to sensuous reality? Why do we take it for granted, Bion adds, that a person is really playing the violin and that this view is the only correct one? Psychic reality is infinitely more complex. Can we tolerate the paradoxical reality in which the man is playing the violin *and* masturbating in public?

While sensuous reality is perceived through the five basic senses, psychic reality is *intuited*. Intuition is an unmediated knowledge or understanding of truth, not supported by any information derived from a familiar sensual source. Since it cannot be communicated to another and cannot be corroborated by a rational method of scientific knowledge, it is often seen as close to mystical revelation (de Bianchedi, 1991). Hence, for example, the analyst 'sees' an internal world, inhabited by internal objects, and has no doubt of their existence, even though he has no sensuous evidence for it.

The intuition of a non-sensuous realm appears throughout Freud's writings beginning with the very fact that the free associations are connected to each other with *apparently* invisible, unconscious threads which are sensuously non-existent. It is realized pre-eminently in the creation of an analytic setting negativizing perception as an indispensable means of approaching the psyche (Botella and Botella, 2005). And what appears in the space that is generated, is not only that which was repressed or the return of something that was once represented in the mind, but rather an encounter with the *irrepresentable*.

Winnicott (1969) writes of the 'non-event'. He 'hears' the scream which the patient is always not experiencing. The great non-event of the session is the screaming that the patient does not scream. This seems to be an illustration of Winnicott's intuition of the negative as described by Green (1997), who himself wrote widely of the negative, emphasizing that he does not use the word absence, because in the word absence there is the hope of a return of the presence. It is also not a loss because this would mean that the loss could be mourned. The reference to the negative is to the sensuously non-existence, the void. Winnicott's contribution, according to Green, is to show how this negative, the non-existence, will become at some point, the only thing that is real. This might be the sensuously undetectable *invariance*, the innermost essence that the analyst must be able to intuit.

Bion (1974) illustrates this further by describing the observation of a game of tennis, looking at it with increasing darkness, while dimming the intellectual illumination and light. First, we lose sight of the players, and then we gradually increase the darkness until only the net itself is visible. If we can do this, it is possible to see that the only important thing visible to us is a lot of holes which are collected together in a net.

Botella and Botella (2005) speak of the negative of the trauma which has its origin not in a quantifiable positive, but in the absence of what, for the child's ego, should have occurred as a matter of course. Something fundamentally evident for the subject that should have happened did not happen, even though he is not aware of it, let alone form an idea of what this negative is. These authors, too, argue that the negative of the infantile trauma is not a product of the abolition of a representation, but the consequence of a lack at the outset, a missing inscription, at any rate in the form of a representation.

All these lead up to Sandler's (2011) conceptualization of the realm of Minus,

> a non-concrete, immaterial realm that complements the positive 'senseable' realm of the material reality . . . [T]he realm of Minus cannot be equated to denial; It contemplates the possibilities of

> impossibility and its propositional content cannot be seen on the same level . . . as the 'Plus realm', what is affirmative; in other words, what occupies a position in space-time. Therefore, since it indicates 'what is not' . . . it cannot have the properties assigned to what would be the opposite of 'what is'. It is ineffable.
>
> (pp. 13–14)

An uncharted mental life

Bion (1977) describes an unconscious mental state that has never been anything else, has never been conscious. He suggests that in addition to unconscious and conscious states of mind there may be another state of mind, one that might provisionally be called an *inaccessible* state of mind. Bion tries to address this inaccessible part that has remained as a meaningless franticness in the psyche. He thus tries to approach "a mental life unmapped by theories elaborated for the understanding of neurosis" (Bion, 1962, p. 37).

I suggest that this unmapped mental life is to a large extent congruent with an *unrepressed* unconscious, a term never used by Bion himself, but only elaborated by those inspired by him. Bion (1962) seems to refer to this unmapped mental life primarily when describing the so-called psychotic part of the personality. Yet I would like to emphasize that Bion distinguishes between being *psychotic* and being *insane*. The psychotic part of the personality is a part of being human. About himself, he is said to have claimed that he may be psychotic, but not insane (Mason, 2000).

To my mind, the notion of the psychotic part of the personality was elaborated by Bion differently from Klein's depiction, and even differently than was initially described by Bion himself in his earlier, so-called schizophrenia papers. I suggest that in addition to describing a part of the personality where thought is fragmented as a result of destructive attacks on the mind, Bion is referring to what would probably be conceived of today as a primal, pre-natal, unborn mental state, perhaps akin to an autistic part of the personality, as was in fact delineated by clinicians and authors inspired by Bion such as Donald Meltzer and Frances Tustin (Bergstein, 2018).

Thus, what was initially referred to as 'psychotic', is later elaborated by Bion to contain undreamt and undreamable, primordial, emotional experiences. This, in its turn, will be further elaborated by Bion to encompass its counterpart in an unknowable, ineffable psychic reality which must be borne by the individual and which comprises the essence of psychic life. These may in fact be two sides of the same coin, where on the one hand we are faced with undreamable things-in-themselves due to an impaired or deficient capacity for 'dreaming' and on the other is the irreducible, invariant, unknowable ultimate reality of the session which can only be intuited. The analyst must sharpen his skills so as to be in contact with both.

Much like Melanie Klein's investigations into the minds of young children, delving into the psychotic mind has led Bion too, to hone the psychoanalytical tools required for the apprehension of psychic reality. It has capacitated the exploration of a non-sensuous psychic realm as well as of the state of mind required of the analyst in order to approach it. These explorations help to appreciate that which lies at the foundation of Freud's plea in favour of lay analysis: the distinct nature of psychoanalysis which strives to get in touch with this undreamt and undreamable psychic reality, which is the marrow of the so called psychotic part of the personality as well as of the *unrepressed* unconscious. However, in order to substantiate this notion, it may be necessary to briefly rehearse Bion's contribution to the understanding of the psychotic part of the personality.

Bion describes an inchoate layer of psychic functioning, undeveloped and lacking crucial mental capacities. It is a part of the personality where thought is severely disordered and the capacity for mental transformation is deficient, hence experience remains non-mental, as an overwhelming frenzy of stimuli inside the mind and body. Yet, it may also be the result of an internal attack on these mental capacities as a way to avoid pain.

Unfolding his theory of functions, Bion describes an alpha-function, or 'dreaming', as unconscious emotional thinking required to transform the primordial emotional experience, perceived as sense impressions from within and from without, into something that can be thought, known, felt, suffered, and ultimately – repressed. Bion is referring to patients in whom the capacity for alpha-function is deficient; hence they cannot dream or think and so cannot repress. They are thus rendered in a psychotic state of being, overwhelmed by undigested and indigestible sense impressions he calls beta-elements. To paraphrase Freud's (1915) depiction of the instincts, one might say that beta-elements can never become an object of consciousness – only the idea that represents the beta-element can. Even in the (repressed) unconscious, moreover, a beta-element cannot be represented otherwise than by an idea. If the beta-element did not attach itself to an idea or manifest itself as an affective state, we could know nothing about it. Lacking a capacity for alpha-function, these beta-elements cannot be worked upon and tranformed, hence they carry almost no symbolic meaning. Alpha-function, or 'dreaming', is thus equivalent to the mind's capacity to deal with the emotional experience and to bear its turbulent implications on the personality. Much like "the instincts in the id press for immediate satisfaction at all costs, and in that way they achieve nothing or even bring about appreciable damage" (Freud, 1926, p. 201), so do beta-elements, when accrued, press for evacuation. An inability to dream the emotional experience renders the personality in an intolerable emotional storm that has to be acted out and evacuated through projective identification, somatic disorders, addictions, perversions, etc. The personality is thus under the sway of the so-called psychotic part of the personality, entailing an intolerance of the live, unpredictable, and uncontrollable aspects of the object.

As a model, Bion (1962) suggests that when the emotions aroused are too strong or intolerable for the infant, and so cannot be worked upon mentally, it may withdraw from the nourishing breast so as to avoid the complications inherent in the awareness of life and of live objects. However, hunger and fear of death through starvation force the infant to resume feeding. The infant is thus compelled to split the material milk from the psychical breast, so that it can resume feeding with no need to acknowledge its emotions in the face of the animate, feeding object. The need for love, understanding and mental development is now deflected into the search for material satisfaction. This is a state originating in a need to be rid of the emotional complications inherent in life and to deaden emotion. Hence, the individual lives in an omniscient world of allegedly predictable, emotionless, inanimate objects, much like the use a child with autism makes of autistic objects. This is a delusional world dominated by causal thinking which is not suited for a live, animate, often capricious, emotional world where almost nothing is predictable.

The personality's inability to dream and become emotionally engaged thus creates a state of mind that is one-dimensional and "substantially mindless, consisting of events not available for memory and thought" (Meltzer, 1975, p. 225). It is a world furnished with inanimate objects and a frenzy of beta-elements. It is a primal area of the mind of things-in-themselves, which are beyond our capacity to know or to verbalize except through their phenomenological derivatives.

Since beta-elements do often accumulate, they may appear indistinguishable from a confused state resembling a dream, or a dreamable narrative, deluding the analyst who adheres to a positivistic, (pseudo)scientific outlook, seeking order where disorder reigns. This may be illustrated pictorially if one imagines a mass of flies that may seem from afar as a black curtain, but with the wave of one's hand they are scattered, leaving no trace. This is different from a dream made up of alpha-elements which connect to each other through a network of associations, thus forming a "curtain of illusion" (Bion, 1965, p. 147), a narrative that can be communicated, stored in the mind and made use of as a transitional object.

Even though a patient may seem to be talking and free associating, when unable to dream his words do not cohere and do not evoke an integrated emotional response other than perhaps feelings of confusion, irritation, impotence or boredom. This in its turn may evoke an emotional response from the analyst who may become critical, or even praiseful, thereby colluding with, or perhaps one should say *reflecting*, the psychotic part of the personality assuming moral superiority and omniscience. The patient evacuates masses of words with which the analyst may try futilely to connect and find meaning to, thereby missing the fact that the patient cannot think or dream. Rather, the patient is discharging verbally an excess of tension or distress that has been harboured within him as a result of not being able to do anything mental with them. This requires *the analyst* to 'observe' and 'dream', through the exercise of analytically trained intuition, an emotional experience which is unobservable or undreamable by the patient. This often amounts to suffering long periods of painful distress, helplessness, despair, persecution, not knowing where we are headed to or what we are actually doing. It seems to me that this is a vital part of what Bion means by the notion of 'dreaming the patient'.

The analyst may often be tempted to work at a more symbolic, insight-giving level, assuming higher psychic and mental integration. However, interpretations focusing on conflicting desires, or linking repressed and displaced parts of the personality with the defences against them, or interpretations adding alternative symbolic meanings, do not reach these patients in whom alpha-function is predominantly disturbed and inoperative, in a way that facilitates psychic change (Alvarez, 2010; Bergstein, 2016).

Bion emphasizes the hazards of treating the non-symbolic, undreamt, psychotic part of the personality as non-psychotic. Moreover, in its attempt to protect the personality from psychic pain, the psychotic part of the mind is always stimulating the analyst's memory (past) and desire (future), misleading him to think in a linear, positivistic way. It thus serves as a barrier to encountering, and bearing, the infinite and jarring complexity of the emotional experience. Analysis may then go on indefinitely with the patient alledgedly knowing more and more *about* himself but with very little psychic transformation towards *becoming* who he is.

As mentioned, inasmuch as beta-elements cannot be mentally elaborated and transformed into alpha-elements and dream thoughts, they cannot in effect be repressed. It is not possible to repress something that has not yet been represented through some mental process. The capacity to repress thus seems to be a psychological accomplishment. When deficient, the individual is confronted with experience which is unconscious *but not repressed,* often experienced as psychotic franticness.

An unrepressed unconscious

The unrepressed unconscious has been hinted in Freud's writings. At the beginning of *The Unconscious* Freud writes: "Everything that is repressed must remain unconscious; but let us state at the very outset that the repressed does not cover everything that is unconscious. The unconscious has the wider compass: the repressed is *a part* of the unconscious" (1915, p. 166, italics added). Freud will further elaborate this notion only slightly in *The Ego and the Id* and say that

> we recognize that the *Ucs.* does not coincide with the repressed; it is still true that all that is repressed is *Ucs.*, but not all that

> is *Ucs.* is repressed. A part of the ego, too – and Heaven knows how important a part . . . undoubtedly is *Ucs.* And this *Ucs* . . . is not latent like the *Pcs.* . . . [W]e find ourselves thus confronted by the necessity of postulating a third *Ucs.*, which is not repressed[1] . . . Pathological research has directed our interest too exclusively to the repressed.
>
> (1923, pp. 18–19, italics in the original)

At the beginning of his writing, describing the anxiety disorder, Freud (1895) was aware that the anxiety does not derive from a repressed conflict but rather from primal, almost biological experiences. It seems that we can already find here the buds of the notion of an unrepressed unconscious, and yet, at this phase of his thinking, Freud had left that which was not repressed outside the realm of psychoanalysis. He writes: "the affect does not originate in a repressed idea, but turns out to be *not further reducible by psychological analysis, nor amenable to psychotherapy*" (1895, p. 97, italics in the original). However, the anxiety disorder seems to have continued to occupy his mind. He wrote quite a bit about it and seems to have had the intuition that it would *not* be possible to place it outside the realm of psychoanalysis. Without formulating it in so many words, it seems he may have laid the foundation for a differentiation between neurosis originating in the repressed unconscious and a state originating in an *un*repressed unconscious. In a letter to Fliess he writes: "in hysteria it is *psychical* excitation that takes a wrong path exclusively into the somatic field, whereas here [anxiety neurosis] it is a *physical* tension, which cannot enter the psychical field and therefore remains on the physical path" (1894, p. 195, italics in the original). He goes on to suggest that anxiety disorder is related to an accumulation of excitation and one cannot find traces leading to a psychical conflict. Freud seems to suggest that in the absence of an appropriate mental capacity, the somatic excitation (beta-elements?) could not be transformed into the psychical sphere and remained as intolerable excess. It has remained in the somatic field and not entered the psychical field. Hence, as Bion (1970) suggests, the patient *feels* the pain but will not mentally *suffer* it.

The painful situation then, seems to be an excess of excitation, unable to be transformed even in the form of a neurotic symptom. The individual remains as a 'slave of quantity' (de M'Uzan, 2003) condemned to the dominance of quantities of excitation he cannot monitor or elaborate mentally. The individual is left in extreme helplessness, perturbation, agitation and confusion which can only acquire meaning *in retrospect* through the mind of an analyst able to suffer these emotional experiences (Bergstein, 2014).

Beyond the spectrum

In his discussion of *The Question of Lay Analysis*, although acknowledging the notion that "neuroses and psychoses are evidently intimately related" (p. 204), Freud does seem to remain largely in the sphere of the transference neuroses and of the non-psychotic part of the personality. He is primarily engaged in explaining the origin of neurosis due to "the circumstance that the ego has made use of the inefficient instrument of repression for dealing with the conflict [between the ego and the id]" (ibid.).

Bion's elaboration of Freud's thinking, as well as his own radical propositions, seem to have once more threatened to disrupt the institutionalized psychoanalytical establishment – this time not with regard to who should practice psychoanalysis, but rather as to what patients could or could not be analyzed. Bion demonstrated the possibility of working analytically with psychotic patients and with the psychotic parts of the personality. He illustrated the prospect of listening analytically to the communicative potential in those parts of the personality that seemingly attacked and rejected communication (Bergstein, 2015).

Bion (1967c) makes use of the spectrum of the electromagnetic waves as an analogy for emphasizing the limits of our sensory apparatus which receives only a small part of the spectrum. The wavelengths visible to us fall in a narrow strip of visual perception in between the infrared on the one end and the ultraviolet on the other. We cannot see the ones that fall off these ends, but they are nevertheless there. Using that as an analogy, Bion suggests that thanks to verbal capacity, there is a certain realm of mental life, which we can speak of in terms like personality, mind and so forth. This is the small part of the spectrum, in which one could talk about it as being verbally communicable. However, the psychoanalytic encounter compels us to observe and meet those areas of the mind that lie beyond that narrow sphere. We see a patient who seems an ordinary neurotic patient, Bion says, but as the analysis goes on, he seems to have what one might call a psychotic breakdown. "The illness may have an innocent appearance for a considerable time, till in the end it after all displays its evil character" (Freud, 1926, p. 240). Alternatively, the analysis takes a turn in that what we are accustomed to regard as psychotic elements, become much more visible. "Can we make some corresponding extension of our . . . mental capacity, to take in a little bit more of . . . the invisible aspects of the spectrum?" (Bion, 1967c, p. 60).

Bion is thus steering us towards an ineffable, irrepresentable part of the mind, the unknowable navel of the dream, the noumena beyond the phenomena. This is an ineffable psychic reality which cannot be represented; it is only its phenomenological counterparts that can appear in dreams, slips of the tongue, symptoms and so on and brought into consciousness by interpretation.

Perceiving this psychic realm requires a different kind of skill from the analyst.

How then, can we approach this psychic reality? How do we get in touch with this ineffable, unrepressed unconscious? What is needed of the analyst's mind in order for this irrepresentable emotional experience to acquire meaning? The analyst, Freud says,

> must turn his own unconscious like a receptive organ towards the transmitting unconscious of the patient. He must adjust himself to the patient as a telephone receiver is adjusted to the transmitting microphone. Just as the receiver converts back into sound waves the electric oscillations in the telephone line which were set up by sound waves, so the doctor's unconscious is able, from the derivatives of the unconscious which are communicated to him, to reconstruct that unconscious, which has determined the patient's free associations. But if the doctor is to be in a position to use his unconscious in this way as an instrument in the analysis, he . . . may not tolerate any resistances in himself which hold back from his consciousness what has been perceived by his unconscious.
>
> (1912, pp. 115–116)

Bion might say "by his *analytically trained intuition*" (1965). The analytic stance capacitating the approach to these ineffable psychic realms is described by Bion (1970) as "an 'act of faith' [that] has as its background something that is unconscious and unknown *because it has not happened*" (p. 35, my italics). It has not yet happened in the sense that it has not yet been worked upon by an experiencing self; something that has never been registered "for want of a poet . . . [and since] as yet the poet hadn't turned up, so the recording tape was a blank!" (Bion, 1975, p. 120). For Bion, 'faith' is a scientific state of mind; faith that truth exists.

Bion implores that we listen to what is apparently blank, listen beyond what is being said, and hear beyond the 'noise' of the words being uttered. The patient's words refer to the past and to the future, and so he avoids being in touch with himself and with the pain and turbulence of being in touch with himself in the present. However, in order to hear beyond that which is *spoken* in the session, the analyst must live *in the present*, in the here and now of the session, and listen with his intuition. Intuition is thus a process by which a second mind can realize what the first no longer can (Boris, 1986). This may be the embryonic intuition we all once possessed, and whose potential we all carry and which must be restored to us and our analysands. For this to happen, we must 'blind ourselves' to the evidence of engaging in a conversation seemingly between two adults, and loosen the grip on familiar anchors of mature thought, so as to hear "the incomprehensible, inaudible, ineffable . . . from which will come the future interpretation" (Bion, 1974, p. 127).

> The attitude which the analytic physician could most advantageously adopt was to surrender himself to his own unconscious mental activity, in a state of *evenly suspended attention*, to avoid so far as possible reflection and the construction of conscious expectations, not to try to fix anything that he heard particularly in his memory, and by these means to catch the drift of the patient's unconscious with his own unconscious.
>
> (Freud, 1923, p. 239)

This is referred to by Bion as suspension of memory, desire and understanding, which promotes the analyst's 'Negative Capability' – the capacity "of being in uncertainties, mysteries, doubts, without any irritable reaching after fact and reason" (Bion, 1970, p. 125, citing the poet John Keats). Bion is very clear when he says that what is known about the patient is of no further consequence: it is either false or irrelevant. It is always misleading since it is distorted by the influence of unconscious forces. The only point of importance in any session is the unknown. Nothing must be allowed to distract the analyst from intuiting that.

Still, these are not the requirements from a medical doctor. This may be why Freud is quoted as saying that "a medical man cannot practice psychoanalysis because he always has medicine on his mind" (in Gay, 1988, p. 493). However, Bion warns that an analyst maintaining a state of ignorance about the patient may be subjected to accusations of malpractice and inappropriate conduct as expected from a psychiatric doctor. This in itself puts the analyst at great risk, evoking a great deal of anxiety in the analyst, threatening to steer him away from the emotional truth of the session.

Moreover, as Bion writes, the more the analyst becomes skilled in eschewing memory of past events, analytic theories, desire for cure, alleviation of pain, success, understanding, etc., the more he is likely to experience painful emotions and anxieties, many times of a psychotic, maddening nature. Bion highlights the need for the analyst to get in touch with the psychotic part of his own personality and to develop the capacity for dialectic interplay between this and the non-psychotic part of his personality. Failure to encompass the psychotic part of the personality renders the individual, be it patient or analyst, as "a total character *minus* . . ." (Bion, 1977, p. 52). As emphasized both by Freud and Bion, it is primarily the analyst's own analysis that can equip him with tools adequate to deal with the psychotic, irrepresentable part of his personality. No amount of medical or other education can serve as a substitute for that.

A psychotic state of mind?

As aforementioned, the 'scientific' method characterizing the medical doctor leans on a sensuously apprehensible reality. Bion writes that "it appears that our rudimentary equipment for 'thinking' thoughts is adequate when the problems are associated with the inanimate, but not when the object for investigation is the phenomenon of life itself. Confronted with the complexities of the human mind the analyst must be circumspect in following even accepted scientific method; its weakness may be closer to the weakness of psychotic thinking than superficial scrutiny would admit" (1962,

p. 14). Bion naturally differentiates between the scientist and the psychotic patient, yet he suggests that adherence to scientific thinking characteristic of medical thinking, may lead us to a model of a mind which is mechanical, lacking emotional resonance, and saturated with (omniscient) knowledge.

Allegiance to a positivistic (pseudo)scientific state of mind, not taking account of the mind's infinite complexity, often provides an illusory bulwark against fear of the unknown and the feeling of going mad. However, as Bion writes in his *Commentary* to *Second Thoughts*, "[t]he proper state for intuiting psycho-analytical realizations . . . can be compared with the states supposed to provide conditions for hallucinations. The hallucinated individual is apparently having sensuous experiences without any background of sensuous reality. The psycho-analyst must be able to intuit psychic reality which has no known sensuous realization" (Bion, 1967b, p. 163). Furthermore, he writes,

> Receptiveness achieved by denudation of memory and desire . . . is essential for experiencing hallucination or the state of hallucinosis. . . . This state I do not regard as an exaggeration of a pathological or even a natural condition: I consider it a state always present, but overlaid by other phenomena, which screen it . . . [T]o appreciate hallucination the analyst must participate in the state of hallucinosis . . . by which alone he can become at one with his patients' hallucinations.
>
> (Bion, 1970, p. 36)

Bion (1975 in Aguayo, 2013) contemplates the possibility of daring to use some kind of hallucination on the off-chance that it may be non-pathological. This might refer to the caesuras between dreaming, intuiting and hallucinating, acknowledging the similarity between them without denying the difference. Essentially, the purpose of the analyst's partial severance with external reality differs from the purpose of the psychotic manoeuvre. *The psychotic wishes to destroy contact with psychic reality whereas the analyst wishes to establish it* (Bion, 1970).

Many patients, Bion adds, are afraid of ideas that may appear irrational and mad. However, I would like to take Bion's words as being directed to the analyst, for he too is afraid. Receptiveness to the psychotic parts of the patient's psyche, exposes the analyst to the psychotic parts of his own psyche, just as the mother, through her receptiveness to the infant's fear of dying, actually feels the dread of dying herself.

It is the analyst who must be able to be in touch with his psychotic part of the personality, in order not to fall prey to its mind-deadening effect. "His own analysis should have made it possible for him to tolerate this emotional experience though it involves feelings of doubt and perhaps even persecution" (Bion, 1963, p. 102). Letting his mind roam freely, and with the aid of his analytically trained intuition, the analyst can begin to 'see' with his mind's eye that which is "invisible to mortal sight" (in Bion, 1975, p. 225, after Milton, *Paradise Lost*, Book 3).

Bion (1978) illustrates this in an example:

> A young man of twenty-five complains of having an unsatisfactory family life; I am not sure what family he is talking about, and in the course of a preliminary discussion I ask him his age and he says forty-two. Forty-two? But I said twenty-five just now. As I see him more closely I notice lines on his face, and every now and then I think he looks more like sixty-two than forty-two or twenty-five. Well, what is his age? . . . I suggest that behind this forty-two-year-old man is hidden a person, and that person has roots, an unconscious which, like the roots of a tree, is hidden from sight. . . . So when this person comes into your room, what do you see? I am not asking simply what do you see with your eyes, but also what does your intuition enable you to see?
>
> (p. 205)

***

All this readily draws to the question of cure. Psychoanalysis, as Freud writes, was believed to be a procedure for curing or improving neurotic symptoms (or nervous disorders, as it was sometimes described). Bion (1967a) contends that we have been saddled with doing a cure. We are put under pressure to take over the role of magicians who do cures. I suggest that this idea of 'cure', may have been initially produced in order to act as a container for psychoanalysis, its *raison d'être*. However, "the tendency to equate psycho-analysis with 'treatment', and 'cure' with improvement, is a warning that psycho-analysis is becoming restricted; limitation is placed on the analysand's growth in the interest of keeping the group undisturbed" (1967b, p. 157). The psychoanalytic quest does not strive to arriving at safe harbour, but is rather aimed at widening the capacity for (e)motion and free flowing between the different parts of the personality. It strives to expand our contact with remote, irrepresentable parts of our personality. Too often we restrict the psychoanalytic action to that of allowing the analysand to develop his capacity for thinking, dreaming and mentalizing, in the sense of facilitating the formless, undifferentiated, unrepresented and unthought to acquire a represented, differentiated form. This is a positivistic, linear description of psychoanalysis. I suggest that the mere movement and transition is what matters and not its direction, hence there is no notion of moving forward towards a goal, or cure. *The movement itself* is what expands the mind and facilitates its capacity to bear the emotional turbulence entailed in living. Hence, it promotes psychic aliveness (Bergstein, 2013).

Freud too was saddled with having to be 'scientific'. In the *Postscript* to *The Question of Lay Analysis*, Freud clearly attests to the influence of Ernst Brücke, the most eminent positivist in 19th-century Vienna, "who carried more weight with me than anyone else in my whole life" (1927, p. 253). However, he would apply his mentor's principles in ways Brücke could not have easily foreseen, nor wholeheartedly have applauded (Gay, 1988). It seems that his 1926 paper carries the intuition that psychoanalysis would not be able to remain a purely positivistic science. In fact, Freud *was* scientific in the sense that science is the pursuit of truth, yet in a state of mind different than the one acceptable in the naturalistic sciences demanding empirical evidence based on the senses. As Hanna Segal said, all the sciences pursue truth, but only in psychoanalysis is truth therapeutic, that is, it has a capacity to heal. It awaited thinkers like Bion to dare to add that

> it is very important to be aware that you may never be satisfied with your analytic career if you feel that you are restricted to what is narrowly called a 'scientific' approach. You will have to be able to have a chance of feeling that the interpretation you give is a beautiful one, or that you get a beautiful response from the patient. This aesthetic element of beauty makes a very difficult

> situation tolerable. It is so important to dare to think or feel whatever you do think or feel, never mind how un-scientific it is.
>
> (Bion, 1978, p. 211)

***

However, a caveat might be necessary in order to not to fall into the trap of a moralistic split between medicine and psychoanalysis. The emphasis on a non-positivistic science is placed in order to counterbalance the prejudice we have, as Bion says, in favour of the post-natal, waking, conscious, differentiated state. Confronted with the unknown, "the void and formless infinite", the personality tends to fill the void, provide form and give boundaries to the infinite. Our mind, as Kant might say, is discursive and not intuitive. We learn in a roundabout way, one thing from another, through deductions, judgements and general concepts and do not capture the emotional experience wholly and directly. Yet, as analysts, we are always required to work counter to our human nature, counter to our tendency to think linearly in terms of cause and effect, judgements, desires, holding onto past memories as an anchor. We must as Bergson (1903) says, direct a painful effort to the unmaking of our previous habits of thinking and perceiving. We are required to reverse the usual pragmatic work of the intellect so as to sharpen our intuition in order to approach, experience and perhaps even make fleeting contact with the elusive dynamic reality.

We must also remember that medicine is only used as *a model* representing a positivistic state of mind. As aptly expressed by Atul Gawande (2002), an acclaimed New York surgeon and writer,

> We look for medicine to be an orderly field of knowledge and procedure. But it is not. It is an imperfect science, an enterprise of constantly changing knowledge, uncertain information, fallible individuals, and at the same time lives on the line. There is science in what we do, yes, but also habit, intuition, and sometimes plain old guessing. The gap between what we know and what we aim for persists. And this gap complicates everything we do.
>
> (p. 7)

***

In November 1928, Freud wrote to his close friend Pfister, a Swiss pastor and lay analyst: "I do not know if you have detected the secret link between *Lay Analysis* and the *Illusion*. In the former, I wished to protect analysis from the doctors and in the latter, from the priests. I should like to hand it over to a profession which does not yet exist, a profession of *lay* curers of souls who need not be doctors and should not be priests" (Meng and E.L. Freud, 1963, p. 126, italics in the original). Freud may be alluding to the essential requirement of an analyst, that of having an unsaturated mind. The state of mind represented by 'doctors' is saturated with memory; the one represented by 'priests' is saturated with desire.

Note

1 This is sometimes referred to as primal repression in which "the mechanism . . . of withdrawal of preconscious cathexis would fail to meet the case; for here we are dealing with an unconscious idea which has yet received no cathexis from Pcs. and therefore cannot have that cathexis withdrawn from it" (Freud, 1915, p. 181, italics in the original).

References

Aguayo, J. (2013). Wilfred Bion's 'Caesura'. In: H.B. Levine and L.J. Brown(Eds.),*Growth and Turbulence in the Container/Contained: Bion's Continuing Legacy*(pp. 55–74). London: Routledge.

Alvarez, A. (2010). Levels of Analytic Work and Levels of Pathology: The Work of Calibration. *International Journal of Psychoanalysis*, 91: 859–878.

Bergson, H. (1903). *An Introduction to Metaphysics*. Cambridge: Hackett.

Bergstein, A. (2013). Transcending the Caesura: Reverie, Dreaming and Counter-Dreaming. *International Journal of Psychoanalysis*, 94: 621–644.

Bergstein, A. (2014). Beyond the Spectrum: Fear of Breakdown, Catastrophic Change and the Unrepressed Unconscious. *Rivista di Psicoanalisi*, 60: 847–868.

Bergstein, A. (2015). Attacks on Linking or a Drive to Communicate? Tolerating the Paradox. *Psychoanalytic Quarterly*, 84: 921–942.

Bergstein, A. (2016). Obsessionality: Modulating the Encounter with Emotional Truth and the Aesthetic Object. *Journal of the American Psychoanalytic Association*, 64: 959–982.

Bergstein, A. (2018). The Psychotic Part of the Personality: Bion's Expeditions into Unmapped Mental Life. In: *Bion and Meltzer's Expeditions into Unmapped Mental Life: Beyond the Spectrum in Psychoanalysis*. London: Routledge.

de Bianchedi, E.T. (1991). Psychic Change: The 'Becoming' of an Inquiry. *International Journal of Psychoanalysis*, 72: 6–15.

Bion, W.R. (1962). *Learning from Experience*. London: Karnac, 1984.

Bion, W.R. (1963). *Elements of Psychoanalysis*. London: Karnac, 1984.

Bion, W.R. (1965). *Transformations*. London: Karnac, 1984.

Bion, W.R. (1967a). Second seminar. In: J. Aguayo and B. Malin (Eds.), *Wilfred Bion: Los Angeles Seminars and Supervision* (pp. 33–54). London: Karnac, 2013.

Bion, W.R. (1967b). *Second Thoughts*. London: Karnac, 1984.

Bion, W.R. (1967c). Third Seminar. In: J. Aguayo and B. Malin (Eds.), *Wilfred Bion:Los Angeles Seminars and Supervision* (pp. 55–79). London: Karnac, 2013.

Bion, W.R. (1970). *Attention and Interpretation*. London: Karnac, 1984.

Bion, W.R. (1974). *Brazilian Lectures*. London: Karnac, 2008.

Bion, W.R. (1975). *A Memoir of the Future*. London: Karnac, 1991.

Bion, W.R. (1977). Caesura. In: *Two Papers: The Grid and Caesura* (pp. 35–56). London: Karnac, 1989.

Bion, W.R. (1978). A Paris seminar. In: C. Mawson (Ed.), *The Complete Works of W.R. Bion, IX*. London: Karnac, 2014.

Bion, W.R. (1979). Making the Best of a Bad Job. In: *Clinical Seminars and Other Works* (pp. 321–331). London: Karnac, 1994.

Boris, H.N. (1986). Bion Re-visited. *Contemporary Psychoanalysis*, 22: 159–184.

Botella, C., and Botella, S. (2005). *The Work of Psychic Figurability*. New York: Brunner-Routledge.

Freud, S. (1894). Draft E. How Anxiety Originates: From Extracts from the Fliess Papers. *SE*, 1.

Freud, S. (1895[1894]). On the Grounds for Detaching a Particular Syndrome from Neurasthenia Under the Description "Anxiety Neurosis". *SE*, 3.

Freud, S. (1912). Recommendations to Physicians Practicing Psycho-Analysis. *SE*, 12.

Freud, S. (1915). The Unconscious. *SE*, 14.

Freud, S. (1923). The Ego and the Id. *SE*, 19.

Freud, S. (1926). The Question of Lay Analysis. *SE*, 20.

Freud, S. (1927). Postscript to *The Question of Lay Analysis*. *SE*, 20.

Gawande, A. (2002). *Complications: A Surgeon's Notes on an Imperfect Science*. London: Profile Books.

Gay, P. (1988). *Freud: A Life for Our Time*. London: JM Dent & Sons Ltd.

Green, A. (1997). The Intuition of the Negative in *Playing and Reality*. *International Journal of Psychoanalysis*, 78: 1071–1084.

Laplanche, J., and Pontalis, J.B. (1967). *The Language of Psychoanalysis*. Trans. D. Nicholson-Smith. New York: W. W. Norton and Company, 1973.

Mason, A. (2000). Bion and Binocular Vision. *International Journal of Psychoanalysis*, 81: 983–988.

Meltzer, D. (1975). *Explorations in Autism*. Strath Tay: Clunie Press.

Meng, H., and Freud, E.L. (1963). *Psychoanalysis and Faith: The Letters of Sigmund Freud and Oskar Pfister*. Trans. E. Mosbacher. New York: Basic, 1964.

de M'Uzan, M. (2003). Slaves of Quantity. *Psychoanalytic Quarterly*, 72: 711–725.

Sandler, P.C. (2005). *The Language of Bion*. London: Karnac.

Sandler, P.C. (2011). The Realm of Minus and the Negative. In: *Analytic Function and the Function of the Analyst* (pp. 13–34). London: Karnac.

Winnicott, D.W. (1969). Additional Note on Psycho-Somatic Disorder. In: C. Winnicott, R. Shepherd, and M. Davis (Eds.), *Psycho-Analytic Explorations* (pp. 115–118). London: Karnac, 1989.

12

Enduring questions

Who is the lay today? Are today's judges impartial persons?

Paulo Cesar Sandler and Gley Pacheco Costa

The question of lay analysis became a leitmotiv that deeply affected the obtrusion of the psychoanalytical technique in our encircling social environment, embedding the history of the International Psychoanalytic Association (IPA).

Psychoanalytic movement and psychoanalysis proper

It seems to us that there is an absolute need to achieve the most precise possible discrimination between the psychoanalytic movement and psychoanalysis proper. This first is a social fact; the second, a scientific discipline, as far as the knowledge of the editors of this book is concerned.

Socially speaking, the question of lay analysis forged a question that motivated, and still motivates, a host of heated claims, protests and their correspondent defenses, under the form either of written or spoken words. It has to do with the old question of the relationships of quantity and quality, reviewed in the end of this chapter (Russell, 1903, pp. 162, 171, 195).

At first, and for eighty years, the distrust assumed the form and content of illegal practice under the rules of the judiciary system in many countries. In other terms, it was not dealt with the psychoanalytic vertex. Such a distrust contributed to an ever-growing formation of "warring" parties within the psychoanalytic movement. Either inside or outside the boundaries of the IPA – the question lurks.

It is possible to observe that this continuous unresolved question increased the occurrence of a destructive fact that can be briefly described under a psychoanalytic vertex in the discipline of group dynamics – the observation and dealing of human beings' behavior in groups. Groups can be quantitatively regarded as masses with more than three hundred gathered individuals; medium and small groups are less than twenty people. The psychoanalytic vertex allowed scientists to observe some "basic assumptions" governing the mindless behavior of any group in which either most or a minority of its members are under the sway of each member's narcissistic and paranoid tendencies. It is a well-known fact that in this case, the psychotic personality traits prevail at the expense of the non-psychotic traits. In large groups, those psychic tendencies tend to the infinite, displaying one of the most complex results of the previously mentioned relationships between quantity and quality (more detailed information on page 266). In the view of those authors, this constitutes a state of shared hallucinosis. It is expressed by deluded personal experience of appertaining or not appertaining to a fantasized, ruling elite – self-styled and socially empowered – within the whole, encircling group. The issue was investigated by one of those authors elsewhere (Mackay, 1841; Le Bon, 1895; Trotter, 1919; Freud, 1922; Jaques, 1960; Bion, 1961; Thorner, 1973; Pisani, 2000; Sandler, 2013).

Should one expect that the subgroup made up of the members of the psychoanalytic movement could be immune to act out such behavior? (Fenichel, 1945). After all, for a matter of principle, those members could be submitted to the suffering, rather than feeling, of a very specific painful experience: psychoanalysis (Bion, 1970, p. 29), which supposedly helps one individual to deal with, and at least to discipline, one's narcissistic and paranoid tendencies, as well as one's good enough elaboration of one's Oedipus complex – the most fundamental basis of any group's "basic assumptions". Nevertheless, reality has nothing to do with our expectations – mostly stemming from an infantile prospect or longing. The subgroups composed of members of the psychoanalytic movement display a behavior that has a striking similarity to the overall behavior of the encircling social groups from which they are derived. Is it a matter of hoping for more development of our technique? Or does this fact vouch for its limitations as a therapeutic technique?

Or, more seriously, does it reflect persisting problems in the formation of analysts? Which would be the psychoanalytical society that is reminded of Freud's suggestion that analysts should undergo a "re-analysis" in a five-year span of time? (Jaques, 1986; Sandler, 2001, 2013a; Freud, 1937a).

Real facts

Today it would be difficult to read a letter published in 1929 in *New Freie Presse*, in July, signed by Dr. Sigmund Freud. This would not be the case for knowledgeable and progressive Austrians in 1926. This letter brought a clear statement: a non-doctor could be a psychoanalyst. Freud gave as an example his daughter Anna, and also Dr. Theodor Reik, to whom he sent the cases that were not serious or were without any somatic complications (Perron, 2002). In hindsight, it seems that Freud made an apt choice in the media he chose. This newspaper (in a rough translation, "The New Free Journal") replaced, in the morning reading of cultured Viennese, *Die Presse*, or "The Journal". After all, whole issues could be subsumed by a single word: freedom.

Following this episode, Freud wrote the well-known and controversial exposé, published two months later: *The Matter of a Lay Analysis: Dialogues With an Impartial Person* (*Die Frage der Laienanalyse: Unterredungen mit einem Unparteiischen*) (Freud, 1927). What would be the "impartial person"? A judge in a law court? Written in a rush – less than a month – it had a number of purposes. Among them, Reik's defense. Reik had been accused of charlatanism and of practicing psychoanalysis without having the degree of a physician.

The quest did not include any kind of personal vanity or megalomania. In that time, it was not only common, but it was a necessity that newspapers furnished a considerable space and attention to letters from readers – especially those from distinguished ones.

It became obvious to Freud that the attack was not directed exclusively against his then young pupil in the University of Vienna, Professor Theodor Reik. This does not mean that such events did not reveal a strong and complex affective relationship between Freud and Reik, which started in 1910. Reik had just presented a thesis to obtain a doctorate in the University of Vienna. In fact, he was the first person to obtain a doctorate in psychology in what was a very prestigious school. A year later, as mentioned by Natterson (1966), Freud advised him not to pursue the idea of becoming a physician but to begin the Analytic Graduation course. Reik didn't have the financial resources, so Freud managed to get Abraham to analyze him for free. Throughout his two-year stay in Berlin – from 1913 to 1915 – he got a monthly stipend of two hundred marcs. Back in Vienna, Reik became a member of what came to be known as the "Wednesday group", gathered around Freud – the embryo of what would become the IPA.

It seemed to Dr. Freud that such an attack needed an "impartial person" to tolerate a serene, technical defense and also its "public action". We suppose that, in hindsight, one may have an enlightened view about both the attack and its defense, if one considers a contribution to psychoanalysis from a later contributor:

> Megalomania. Common sense produces, from this point of view, a restrictive state of mind; it conflicts with megalomaniac narcissism. Without common sense, phantasy can be felt as a fact. Indolence can be the need to remain free to indulge phantasy: again, common sense is the obstructing force.
>
> Public-action is an essential of scientific method, as this means that common sense plays a vital part. If it is inoperative for any reason, the individual in which it is inoperative cannot publish, and unpublished work is unscientific work.
>
> (Bion, 1959, p. 24)

When the editors of this book read Freud's paper for the first time, in the late seventies of the last century, they made a hypothesis: Had Freud fully realized that it was an attack against the whole psychoanalytic method and the social movement it evoked, now put into the form of a breaking of the law? One decade later, we found hard factual evidence that confirmed this hypothesis. In an excerpt of a letter from Freud to Max Eitington, we read:

> The movement against lay analysis seems to be only an offshoot of the old resistance against analysis in general.
>
> (Jones, 1957, p. 314)

Could it be a coincidence that this letter was directed to the main organizer of the most complete program of analytical formation?

On the other hand, the exposé brought much more than just decisive statements by a most influential practitioner. According to James Strachey, a lay analyst, who was both the translator and editor of Freud's complete works,

> it is perhaps his [Freud's] most successful non-technical account of the theory and practice of psychoanalysis, written in his liveliest and lightest style. The theoretical part has the advantage over his earlier expository works of having been composed after the great clarification of his views on the structure of mind in *The Ego and the Id*.
>
> (Strachey, 1959, p. 181)

Once upon a time . . . are biographies a reliable source of data?

If one considers the overall sales in book trade, one may easily conclude that the genre of biography is much sought after. There is no secret about the spread of this interest among the vast majority of members of the psychoanalytic movement. Moreover, some members of the psychoanalytical movement suppose that an important part of our intra-movement communication between peers, the written reports of clinical cases, must include a detailed study of our patients' biographies. This is independent of some controversies. For example, some members of the movement entertain restrictions about the way one deals with biographical details. They suggest restrictions, due to the fact that any patients' biographies are just products of their memories. After all, was it not Freud who noticed that "neurotics suffer from reminiscences"? Was not this a noticeable, main factor in his discovery of psychoanalysis? (Freud, 1909). Quite independent of those controversies among members of the psychoanalytical movement, one may see that the existence of the controversy is a real fact. It exemplifies, at least in part, the importance given to biographies by perhaps all members of the psychoanalytical movement. In contrast to the heavy interest of the members of the psychoanalytic establishment, Freud was absolutely against the writing of biographies, with the possible exception of three, by Leonardo da Vinci, Daniel Paul Schreber and Woodrow Wilson. However, the priority was not the autobiography itself, but as a means to profit from some special data to construe a written exercise from the psychoanalytic point of view – rather than "analyzing deceased people" – profiting from autobiographical data furnished by Leonardo da Vinci's report of a dream; Judge Paul Daniel Schreber's periods of illness; Woodrow Wilson's behavior and previous personal development, as recounted by a close collaborator, Ambassador Bullitt; as well as some hypothesis about Goethe. One may discern that Freud based his psychoanalytical exercise about those historical figures in a rather specialized mode of this writing genre: not just biographies by other people, but by autobiographies. According to Young-Bruhel (2008), Anna Freud's father severely warned and even forbade his close friend Arnold Zweig, a writer, who was willing to write a biography about Freud. The discoverer of psychoanalysis is reputed to state that biographies are a huddle of lies; who could be wholly truthful if the case was to display his life to other people? He would have quoted to Zweig Shakespeare's *King Lear*: "truth's a dog must to kennel; he must be whipped out" (Shakespeare, 1603–1606, p. 33).

After his death, many who had presented themselves as his friends committed biographies purportedly about him. Starting from his own doctor – who had helped him to die more peacefully. Was their attitude a question of their own physical survival? Did they have any qualms about doing something strongly disapproved of by Freud?

Ernest Jones waited almost a decade to seek Anna Freud's authorization to publicize his own version about Freud's life. He allowed himself to repeat many metaphors that he adequately attributed to Freud. In what is relevant to the heated question of lay analysis in the United States, Jones quotes a letter from Freud to Max Eitington: the former felt as if he was a "commander without an army" inside this fight. But not for this reason, less fierce in making an accusation: Americans were against lay analysis. Jones also quotes a letter from Freud to Mr. Jacques Schneier, a San Franciscan sculptor devoted to analysis: "I insist on them [Freud's favourable ideas about lay-analysis] even more intensely than before, in the face of the obvious American tendency to turn psychoanalysis into a mere house-maid of psychiatry" (Jones, pp. 320, 322).

Those metaphors of Freud's were not coming from direct conversations between Freud and Jones, albeit they are true and well-documented. The editors of this book observed that many biographers speak about the subjects of biographies, but what is at stake? In many instances, it is the biographer's feelings and views. In addition, most times, the motivation to write biographies is idolatry. From the psychoanalytic view, there is no idolatry without its opposite, hidden side, the iconoclast. This side was illuminated through the psychoanalytic vertex: "And it is not only the vehemence of the subject's uncontrollable hatred but that of his love too which imperils the object" (Klein, 1934). This illuminates the surge of too many iconoclasts, always centered in personal interpretations of purportedly "biographical" data: Sulloway, Grunberger and lesser known persons, as (Warner, 1989) Jones, whose love of Freud and psychoanalysis cannot be put into question, left many marks of the hidden iconoclast within him; for example, when stated, the future prospect of a young Freud was that of a "public menace". This was a false accusation, or, in its better face, "post-occupation", for it never could be a real preoccupation from a friend: Jones did not know Freud when the later used cocaine. It seems to us that it is fair to state that in those cases – Freud as a commander without army and a public menace – both were at least identified. It is known that too many people – friends or foes – felt that Jones commanded the British Psychoanalytical Society like an iron-fisted army commander. This is not a criticism of Jones; for example, it is highly probable that Melanie Klein could have faced expulsion if it were not the case, and, in this case, his attitude had a constructive effect. Did Jones learn from Freud's bad experiences in what is of concern to people around him? In what is relevant to being a "public menace", Jones had his own share of lawsuits, which forced him to get out from Canada.

As a kind of habit in the psychoanalytical movement, most members who did not know Freud and his collaborators personally tried their hands in issuing interpretations about historical attitudes adopted by those pioneers, profiting from biographies and, too many times, hearsay. Especially when the pioneer is the discoverer of our discipline, called by him psychoanalysis, and also deep psychology and psychodynamics:

> Freud liked so much this neurotic man always in search for a father, that he adopted him as a son. After the end of the First War, Reik got very sick, and Freud agreed to take him as

> a patient, thus starting, as it had been put forward by those authors an "endless" treatment. There were good reasons to be admired by the "Father of the Psychoanalysis": besides being a doctor in languages and philosophy, Reik had a solid basis in psychology, music and anthropology, becoming along his life a profitable and creative writer. His devotion to Freud got him to copy him in all possible aspects, inclusive of growing a beard, his attire, and, impossible to omit, the habit of smoking cigars, which made him well known among his peers by the nickname "simile Freud".
>
> (Roudinesco and Plon, 1997, p. 655)

Sometimes, lack of information is conducive to hurried interpretations: physical resemblance, as it occurs with doppelgangers, is a genetic endowment, even though the use one makes of such similarities is wholly at one's will. His biographer, Natterson, makes clear that Theodor Reik had a beard just in his old age. In any case, besides the admiration, it's possible that Freud had also become identified with Reik by his being a Jew of poor background who had lost his father at eighteen. After less than ten years following Freud's death, now working in the United States, where he had emigrated to escape from Nazism, Reik wrote:

> Let me freely admit that in these thirty years of psychoanalytic practice, I had this wish [to change my career] more than once. I have had moods in which being a psychoanalyst appeared to me less a profession than a calamity.
>
> (Reik, 1948, p. viii; the same appears in a slightly different grammar in Natterson, 1966, p. 285)

It is not difficult to perceive that the psychoanalytic model conceived by Freud in the article on lay analysis matches with some information about this man – including those furnished by himself. It is safe to state that Freud was his godfather, his counselor, and eventually his analyst, getting from him an acknowledgment on the book *From Thirty Years with Freud* (Reik, 1940), where he speaks rather about himself than about his professor. Likewise, one is allowed to offer a hypothesis, even if it cannot be proved for the lack of reliable empirical data: might Freud have felt guilty of the accusation towards Reik for having put him down regarding studying medicine? According to Peter Gay, the American physician Dr. Newton Murphy desired to have an analysis with Freud, who turned him over to Dr. Reik. Referrals in medicine may be a problem: How can the referee, always a partisan, warrant the good results or be responsible for bad results, which are, in the long run, the responsibility of the therapist? Under the psychoanalytic vertex, one may emphasize the presence of the phenomena of transference – not for a mere coincidence, another discovery we owe to Freud. Now the problem is logarithmically heightened (Freud, 1912a). We have no hard data that could back or not those hypotheses that may have the value of a psychoanalytical exercise about historical data. In any case, Dr. Murphy sued Dr. Reik for quackery, with the probable backing of Dr. Wilhelm Stekel (Gay, 1998, p. 490) – one among the early idolaters of Freud who, as any idolater, sooner or later displays his previously hidden iconoclast side (Sandler, 2015a, p. 46). In contrast, Reik, in many instances idealized Freud, but in other moments, he denigrated him in frequent quarrels with other psychoanalysts, particularly doctors, up to a point that, according Natterson, Freud had to warn him in 1928:

> Your hostility by-passes all justifiable limits.
>
> (Natterson, 1966, p. 293)

Today one may safely state that all of us living analysts can learn from Freud's errors; psychoanalysis takes much more time to be accomplished than the "vain philosophy" of that era thought was needed. At least, according the data at our disposal from Natterson, it was not a question of gossip: Freud told this directly to Reik.

Freud, according himself, was not a *menschen kenner* (Young-Bruhel, 2008) – a man who knows other men at the first sight – a statement that surprised a lot among his contemporaries. Instead, he really needed too much time and observation to get to some conclusions. There are evidences of it, as the troubled, rivalry-ridden actions from all of his first followers, who angrily abandoned not only the psychoanalytic movement, but accused him with many epithets, some of them utterly disrespecting: "pan-sexualist", "Victorian", "anti-German", "plagiarist", "scientifically dishonest" and the like. Some of his early collaborators met violent death by suicide.

Nevertheless, in Dr. Reik's case, one may vouch that Freud did not err. After Freud's death, and already living far from his homeland, struggling for his existence with inadequate economic means, but under as stimulating an environment as the one provided by post-war America, Dr. Reik wrote fifty books. From which *Listening With the Third Ear* turned out to be a classic – if nowadays being submitted to neglect among many institutes. Theodor Reik's writing, not dissimilar to Freud's, was noticeably clear, direct, objective, free of jargon and full of aphorisms and metaphors. He was able to elicit clearly that analysts must use "creative intuition", something that he conveyed through a metaphor, "the third ear", to sense the unspoken but told by other means (via free associations, demeanor, dreams, etc.) in order to turn this data into verbal formulations, to benefit the patient. In this sense, Reik can be seen as the unrecognized rescuer of Freud, and predecessor of Winnicott and Bion's contributions. His other works made invaluable contributions to the dealing of masochism – he seems to be the first to notice it as a pleasure-ridden source – adding to the psychology of love.

Freud's posture about the existence of lay analysis

Far beyond this clash, still actual nowadays, we must pay due attention to the professional, ethical and legal aspects that make it difficult to universalize lay analysis. This adds to the widespread acceptance of "non-lay analysis" coinciding with the many, albeit most unduly, criticisms against our activity from the overall encircling milieu, as we will see later.

One may consider two facts, namely (1) the existence of lay analysts if one uses the nomenclature adopted by Freud, which is an individual situation, which must be dealt with in a psychoanalytical setting; and (2) currently, what would merit to be called "lay analyst", besides the former idea, which dates from Freud's time? Is this now just a social fact, appertaining to the realm of groups, belonging to the existence of the psychoanalytic movement? This movement is made by people gathered for many motives; in Freud's time, just to the study of psychoanalysis. It would be imprecise to state that today the motives are limited to those from Freud's time, in social terms. Other motives were adjoined as time passed by and the movement grew numerically. For example, now we have more difficulties between the relationships of the political meritocracy and the scientific meritocracy that befall in any kind of group (Sandler, 2012; 2015b, pp. 218, 301; 2016, p. 89). There is no judgmental value in this observation: for example, when the political meritocracy prevailed over the scientific meritocracy in the final decision of the German dictatorship by Adolf Hitler to not pursue the building of a nuclear bomb (Bracher, 1968; Heisenberg, 1958).

The truth is, we need to acknowledge that the defense of lay analysis by Freud did not start with Reik's episode, but it was from it that the topic became the target of a wide and fierce debate by most members in the psychoanalytic movement around the world, bound to disagreement among many from the most varied societies and also inside the same society.

Freud occupied a central position in this contention, moved by a radicalism unknown till then, up to a point where he weighed in against the considered and responsible position in relation to his friend Ernest Jones, engaged in avoiding an imminent rupture within the IPA by an expressive group of psychoanalysts, formed by North American and European members.

> Analytic training, it is true, cuts across the field of medical education, but neither includes the other. If – which may sound fantastic to-day – one had founded a college of psycho-analysis, much would have to be taught in it which is also taught by the medical faculty: alongside the depth – psychology, which would always remain the principal subject, there would be an introduction to biology, as much as possible of the science of sexual life, and familiarity with the symptomatology of psychiatry. On the other hand, analytic instruction would include branches of knowledge which are remote from medicine and which the doctor does not come across in his practice: the history of civilizations, mythology, the psychology of religion and the science of literature. Unless he is well at home in the subjects, an analyst can make nothing of a large amount of his material. By way of compensation, the great mass of what is taught in medical school is of no use to him for his purposes.
>
> (Freud, 1927, p. 246)

The psychoanalytical movement was precociously fated to be violently divided by and among his earliest collaborators, as Freud painfully learned. This internal (to the group) violence had at least one "too human" factor: rivalry fueled by omnipotence and omniscience – two expressions of what Freud termed as "narcissism". By itself, an expression of difficulties subsumed by the "Oedipus complex". Nevertheless, Freud's psychoanalytic achievements did not evoke just rivalry. They provided a fertile soil to real collaborators, such as Karl Abraham, among others, who prepared the ground for further discoveries by following generations, exemplified by Fairbairn, Klein, Winnicott and Bion. It seems that Freud did not anticipate that the psychoanalytical movement was also fated to be subjected to later divisions, adjoined to rivalry, albeit he had clear signs of them. His awareness of this risk can be seen in his identification of basic issues that precluded a good enough apprehension of reality, whose study can be made through the theory of science. He left some warning about those basic issues, mostly linked to a tendency to make supportive, superficial psychotherapies – for this reason he also named psychoanalysis as a depth psychology – as the influence of religious beliefs, alien to science. In his last lecture on psychoanalysis, he warned about another human destructive, paranoid tendency: "solipsism" (nowadays called "subjectivism", "idealism" and "relativism"; Freud, 1933–36, p. 158 and followings). Immanuel Kant was one who named two among those basic issues in human processes of thought. Probably there are more. He proposed the qualification "naïvetés". The prevalence of those naïvetés precludes the advancement of any scientific discipline hitherto known. The warring parties under the sway of those naïvetés can be named as the naïve realists versus the naïve idealists (Sandler, 2001b). People that put too much emphasis on just one of the two sides can be easily found either in medicine or in the other disciplines quoted by Freud. The result is a group that cannot profit from two mutually enriching sources; the group uses them as mutually destructive weapons to prove the superiority of one over the other.

Ernest Jones, who quoted Freud almost *verbatim*, was worried about this possibility, especially when it was not any more just an enlightened premonition, but when it occurred. Therefore, he wrote under his own learning from an experience that Freud probably did not have:

> no motive has yet been discovered, or is likely to be discovered in the future, making possible the investigation of the deepest layers of the mind beside of personal *suffering*. That awesome

> fact irrevocably binds psychology, and all the sciences ancillary to it, to psychopathology. So an anthropologist, for example, desirous of applying psychoanalytical doctrines in his special field would first of all, at least for a time, have to become a psychotherapist . . . those coming from other fields of education, anthropology, art, literature, invariably wish to become practising analysts for the rest of their lives, a decision which necessarily limits their usefulness in applying their newly acquired knowledge in their precious field of work. The recognition that psychoanalyst insight into the deep layers of the mind is not something acquired once and for all at a given phase of study. But has to be refreshed and extended by continuous contact with the raw material of observation, i.e. the analysis of patients. Such a person is then termed a lay or non-medical psycho-analyst.
>
> (Jones, 1957, p. 310)

What should we do with members of the psychoanalytical movement who have achieved the "official" status of analysts, given by any accredited political institutions – if those members too much times replace psychoanalysis – wittingly or not – under the spell of other disciplines?

The doctorate in mental health

Freud's project proved to be feasible when one considers just individuals – after all, the purpose of any psychoanalysis, a "two-body" psychology (Rickmann, 1950). Most analysts, individually, look for information and sometimes formation in some of those disciplines. Some – not most – "lay analysts", today, look for work in general hospitals. Conversely, one must be reminded that what Freud felt as a "fantastic project", in terms of groups, proved hitherto to be so. The insertion of psychoanalysis in universities has been met with controversy. One program wholly similar to Freud's "fantastic project" proved to be short-lived: the troubled "Doctorate in Mental Health" at the University of San Francisco. Initiated by Dr. Lawrence Kubie and continued, up to a point, by Dr. Robert S. Wallerstein (1990). At the very same time, Wallerstein faced serious pressures that ended with a lawsuit – promoted by the establishment of American psychologists. Wallerstein arranged the sponsorship of Jimmy Carter's Presidential Commission on Mental Health

(Grob, 2005) to put forth the project. As probably anything that was linked to the backing of that administration, it implied that such a doctorate lasted for a few years: a handful of hopeful pupils got their certificate. That now serves for . . . ? It is difficult to say. The whole program, marked by bureaucratic disorganization, proved to be submitted to the principle of pleasure and displeasure – typical of any kind of good-willed wishful thinking, with no foundation in real life (Freud, 1911a). Taking into account Freud's appreciation about Woodrow Wilson, the historical predecessor of Jimmy Carter's presidential ideas, one may ask: What could be his idea about such a complete but impossible program?[1]

Social empowerment

The tendency to label people under the idea of "superiority" and "inferiority" – individually or gathered in groups – is a human tendency, questioned by Freud under the psychoanalytic vertex (Freud, 1913). Nevertheless, considering social life as it is, this still is an unavoidable fact. It is clear that the qualification, lay analysis, is a verbal formulation precociously embedded with this kind of tendency. The lawsuit against Reik had a clear denigrating sense. A factor in such a denigration is a social and individual empowerment of the medical profession. Socially, it includes especially those people gathered in academia. Again and again we face a millennia-old social fact, fundamentally based in a too-human trait – our basic helplessness before a hostile environment. Each one of us, human beings, must face it as soon as we are born, despite the resistances, denials and rationalizations stemming from the principle of pleasure–displeasure. The empowerment of the medical profession can be seen, under the psychoanalytic vertex, as one among the many phenomenal expressions of the prevalence of this principle. It is not the real physician that is empowered. Rather, it is a transference-based delusion (Freud, 1912a) – too many times shared by physicians and patients – in our days, by lay analysts and clients. It is best displayed by the beliefs strongly favored by sacerdotal authorities (Porter, 1999). A need in religious practices, but not in scientific research, in which there is a tendency to accept and thus to achieve the principle of reality (Freud, 1911a, 1912a, 1913a).

Any living human being is able to get such an achievement. It is a question of survival. In terms of groups, authoritarian empowerment of a given class or profession is based on delusion and prejudice; real authority is based in the obtrusion of the principle of reality. As a further complication, the same principle of pleasure–displeasure is the nest of a most destructive human trait, expressed by the splitting of thought processes, leading to individual mindlessness. A most destructive phenomenal expression of it can be named: prejudice (Klein, 1946).

One may take fundamental, basic human facts, expressed materially and immaterially: love and hate, as they are displayed in many myths. For example, the family myth about Esau and Jacob in *The Book of Genesis* (25:28); or the various sagas of Ulysses, Achilles, Ajax and Hector, as described in the *Iliad*. All of those characters embody a prejudiced empowerment, as well as different ways to deal with it, both as individuals and in groups. If one examines the myth from the psychoanalytic vertex, one may observe the preponderance of narcissistic, paranoid fantasies expressed phenomenically by the deluded idea that some people are better – superior – than other people. Superiority/inferiority are two different transformations – mere appearances – of the same underlying invariance. May it be named, "difference"? (Bion 1965; Sandler, 2015c, 2018). In a group formed by one family linked by genetics, this fantasy expresses itself by prejudices about the ordinal position of children in the offspring. Some cultures favor the first born; others, the last born.[2] A psychological tale supposed that the middle-born could be submitted to disfavor and thus could develop mental illnesses – an idea unsupported by statistical evidence. In larger groups, the prejudice is against people who do not belong to the same ethnic group, or herd, or family (Freud, 1938).

Notions furnished in the past three millennia, according historic and anthropologic studies, including those specialized in the history of medicine (Porter, 1999) show that it occurs an authoritarian, deluded empowerment to the medical profession in innumerable ethnical groups. Is this a normal feature of humankind?

In Freud's time, there were audible grumblings, here or there, explicit or subliminal. Hints of envy-motivated discontent abounded. Social pressures both stimulated and increased what was a two-century-old prejudice among the medical professionals against what was seen as pseudo-science, echoing attacks on Hippocratic and Galen's medicine in the Hellenic-Greek culture. In some cases, the brand "pseudo-science" could be safely applied.

Nevertheless, as it often occurs, pure prejudice found a good enough container in limited individual experiences, gaining the status of absolute truth in hallucinosis and delusion.[3] It is a known fact that psychoanalysis faced resistances as well as misappropriation (the purest form of resistance) from *part* of the medical milieu in Vienna – despite more recent denials from people without psychoanalytic training (Popper, 1963; Ellenberger, 1970; Sulloway, 1978; Grunbaum, 1984; Eysenck and Eysenck, 1985), which we will briefly review later in this text.

One may emphasize the following social facts that took two centuries to evolve, embedded and concentrated in the legal case against Reik: (1) The rise and fall of mesmerism (Castiglioni 1941; Porter, 1999); (2) the decaying of Goethe's Naturphilosophie into mysticism, then called by philosophers and physicians alike, "metaphysic"; (3) the surge of other quackeries, as the spectacles of "public hypnosis" in which trained artists feigned illnesses; many times, not just artists but also hysterics; (4) the diatribes between the new-formed "schools" to study hypnosis, highly influenced by nationalisms; (5) the realization that phrenology was a false science; (6) the overall attitude of the medical establishment about the work of Freud, a neurologist that even before his discovery of psychoanalysis (Freud, 1891) never, and ever, was at peace with the beliefs of the Positivist Religion invented by Auguste Comte (1896), while the establishment was.

A case of social empowerment: the positivist religion and false medicine

Positivist religion claimed to be the only science possible, albeit it never made scientific hypotheses – rather, it profited partially from past achievements – today dismissed as "the English empiricism"! As any religion, it ruled, as if its rules could be unquestionable, absolute truths. One may summarize those rules: (1) a scientist would be "neutral", meaning he or she would never interfere in his or her observations; (2) the scientist must look for materialized, concrete localization of events rather than immaterializable functions; (3) the scientist must use just, and exclusively, his or her sensuous apparatus, enhanced by technological discoveries or not, to make science; (4) the scientist must be "rational", meaning, he must make discoveries through formal (Euclidean) logic reasoning (deduction or induction); (5) the scientist must find causal chains: to each "cause" would correspond "an effect"; (6) the scientist could aptly formulate previews of events.

The same prejudice exists within the medical profession. In Freud's time, it resulted in a lower status vis-à-vis other medical specialities in the eyes of physicians, either internists or surgeons, to those who were called alienists, neuropsychiatrists and psychiatrists. Politically influential physicians who achieved power in the medical establishment in many countries – the Austro-Hungarian Empire was no exception – rationally based their abhorrence to neuropsychiatrists due to the latter's lack of adequate tools to make diagnoses and therapeutic procedures: concrete maneuvers, mandatory to other medical specialities, made through the use of our sensuous apparatus, including our hands. Alienists could not examine their patients' psychic apparatus without acoustic and/or optical instrumentation that already had enhanced the physician's sensuous apparatus in that time: stethoscopes, sphygmomanometers, smoke-drums, microscopes. It made part of the prejudiced empowerments that false physicians always made heavy use and overabused of technical expressions in their communications with the laymen and laywomen. Few among the public noticed that

> *Such labour'd nothings, in so strange a style,*
> *Amaze th'unlearn'd, and make the learned smile*
>
> (Pope, 1711)

Today, it contributes to the psycho-babble that still persists among laymen and women.

In Freud's time, Galton's "eugenics", Lombroso's forensic "medicine" and Wagner-Jauregg's "malariotherapy" were bandied about the real saviors of humanity (Gilham, 2001; Wolfgang, 1961; Karamanou et al., 2013). They proved to be a sad destructive practice, due to disappointments as a result of lack of knowledge and a striking lack of therapeutic results. The three fashionable pseudo-theories – complete with their rationalistic cause-effect ethos – proved to be concretized delusions, with utterly destructive social consequences. A shared hallucinosis, manifested by a collusion between academia and the public, mistook the Positivistic reasoning's limited successes in very limited inanimate, less complex realms – as engineering or in the heavy bodies physics – with false promises that tried to apply the same reasoning to incomparably more complex realms. Most people, either in that time and also today, do not give a damn about Pope's poem about the "*Bookful Blockhead, ignorantly read/With loads of learned lumber in his head*" who could not fathom that "*fools rush in where angels fear to tread*" (Pope, 1709, p. 351).

Neurologists, inspired by cardiologists who already counted with a powerful electrical device, the electrocardiograph, could use a tool first devised in 1924 by Hans Berger: the electroencephalograph. Neurologist's materialized armamentarium now includes echographs, tomographs and magnetic resonance devices. Too many times, those inanimate devices are submitted to inadequate use, serving to perverse fringe benefit: as if they could be buffers to preclude human contact. Together with economic interests, it increased the deluded empowerment of the medical profession. Computerized screens replace what once was called the patient–physician relationship. Those are distortions, not real medicine: those tools, adequately used, helped to improve the Hippocratic method to make reliable diagnoses and a good enough dealing with diseases. Nevertheless, the advent of newer technologies also increased the abhorring of the mere use of the expression, "medical intuition" – a skill mounting from the Hippocratic and Galen's tradition. Rationalized approaches, complicated by denial – expressed by abhorrence to the unknown, the begetter of absolute rules – have no place in the study of human nature and its sufferings.[4] The making of rules – an unavoidable fact in other fields, such as law, pedagogy and government – have no counterpart in real life: "for there is nothing either good or bad, but thinking makes it so" (Shakespeare, 1601–1602). Real mathematics, biology, physics, psychoanalysis and art are neither "positive" nor "negative". All of them include paradoxes, which demand to be tolerated, not resolved. Medicine proper, outside its socially deluded empowerment, is not authoritarian-by-itself. Again, it seems to be needed to discern the scientific discipline from the human beings that try to practice it, and a fortiori, the social groups in which it is practiced. The authority of medicine is based in its scientific ethos and as a consequence of it, its real achievements in dealing with the sufferings and vicissitudes of human nature.

When false medicine and false science enjoy periods of social empowerment, medicine proper is subjected to a strikingly similar social distrust which psychoanalysis always had and still has to endure. Both have been accused of pure quackery. The medical establishment is many times seen as if it is a "white Mafia", a self-protecting network unwilling to recognize and to learn from its errors. Medical doctors would be just profiteers, hyenas nourished by other people's miserable conditions. How many among us suppose that physicians are not human beings? Either because they are seen as if they are the devil incarnate or if they must be disembodied beings, not needing any kind of concrete resources to earn a life and to get food or shelter to survive. In truth, some medical specialties, such as emergency care, obstetrics and pediatrics, know no time to be available and seem to some patients of not being endowed of a circadian cycle.

Freud observed a social feeling about psychoanalysis: it is an offense to human omnipotence. Is it true? If it is, then it would not be a surprise that the activity that deals with death, illness, dejection and suffering – real medicine – is met by the encircling milieu from which it is born both with deluded empowerment and its dialectic pole, dismissal and abhorrence when this empowerment proves to be deluded. If one pays attention to the overall death rate, as well as a proneness to addictions in physicians, and compares it with the whole population, one would be surprised about the price one pays to practice medicine. One cannot deny, under a psychoanalytical vertex, that members of the medical establishment share with their patients the omnipotent and omniscient delusions of superiority, of achieving fame and immortality. Part of the medical establishment acknowledge the existence of iatrogenic, placebo and nocebo effects. In psychoanalysis, a more limited realm and paradoxically more ample in its insights, it is possible to state that:

> Having two sets of feelings about the same facts is felt as madness and disliked accordingly. This is one reason why it is felt necessary to have an analyst; another reason is the wish for me to be able to be regarded as mad and used to being regarded as mad. There is a fear that you might be called an analysand, or reciprocally, that you may be accused of insanity. Should I then be tough and resilient enough to be regarded and treated as insane while being sane? If so, it is not surprising that psycho-analysts are, almost as a function of being analyst, supposed to qualify for being insane and called such. It is part of the price they have to pay for being psycho-analysts.
>
> (Bion, 1975, p. 119)

Medicine, psychiatry, psychology

The social empowerment of medicine has at least a factor elicited by psychoanalysis. In the lack of a better name to study this factor, which has a real counterpart in the realm of phenomena, Freud coined the name "transference" (Freud, 1912a). Under the psychoanalytical vertex, to take actions under transference fantasies is a tendency of the "psychotic personality" (Bion, 1957).

Albeit mostly unknown in its wholeness, fragmentary hints about origins and formation of authoritarian societies can be found in historic, biologic, anthropologic, sociologic and transdisciplinary studies (Darwin, 1871; McNall Burns, 1949; Toynbee, 1934–1961; Arendt, 1958, 1979). This was the case of the European soil that reached (until now) its destructive climax in the nineteenth and twentieth centuries, reaching what was recently called "bloodlands" (Snyder, 2010). Under the psychoanalytical vertex, one may spot a fundamental immaterialized fact which is materialized in the form of idolatric transference phenomena (Freud, 1912a,b; Adorno et al., 1950). At least as it goes our experience, this effect is maximized in science, medical and political activities: idolatry is one form of transference toward the figure of a physician, but not to a real physician, just its figure as it stands in each one's mind. Idolatry is tenuous and tenacious; it has a twin-track base: promises (fulfilled at short time, or not) of command over disease, coupled with the individual or group's subservience to the principle of pleasure–displeasure. In Freud's time, there was little public awareness about transference phenomena as well as about its multiplied, corresponding consequence in the encircling society – authoritarianism. Its enlightenment had to wait for better times to prevail – and had a striking cost. It needed the surge of murderous political regimes that killed around ninety million people in a mere twenty-four years – from 1921 to 1945 – to create a mild interest in this individual and social issue.

Paradoxically, it seems to the editors of this book that there is another important, double-tracked factor elicited by psychoanalysis in the social empowerment of medicine: gratitude and reparation (Klein and Riviére, 1936; Klein, 1957). It can be better observed in people who met with real suffering, death-provoking or with a high probability to meet death, and underwent to a medical and/or psychoanalytical treatment, getting out from it alive and/or enlivened. This factor has been socially and individually enhanced due to advancements – always through learning from experience of explicitly errors – of the medical discipline in the last two millennia. One may quote Aristotle, the physician who made the most complete physiological studies in the Antiquity: part of his achievements, kept in good order under a clinical practice by Galen; and under a secluded mode, in the Andalusian Civilization, mainly by Avicenna and Maimonides. When Science was rescued during the Renaissance and Enlightenment periods, one may quote William Harvey, Claude Bernard, Gustav Virshow, Louis Pasteur, Robert Koch. The list is too long; one can make one's own, according his or her knowledge or preferences (Castiglioni, 1947; Porter, 1999; Coelho Fo et al., 2013).

The prejudiced social empowerment goes on unabated today due to technological novelties that reached psychiatry, especially after the inception of mildly successful and still controversial "psychotropic" drugs.[5] Technology exerts fascination and amazement to some professionals and in the laymen's world, always linked with the basic despair of the human race. If "synapsis" – the link that either bridges or precludes the electro-chemical transmission between sections of "nerves", an encapsulated structure, is a real fact – the whole of neurology still depends on a fictitious, theoretical doctrine – that of the "neuron" (Bullock et al., 2005). First summarized by H.G. Waldeyer, over hitherto disconnected histological observations by Sigmund Freud, Camillo Golgi, Albert von Kölliker, Franz Nissl, Santiago Ramón y Cajal and Auguste Forel, the neuron doctrine is just this: still another doctrine. Dr. Waldayer never made any kind of histological study – his bearings were findings from the previously mentioned authors. One cannot state the same about the fundamentals of psychoanalysis: free associations, dream work are not components of a doctrine, but empirically verified, scientific realities. If neurologists do have at their disposal, in their more limited diagnostic and therapeutic scope, electromechanical or electronic devices, such as electroencephalograms, echograms, tomographs, magnetic resonances and positron emission scanning, psychiatrists still do not have them. At least, outside the profit-oriented, make-believe propaganda promoted by large pharmaceutical and computerized devices industries. Those few who are not fooled have not been able to obtain space in the media, specialized or not, to publicize data emphasizing the basic failure of those methods when applied to psychiatric diseases. Take, for example, magnetic resonance: it is just a highly transformed, dead representation that obeys the rules now concocted not by physicians but by engineers specialized in "information technology", a sophisticated name for computers. What appears as "red" or "blue" in echograms, tomographies or magnetic resonance scanners has no real counterpart in the real, *in vivo* situation – in the same way as what happened with histological preparations from dead tissues. The high cost as well as the present impossibility to replicate the results obtained by "brain imagery" are left out from the news – either in respected periodicals or in the laymen's press (Bennett et al., 2009).

The situation is further complicated today with another newfangled social wave: the banal, inadequate use of a very useful scientific tool, statistics, to back what have been bandied as "evidence-based medicine" (Sackett et al., 1996; Hunink, 2004), a thing that, according to the propaganda of its advocates, outdates and must replace millennia-old knowledge. To be under the sway of old or new authoritarian rules is an expression of the French dictum coined by Jean Alphone Karr: *Plus ça change, plus c'est la même chose*. The same applies to the so-called superiority of cognitive psychotherapies invented by Aaron T. Beck vis-à-vis psychoanalysis (Shedler et al., 2015; Fonagy, 2015) – a contemporary version of the first "dissidences". Superficial psychology seems to be much more acceptable to laymen and women. One should ask: Who are the "lay analysts" today?

The psychoanalyst's working tools

In contrast, we analysts have more primitive working tools to perform our double-tracked activity into research and treatment of human nature and its sufferings (Freud, 1930, 1937a, 1937b, 1938a). As Freud (1913), inspired in Frazer and many other anthropologists, showed, "primitive" does not mean "worse" (Frazer, 1890; Malinowsky, 1929; Lévy-Strauss, 1955). One among our working tools can be named "personality"; it performs at least two operational functions that can be described with the aid of Kant's differentiation between objects and methods of scientific study. In psychoanalysis, our object of study and our method of study are the same: the personality (both of a patient and of ourselves). Analysts should not despair about the seeming confusion between our object and our methods. The same question befalls modern physics, biology and other practical scientific disciplines in which the observer participates in the phenomena he or she observes – as noticed by many. First and foremost, Freud. Our other primitive tool can be named "verbal formulations". It is empirically made in the here and now of an analytic session: ours and our patient's verbal formulations, which furnish what theorists of science call "lower-level empirical data" material. Its origins are in the medical practice and must be named as the method of individual cases. Nowadays, the fashionable nonsense looking for the "great data" results in a noxious dismissal of the method of individual cases Charlton and Walston (1988). Until now, little attention to the fact that the looking for "great data", a hyperbolic name for a misunderstood use of statistics and metadata, is responsible, in other "lay" disciplines such as economics, politics and meteorology, for harmful public orientations and decisions. Expressed in the bandwagon of an "evidence-based medicine", it was promptly aped by the psychological establishment.

Those facts helped to better the case against a newborn psychoanalysis, in a time when psychiatrists and neurologists became interested in immaterial facts, for example, hypnosis and seemingly physical diseases with no physical "causes". The same facts still help in the same case. This interest, Phoenix-like, emerges from time to time. In fact, along two millennia, there were and still are "physician psychologists": in Ancient Greece, with Aristotle, and in its revival in the Renaissance-Enlightenment-Romantic times, people today considered as "psychologists" were physicians. For example, John Locke and Wilhelm Wundt, the founder of modern psychology Dennis (1948).

Their work was ever hampered in times of too many beliefs, of too many authoritarian personalities in the role of false physicians rather than in the function of real physicians. As we tried to see, empowered by delusional transference, the false physicians many times belonged and still belong to ecclesiastical guilds rather than to scientific activities – especially when science is institutionalized and what was science turns out to be an elitist political network.

Another built-in feature of this belief-based empowerment is authoritarianship. The foundation of the first universities and institutionalized schools of medicine, performed with the conscious tendency to enhance the formation of real physicians, also contributed, due to the factor of quantity versus quality, to the increasing number of falsities. An effect of what can be named the discontents of our civilization (Freud, 1930), or the destructive effects of the variegated establishments (Bion, 1970, 1975). The final result is invariably another form of a "bloodland" (Snyder, 2010). One may observe that when science and art are more permeable or submitted to the political establishment, the less artistic and scientific their activists will be.

Conversely, Freud already had advanced many of his alternative and different views about this issue before: (1) his warnings about "wild analysis"; (2) his recommendations to physicians who needed to practice the psychoanalytic method – making clear that physicians could be seen as laymen or women in a then novel technique to deal with human nature and its sufferings which he was proposing; (3) his whole life defense of the scientific nature of psychoanalysis. This kind of defense, alas, is in doubt today, especially by those who could or wished not have a scientific or medical formation and, consequently, practice (Freud, 1910, 1912b, 1913b).

The editors of this book suppose that Freud made the "best of a bad job", in making a lasting, transcendent contribution to the psychoanalytic practice, including good-willed warnings and recommendations about the psychoanalytic formation.

The "bad job" can be described as a destructive, violent social action. It was a real fact in which there was a constant conjunction of two underlying complex factors that allowed for at least two vertexes of observation. On one hand, from a macro-vertex, it was possible to elicit social factors; on the other hand, from a micro-vertex of observation, it was possible to elicit psychoanalytical factors: namely, (1) financial factors, studied by historians and economists who cannot be accused to be sympathetic to psychoanalysis – quite the contrary[6]; and (2) a destructive cycle of greed-envy, the nest of rivalry, intra-group or outside from it (Smith, 1776; Marx, 1844; Kahnemann, 2011; Freud, 1905; Klein, 1957).

Human groups

Roughly half a century after the publishing of Freud's paper, most Western countries suffered from renewed fashionable, destructive mass trends disguised as if they were constructive. The trends were real facts in which it was possible to detect underlying, mostly unconscious factors. Born from despair, due to the subservience to the principle of pleasure–displeasure, those desire-ridden trends had and still have unavoidable "too human" companions: mindlessness and ritualistic hate toward truth (Nietzsche, 1878–1880; Freud, 1913).

One may identify still another factor that contributes to heighten mindlessness. It is known at least since the rescue of scientific methods by Renaissance authors such as Spinoza, Thomas Browne and Bacon:

> Solomon said: *There is no new thing upon the Earth.*
>
> So that as Plato had an imagination, that *all knowledge was but remembrance.*
>
> So Solomon giveth his sentence, that all novelty is but oblivion.
>
> (Bacon, 1625, p. 221)

It seems to the editors of this book that a more detailed description of the underlying factors conducive to forgetfulness and mindlessness can be found in Freud's work, even before his discovery of psychoanalysis, but especially after it, for example, with the mechanisms of dream work, from which one may emphasize repression, rationalization and negation (Freud, 1911b). The latter were later seen as the main mechanisms to unleash and construe psychotic states. In the end run, the main goal is to obliterate or preclude cognition, and a good enough access to truth.

In what is of concern to the encircling environment, Freud based his observations in the work of an anthropologist, of a sociologist and of a physician: respectively, James G. Frazer, Gustave Le Bon and Wilfred Trotter. Briefly, one may advance a synthetic, perhaps picturesque definition borrowed from a journalist, Mackay. It may sound rude to laymen and women but not to a psychoanalyst: extraordinary popular delusions and the madness of crowds. Such a mindset has been described in utterly different modes by many authors in different disciplines and activities encompassing millennia. It can be described as a socially shared hallucinosis, which has all the features of what Bion named as an invariance. One may spot it in Ancient myths, in literature and in philosophy. In Freud's time, one may quote people who never had personal contact with him: for example, Friedrich Nietzsche, Max Weber and Elias Cannetti. Also a few that supported him, as his "double nephew", the propagandist Edward Bernays and the sociologist Robert Merton. One may construct one's own roster, according to one's knowledge or personal preferences. Freud's observations, coupled consciously or not with those from other authors, gave rise to the work about groups of social and community psychologists and psychiatrists (Coelho, 1969; Martins and Sandler, 1980; Sandler, 1982). And of some analysts, one may quote Wilfred Ruprecht Bion, Siegmund Heinrich Foulkes and Enrique Pichón-Rivière (Nietsche, 1885–1885; Weber, 1905; Cannetti, 1935; Merton, 1948; Bernays, 2004/1928; Pichón-Rivière, 1980). It is not for a mere coincidence that Bion, who focused on the relationships between the encircling group and the behavior of analysts, named those facts as "catastrophic change". After all, Bion was one who rescued Freud's insights – that were being object of forgetfulness in his time:[7]

> In general it may be said that the cultural background against which analytic work must be done is hardly a matter with which the individual analyst can concern himself; yet the culture may concern him. In the exceptional case, notably Freud himself, psycho-analytic work has profoundly affected the social outlook. Therefore it is a matter of importance to analysts that the public image of our work is not distorted to produce a climate of opinion in which difficulties, already great, are enhanced. That image will be influenced by patients, their analysts, and the societies and groups that analysts form.
>
> (Bion, 1965, pp. 10–11)

In the last century, and in a heightened way in the beginning of our century, one may witness a rebirth of those fashionable trends. One may call those waves resorting to neologisms: medicalization (since the twenties), psychologization (since the thirties) and judicialization of social affairs. One witnesses the transformation of what once was common sense – technical nomenclature – into banal, common place, found easily in careless talk among laymen and women, and occupying a great deal of mass media. There is a community-shared little learning – a dangerous thing, according Alexander Pope in *Essay on Criticism*. If Hanna Arendt was right in pointing out the "banality of evil" (Arendt, 2006[1963]), would it be just a particular case of an ample and still most profound banality: evil-in-itself, disregard for life and truth?

Those trends affected the engineering of most micro-social settings,[8] including the psychoanalytical movement, which never was immune to them. Could it be? If one adopts Freud, Klein and Winnicott's theoretical models about human nature and its sufferings, one may well ask: Is not analysis, a technique to know, and to deal, in the extent it is possible, with one's "narcissism", one's extreme adherence to the "paranoid-schizoid" position, hampering or precluding one's free movement, in tandem, to the "depressive position"; to one's "false-self"? (Klein, 1946, 1957; Freud, 1915; Winnicott, 1955). Was the legal case against Theodor Reik, a case of enthronement of the medical profession, a case of seeing it as the top, the superior one? If there would be one "superior", it is psychologically needed to be an "inferior". In that time, psychoanalysts that had a medical formation composed a majority in the psychoanalytical movement.

For the sake of brevity, we quote a commentary by Bion. It is made in the form of a fictional dialogue between a "priest" named "Paul" and a "Psychoanalyst". Not for a mere coincidence, the same interlocutory technique form was already chosen by Freud in the classical paper under discussion, "The Question of Lay Analysis":

> PAUL (soliloquizing): Anyone would think psycho-analysts never quarrelled. When the Wars of Psycho-analysis start we shall see something – and no holds barred. Santayana feared the day when the scientific beasts and blackguards would get hold of the world. What made him speak of the English as "sweet boyish masters?"
>
> (Bion, 1977, p. 273)

Freud, Murphy and Reik's legal case proved to be the prototype of many following cases, when the hope of Freud and Reik seemed to be that it would be the last one. Nevertheless, we, future members of the psychoanalytic movement (in that time), were fated to witness the obtrusion of too many judiciary interventions, in the form of legal actions, involving private and public institutions, guilds and syndicates, revolving around the life of patients and professionals: "much ado about nothing". Perhaps it is a testimony of a truth stated in one of Marx's observations that history occurs first as a tragedy and then is repeated as a farce. Marx was a controversial historical figure but did not preclude that some of his observations were valid – even though he was, in the whole, a man who wanted to be an economist but, according to many, founded another form of religion (Marx, 1852; Campos, 1994, pp. 155, 911).

In hindsight, any "impartial person" can observe that in the year 1920 history configured itself in the realm of the micro-social phenomena that what was seen as being a "malpractice" by part of the representatives of the Austrian, German and Switzerland's medical establishment and their lawyers could be seen as a fundamentally financial social event.

A mere half century later, history configures itself under the guise of a breach of the United States "equality law", invoked by lawyers at the service of some psychologists, versus the "unlawful" International Psychoanalytical Association – as it was seen, or advertised, by the numerically growing establishment of psychologists. The same fact propagated, as if it was a case of contagion, in a "too human" mode, in less famous countries that already abided psychoanalytical movements. Not so few examples of this occurred in Brazil: the first professor of psychiatry in São Paulo state, Dr. Francisco Franco da Rocha, soon translated Freud's works. His practice, until then that of an alienist, now adopted the psychoanalytic method. As it occurred in other parts of the world, in a kind of aping, some of Dr. da Rocha's heirs dedicated themselves to practice with the psychoanalytic method; and soon inaugurated a local movement. Another portion of his heirs entrenched themselves into an "against" party. As it occurred in Europe and in the United States, this party was called, the "organicists". In the end run, they warred legal wars to extinguish the psychoanalytical movement; unable to do it, they tried to extinguish the method (Franco da Rocha, 1919; Marcondes, 1926; Pacheco e Silva, 1955). In the fifties, two painful examples plagued the psychoanalytical movement in Brazil: one involving Mr. Werner and Mrs. Ana Katrin Kemper,[9] former opportunistic adepts of Nazism who were part of the organization managed by Dr. Mathias Göring. Typical of those unscrupulous people who flatter the official authorities in the government, in order to get prestigious political posts, they tried to hide this fact. If in Germany they defended the Nazi regime, they had no qualms to defend leftist positions as soon as they saw that this was a fashion in Brazil (Roudinesco and Plon, 1997, p. 426). The other case involved the seemingly omnipresent Dr. Pacheco e Silva, a psychiatrist, and Mrs. Virginia Leone Bicudo, a lay analyst. The former was a professor of forensic psychiatry in two universities and in three schools; the latter was a social worker, lay analyst and co-founder of the Sociedade Brasileira de Psicanalise de São Paulo. Since its foundation, in 1921, by the most respected professor of psychiatry in Brazil, the first translator or Freud, Dr. Franco da Rocha, had a then rare, open posture toward lay analysts.

In the 1980s, a series of lawsuits was filed in the United States, a country already overwhelmed by an increasing "lawerization" of its social engineering. It pitted psychologists and their professional bodies against the "unlawful" International Psychoanalytical Association, then presided over by Dr. Robert Wallerstein. According to the most read daily newspaper in the United States:

> the long battle for patients between psychologists and psychiatrists has reached a new intensity, as psychologists try to break down barriers at hospitals and at some psychoanalytical training institutes. Last week a group of psychologists filed a new antitrust suit against the training institutes dominated by psychiatrists. Others have mounted a vigorous campaign to allow more psychologists to admit patients to hospitals. Although the debate ostensibly centres on how best to care for patients, some therapists see the real struggle as one of economic self-interest. The distinctions between the disciplines are at the heart of the dispute. Psychiatrists have medical training with a specialty in treating mental disorders. Psychologists have a Ph.D. and are also trained in treating mental problems but are restricted from prescribing medications. Psychoanalysts can come from any mental health profession and receive extensive training in Freudian techniques.
>
> (Goleman, 1988)

At that time, the same Dr. Wallerstein, together with others, such as Dr. Otto Kernberg, the following president of IPA, reported their worries about a diminishing quantity of younger psychiatrists in psychoanalytic courses (Kernberg, 1984). "Is Freud Dead?" asked an illustrated cover of the then best sold weekly (Gray, 1993) with a questionable content, promptly aped by the competition of a sensationalist printed press. Would it be a mere coincidence that this badly disguised advertisement emerged when "new happiness drugs" were also advertised in the same magazine? Again and again, psychoanalysis proper and the psychoanalytic movement are not adequately discriminated.

Twenty years later, those widely known facts still make part of the common place conversations among members of the IPA and many other organizations with training purposes. New psychoanalytical groups are constantly formed; and open or hidden discontents by disgruntled members abound, fostering the self-styled dissidences. The unabated pace of discontents now encompasses heated discussions about "non-presential" analysis, in an attempt to replace face-to-face contact with electronic means. Now it is increased with claims for a diminishing frequency of weekly sessions, that already is originating in an intra-IPA "war" (Sandler, 2013a, p. 229) in which they resort to laws, bylaws, rules and an authoritarian "majority" represented by a political meritocracy try to deal with relationship issues – as psychoanalysis properly is.

Does the resorting to financial or emotional lawsuits extrapolate the limits of a scientific or of a psychoanalytic interchange of ideas? If members of the psychoanalytic movement cannot resolve their questions, part of them seems to hope that other professionals – lawyers, judges, politicians, economists, sociologists, priests or others – that may appear could. It is outside the scope of this book to put forth a statistically backed scientific study about the numerous studies and claims from many authors who made part of the warring parties "pro" and "against". It seems to the editors of this book that this is the offspring of what was called, in Freud's time, "the lay analyst".

Quantity and quality: who's lay, in what?

Based in previous research, under the psychoanalytical vertex, we suppose that quality and quantity are two forms of presentation of the same existence that interact with each other under a complex manner. The question emerges in infancy; it can be put, for example, as a quasi-philosophical or quasi-mathematical puzzle to test the attention and intelligence of little children: "Consider that a ball coming from the blue falls over your head. What could be more damaging, if the ball was made of a hundred pounds of cotton or a hundred pounds of lead?" One may suppose that this puzzle to test the smartness either from the questioner or the questioned comprises quantity and quality taken as interacting variables by themselves in theoretical or in practical terms. In industry and commerce it is almost impossible, or at least utterly difficult, to deliver industrial products to mass consumption – which presupposes large quantities – without a correspondent loss in quality. This inverse relationship can be shown in those "the need or desire for money is obtrusive" (Bion, 1970, pp. 84, 85). In econometrics used in administration, it is common to measure this inverse relationship in terms of a calculation of a cost–benefit relationship. Those examples display the validity of the following comparison: Quality and Quantity also are two forms of presentation[10] of the very same existence – named by Freud "material reality" (equaled to quantity) and "psychic reality" (equaled to quality). As far as our research goes, the first name, material reality was coined by Immanuel Kant in 1761. One may fairly hypothesize that Freud was inspired by Kant to elicit the second name, psychic reality, in 1900, as an indispensable companion to the first one (Kant, 1781; Freud, 1900, pp. 538–541, 573, 610 and especially 614; Sandler, 1997, 2000).

The work of Kant was just one factor that formed Freud's intellectual environment – a powerful factor functioning together with Freud's individual abilities to give form to something then unknown, and named thereafter as psychoanalysis. As any single word to qualify a scientific discipline, the name psychoanalysis lacks precision. Later, Freud amended other names to it: deep psychology (already adumbrated by Janet and Maynert) and later on, psychodynamics. Freud's contributions to the knowledge of the very complex and mostly unknown processes that form what is usually known as "human nature" and its sufferings included a practical method to operate on it, under a constructive, or useful mode. Such an intellectual environment, usually called by theorists of science as his *zeitgeist* –a term coined by Von Herder (Cassirer (1906–1920), Hartmann (1960), Berlin, 1974). The enunciation of their names form a sizable roster; their contributions to psychoanalysis are reviewed elsewhere

(Sandler, 1997–2003). One must quote Plato, Aristotle, Sophocles, Shakespeare, Goethe, Darwin, Lamarck, Fechner, Von Helmholtz, Virschow and Brentano. The list is too long, as any practicing psychoanalyst knows. Each reader may choose his or her particular list according to his or her preferences or knowledge. Few would argue that the contributions from the previously mentioned authors could not be included in such a list.

A fundamental fact to the elaboration of this present book is that Freud underwent two interlinked experiences: he submitted himself to medical training and thereafter practiced medicine. Human nature and its sufferings were studied by him under the vertex of medicine. Is psychoanalysis therefore an inheritance from a medicine?

Is medicine one among the first manifestations of a "scientific nucleus" of us, human beings?

For "science", the authors of the introduction to this book mean the making of approaches the most possible outside the realm of belief to achieve apprehensions of reality as it is. Science is one of the modes available to us to "realize" in its purest form. Art is another form; one cannot be sure if it is more antique or not. Is "science" a prototype of our appeals to counter the primitive, albeit natural movement that can be seen as an unbroken, chaotic expansion of our psychotic nuclei? Most psychoanalysts that use Freud, Klein, Winnicott and Bion's observations accept that psychosis is a state in which there is severe denial of the existence of reality, and that this denial of reality reaches its climax in the extent that psychotics have a quasi-absolute intolerance of frustration. In other terms, psychotics are enslaved by the Principle of Pleasure–Displeasure. Their attempts to make imperial denials to the inception of the Principle of Reality are doomed to failure, albeit temporarily circumvented in their perception, by hallucinations and delusions.

Wilfred Bion tried to integrate the work of Freud, Klein and theoreticians of mathematics in order to remind us, psychoanalysts, that mathematicians gave us a seminal concept: the number zero – a remarkable achievement of Ancient Greeks, displaying a real growth of our processes of thinking. Bion took his observations mainly from three of Freud's papers: *Formulations on the Two Principles of Mental Functioning*, *Beyond the Pleasure Principle*, and *On Negation* (Freud, 1911a, 1920, 1925). From Klein, Bion took her observations included mainly in a paper and in a book: *Notes on Some Schizoid Mechanisms* and *Envy and Gratitude* (Klein, 1946, 1957); the mathematicians quoted by Bion are Euclid, Plato, Proclus and Gottlob Frege. In doing this, Bion suggested that mathematics also furnished us human beings with a way to deal with what can be named the emotional experience – real or hallucinated – of what lacks; the lacking of anything, which to some people equals lacking everything (Bion, 1962, pp. 103–105; 1963, p. 2; 1965, pp. 55–58; 1970, p. 90).

Would be the conception of the existence of zero a primeval mode to deal with psychosis?

The example given by Bion begins with the struggles to found a name to it, displayed historically in the diatribe between Proclus and Plato and in the discussions between Zenon and Aristotle. The later retracted from his earlier definitive statements about the impossibility of any kind of realization about the existence of a counterpart in reality corresponding to the concept of infinite (Aristotle, 360 B.C., pp. 315, 359; Heath, 1956, Chapter 9; Bell, 1937; Anderson and Zalta, 2004). Social applications of mathematics provided examples about this issue – tolerance to frustration – during the last millennia. For example, the inception of methods of measurement to limit – define – arable properties alongside the Nile. One may imagine the degree of frustration such a limitation possibly caused to Ancient Egyptians. The same happened – and with more historical testimony – in the promulgation of the Magna Carta: an enduring breach to King John's greed that solemnized the dawning of a durable judicious era in England.

The editors of this book resort to a fable, to be amended to Bion's suggestion: before, or together, or after (it is not possible to delimitate it historically) the obtrusion of mathematical thinking, as the prototype of a scientific nucleus in our psyche, we propose to consider another transcendent situation. Namely, when primitive hominids, 100,000 years ago, witnessed that one among their contemporaries had suffered a serious and undoubtful injury. For example, he or she had just lost one of his or her leg, or arm, or other parts of his or her body. In consequence, he or she exposed inner organs. He or she could have been overwhelmed by environmental conditions, such as inclement weather, or sudden, or chronic, geological changes; he or she could have been overwhelmed by environmental conditions, such as inclement weather, or sudden, or chronic, geological changes. One may imagine other probable ailments: he or she could face the attack of a ferocious or cruel animated entity like a dinosaur or a furry saber-toothed tiger in a savannah. The list is rather long: the male or female hominid, still uninformed by previous experience, in a search for shelter, could be forced to enter into a cave to protect him or herself from, say, a snowy inclement weather. But the cave already abided a bear. Or the hapless hominid could have performed a reckless act under an attempt to try to get food and ate a poisonous mushroom. Or, with more probability, had to face another hominid more prone to make a cruel attack. Some of those situations, with most probability, could have been almost self-inflicted – the hominid could have made provocations or evocations in other animated entities, or even inanimate objects, demanding too much from either one of those. In the next moment, an injury ensued from what we today, under the analytic vertex, call an acted out impetus revealing omnipotent and omniscient phantasies. That, for its turn, owe their genesis to a severe disregard to truth. More often than not – for sure, in our current times – and most probably in that time, those were cases of a "self-assault". The unavoidable consequence of being moved preferentially by desire, under the aegis of the principle of pleasure–displeasure.

Another passerby, also a hominid, could find him or herself pulled or pushed by a need to help the hapless injured contemporary. This was a need, not a desire. Someone born in a primitive Indo-European society, called this enterprising fact – to help, to care –as *medeor*. Today it is called "medicine". Etymologically, the words, motion, move, emotion and medicine keep the same origin. They found their correspondents in the reality of human nature. The editors of this book suppose that medicine, or at least the rescue of medicine in the Enlightenment, is the most remote origin of psychoanalysis. This supposition finds bearings in Freud's emphases in the need of development of the psychoanalytic method vis-à-vis the methods used in medicine – including expansions as well as differences.

Those emphases included a kind of technical counsel, made by a mix of direction and warning, in the form of an analogy. Namely, a psychoanalyst should pattern his or her attitude under the model of a surgeon (Freud, 1912b, p. 114). His many references about this pattern, sometimes indicating another medical speciality, different from surgery, such as pediatrics (Freud, 1900, p. 575), would demand a whole book to be described. It seems to the editors that it was not by coincidence that the translation of Freud's paper about lay analysis was made by a lay analyst: Mrs. Joan Riviere.

In the other side, in what concerns to differences, we analysts make heavy use of verbal formulations – what Freud called "word-representation" – as our brain's ability to make images through the aid of our sight apparatus, two of our fundamental working tools. Language formation, symbol formation and dreams were the clinical nest of Freud's discovery of psychoanalysis.

> Nothing takes place between them except that they talk to each other. The analyst makes use of no instruments – not even for examining the patient – nor does he prescribe any medicines. If it is at all possible, he even leaves the patient in the environment and in his usual mode of life during the treatment. This is not a necessary condition, of course, and may not always be practicable. . . . And incidentally do not let us despise the word. After all it is a powerful instrument; it is the means by which words. . . . Words can do unspeakable good and cause terrible wounds. . . . But originally the word was magic – a magical act; and it has retained much of its ancient power.
>
> (Freud, 1927, pp. 187–188)

Those human traits, tendencies and moving actions are displayed in the realm of phenomena and can be represented scientifically by their respective counterparts as verbal formulations in some scientific disciplines. At first, "medicine"; and later, in specializations called "psychology", "psychiatry" and "psychoanalysis". Are those names really useful in real practice? Could those names be seen as useful to the issuing of official certificates legalized by governmental agencies? Is it needed, or even possible to regulate legally what is real? Is truth determined by a higher authority, while this "higher" is dependent of peers which are equals in their innermost aspects – human beings? Personal skills are genetically dependent; and also dependent of social opportunities. Is there a higher authority than nature itself, and probability, that can regulate genetic and social opportunities? Are those opportunities at the service of our will, of our desire and pleasure? Are they subservient to our tendency to avoid displeasure, or to accept it if our pleasure is made by what is, under a common-sense view, displeasure – as one may find in sadism (Freud, 1920)?

If Freud remained deeply interested in his whole scientific life, in researching and describing verbal formulations – we analysts do not have at our disposal chemical formulations, mathematical or musical formulations to communicate with our patients or with our colleagues – he was also deeply interested, in his whole scientific life, in researching and describing the possible relationships between quantity and quality of material and psychic "forces". This issue had a kind of reticent rebirth with the timid acknowledgment about the "prescient" work of Freud by a few "neuroscientists" such as Erich Kandel (2012, p. 520), and in the form of deep, continuing and seemingly insurmountable controversies, as those propitiated by a proposed "neuropsychoanalysis", by Mark Solms (for example, Blass and Carmeli, 2015; Yovell et al., 2015).

In any case, leaving aside delayed and confusing acknowledgments in the form of praises and acceptance, as well as the profiting to launch yet more disciplines with no empiric evidence to base them on, it is possible to notice that Freud mentions a "psychic intensity", in which it seems clear to the authors of this text that he emphasizes the relationship between a quality – "psychic" – and a quantity – "intensity" (Freud, 1900, pp. 575, 583ff.). James Strachey's editorial comments help the reader to find its origin: they are in another remarkable attempt of Strachey to contribute to spreading Freud's word. Strachey – but not Freud – called a writing as a "project for a scientific psychology" (Freud, 1895) what in reality was Freud's unfinished, posthumously published notes of observational inferences he made about our sensuous apparatus and the dynamic responses of us, human beings, as they could be seen and grossly measured in that time, reflecting our feelings, affects, emotions and emotional experiences. Freud decided not to publish it; yet he used parts of it in all his later works; it served as a kind of draft. In Part I, one may vouch that he used the name "forces". It is as common in Freud's work as it was in Gustav Fechner and Herrman von Helmholtz's. Those "forces" were better named as "instincts" – thanks to Freud's introjection of Darwin and Lamarck's contributions to human nature and its sufferings into his own discovery, psychoanalysis. "Instincts", or inner and outer (as an inheritance) push, manifested as "cathexes" seems to be an indispensable hallmark of any animated entity one may consider. Both in those denominations and in their counterparts in reality, one cannot see any kind of split, for example, between "matter" or "energy". Freud did not have available modern genetics or molecular biology, but there are implicit indications of his awareness of Friedrich Miescher's work, who described the existence of a "nuclein", which gave base to later contributions by Mendel, Watson and Crick (Freud, 1920; Pray, 2008).

Ancient Greek's words – *psyche* and *physis* (ψυχή and φυσική) – attempt to describe those inner and outer material and immaterial "pushing" entities without any kind of attempt to split them. Those attempts inextricably linked, in a complex way, the descriptions of two human attributes, with no cleavage between the realities corresponding to those names. This is not a detailed study on Ancient Greek's apprehension about human nature and its sufferings, that can be seen in works made by scholars capable to do it, which is not the case of the editors of this book. Briefly, Ancient Greek's ideas made for a rather complex structure of thought, expressed through a real nomenclature associated to human "material and psychic" or, in Bion's nomenclature, "sensuous and psychic" attributes: *etor*, *nous*, *phrenes*, etc. We refer the reader to the studies of Onians and Jaynes – in the last one, there is a description of the beginning of the formidable splitting between *physis* and *psyche*, called by this author the inception of consciousness with a "bicameral mind" (Onians, 1951, pp. 95, 13, 38, 107–111, 184, 247, 253; Jaynes, 1976, pp. 68–83; the beginnings of the splitting can be seen from p. 84 onwards). Such splitting had a seminal impulse with the work of the young Aristotle; St Thomas Aquinas profited from it, as well as René Descartes (D'Arcy, 1953) at the service of interests of the apostolic branch of the Roman Catholic Church, which reigned all alone in social settings and therefore, in the thought processes of people in Europe for centuries. It was critically focused on by some people who lived before Kant, such as Baruch Spinoza and Blaise Pascal, who were careful about the reactions of the ecclesiastic authorities. Both equated the word "God" to "Truth". A decisive action, in the case of Pascal, that was barely able to avoid the murderous wrath of the authoritarian Inquisition. For example:

> One thought alone occupies us; we cannot think of two things at the same time. This is lucky for us according to the world, not according to God.
>
> (Pascal, 1657)

If it is valid to make a verbal analogy about the ultimately unknowable absolute truth – the numinous realm – with "God", made by many, as Luria, the Sufists, St John of the Cross, Meister Ekhard and other thinkers and poets, as well as the fable that "what therefore God hath joined together, let no man put asunder" (St. Mark's Gospel, 10:9), then it is also true that what man splits asunder, no God yet created could join again. The examples are many: for example, a broken Humpty-Dumpty. Is this the same for "material and psychic reality"? Its apprehension as a oneness proved to be difficult to many; the same applies to quantity and quality.

There are verbal formulations that hitherto proved to endure the test of time: *techné* –known in our times as technology; and also *psyche* and *physis*. The same cannot be said about their correspondents in reality, giving reasons to those who cast doubt about the development of mankind's thought processes:

> Is the supposition that the reptilian age is antecedent to Hitler correct or is it a feature of our thinking process which has become an aberration which has not been considered, but has become part of what is observed?
>
> (Bion, 1975, p. 76)

Probably the only renewing is just an illusion about our ability to apprehend reality, similar to that described in Plato's analogy about shadows in a cave, in the form of a dialogue between two characters, Glaucus and Socrates (Plato, c. 380 A.C., pp. 388–389). Is there a way out? For example, there are indications of the real existence of a cycle, difficult to observe in the extent that the observer makes part of the observed, in which developments are followed by decaying, followed by developments that are mostly the past forgotten and rescued, with the appearance of new developments. In the realm of individuality, there are descriptions of a similar cycle. For example, in the tandem movement between the paranoid-schizoid position and the depressive positions (Klein, 1946). Does what Klein observed in individuals apply to the processes of thought as they can be seen in the history of ideas in Western civilization?

The splitting between *psyche* and *physis* – in the area of human consciousness – seemed to be a tendency that had and still has the upper hand in the mass. It has been manifested under a series of denominations: matter or energy; mind or body; and other dichotomies better studied by philosophers. Graphically, "and" is replaced by "or". Bion's proposal to use the theory of transformations and invariants, akin to the forays into reality made by the mystic tradition, makes possible a discipline over that split:

> My theory would seem to imply a gap between phenomena and the thing-in-itself and all that I have said is not incompatible with Plato, Kant, Berkeley, Freud and Klein, to name a few, who show the extent to which they believe that a curtain of illusion separates us from reality. Some consciously believe the curtain of illusion to be a protection against truth which is essential to the survival of humanity; the remainder of us believe it unconsciously but no less tenaciously for that. Even those who consider such a view mistaken and truth essential consider that the gap cannot be bridged because the nature of the human being precludes knowledge of anything beyond phenomena save conjecture. From this conviction of the inaccessibility of absolute reality the mystics must be exempted.
>
> (Bion, 1965, p. 147)

Lay analysis

Would the practical – social – questions encircling "lay analysis" have been originated in this fundamental, and under our view, utterly serious, distorting (in the realm of apprehension by our thought processes) splitting? A split that some, as for example, in ancient civilizations, especially Greek – did not make? It seems to the editors that Freud also did not make it – as well as many other thinkers and scientists, such as Charles Darwin, Albert Einstein, Max Planck, Erwin Schrödinger, Paul Dirac, Werner Heisenberg and their followers, Isaac Rabi, Stephen Hawking, Peter Highs (Rabi et al, 1939; Planck, 1949; Einstein, 1916/1952; Taylor, 2011).

> The unconscious is the true psychical reality; in its innermost nature it is as much unknown to us as the reality of the external world, and it is as incompletely presented by the data of consciousness as is the external world by the communications of our sense organs. . . . If we look at unconscious

> wishes reduced to their most fundamental and truest shape, we shall have to conclude, no doubt, that psychical reality is a particular form of existence not to be confused with material reality.
>
> (Freud, 1900, pp. 607, 614)

This was already outlines in the provisional, unfinished text that Marie Bonaparte discovered by pure chance and was later named by James Strachey as Freud's Project for a Scientific Psychology (Freud, 1895). It seems to us that too many in the analytical movement read this phrase as if the two forms of existence would be two existences. Until now no one detected and thus described if there is another form, but after Freud, we analysts can know and deal with at least **two forms** – or transformations of the same invariance, if one adopts Bion's borrowing of a mathematical term coined by Sylvester and Cayley (Sandler, 2005, p. 360, 2006). The invariance, or existence – in Freud's terminology – are one and the same: reality itself. For this reason, Freud wrote about material and psychic reality. The issue is clear in the following paragraph taken from "The Question of Lay Analysis":

> Other patients, again, suffer from disturbances in a particular field in which emotional life converges with demands of a bodily sort. If they are men, they find they are incapable of giving physical expression, to their tenderest feelings towards the opposite sex, while towards less loved objects they may perhaps have every reaction at their command.
>
> (Freud, 1927, p. 186)

Even if Freud rarely made the split, and never made it after his discovery of psychoanalysis, influential members in the scientific (or technical) or political meritocracies of the psychoanalytical movement, usually seen by members of the same movement as "-ians" of too many types ("freudians", "jungians", "kleinians", "lacanians", etc.) did and still do what seems to us a serious splitting – as far as our research in published papers and books could go (for example: Sandler, 2005, 2015b, pp. 104, 218, 301). There are too many repeated misreadings, leading to misunderstanding of what Freud wrote. This was conducive, for example, to claims that analysts must promote a "return toward Freud", as stated by Jacques Lacan. Another consequence is wasteful, false controversies about "a Freud" who would be too "physicalist", too "organicist", too "positivist" versus "a Freud" who would be too "psychological", "metaphysical", "unscientific" – the centuries-old quarrel between "idealists" versus "realists". The underlying tendency in the processes of thought remains unconscious, our unknown, motivating new names to the same fact, giving evidence to the popular ditto: old wine in new bottles – what Kant named "idealists", are also known as "subjectivists", "relativists", or, in Freud's time, "solipsists", disagreeing radically with "realists", "positivists", etc.

Those controversies involved members of the psychoanalytical movement moved by certain tendencies and preferences, many times ideological; and theorists of science. In the latter case, too many times with lack of experience in analysis and excess of vanity, promptly profited by large editorial groups whose interest was not the advancement of science but profitable sales (Popper, 1963 Ellenberger, 1970; Sulloway, 1978; Grunbaum A., 1984; Eysenck and Eisenck, 1985).

The result, until now, could be seen as a weird democratic distribution of the same over-simplified misunderstanding of most texts written by Freud. The qualification, "weird democratic" is justified if democracy is seen as a respect toward minorities – as it is practiced in the most successful democracies since its rescue and hitherto final enunciation by John Locke.

It is a known fact that when a social system enshrines the dictatorship of majorities under a mindless group mentality, typical of the masses, this system empowers an armed elite, composing a political meritocracy. This meritocracy is the only minority allowed to survive; all the others are murderously disrespected. In artistic and scientific groups, the disrespect is directed toward the artistic and scientific minorities. The work of the now idolized symbols is co-opted in order to keep reigning in the elite, made by the political meritocracy. The co-optation is made mainly by little learning of what was, in the past, the work of the pioneers and discoverers. There are telling examples of this situation in many places around the world. The European case is probably the most well known: the minorities, with the exception of that forming a political meritocracy, can be almost extinguished. This happened with the Armenians in Turkey; with Jews and other slaves in the Nazi regime; with Germans in the Baltic states, which swiftly passed from conquerors to vanquished. This is an everyday example of the relationship of quantity with quality.

Little learning

The misunderstanding spread over in the psychoanalytical movement, expressed by the various scholastic tendencies, named "-isms" (freudism, etc.), are called "dissidences". Both in its beginnings, and determining its ends, there is a personal factor, manifesting itself as personal tendencies moved by desire, memory and understanding, that is far from the psychoanalytic vertex (Freud, 1937b, 1938b; Bion, 1967a, pp. 127, 137, 143; 1967b, pp. 2, 143–148, 1970, pp. 107, 124). This is a basic feature of erudite scholars – there is no scarcity of them – endowed of **no** psychoanalytic training.

"Dissidences" seem to be a kind of hallmark of the history of the psychoanalytical movement. Many times disguised as "theoretical development", its underlying nature is strikingly similar to what happened in the main religious movements in the last millennia, a fact already noticed by many analysts, such as Freud, Franz Alexander, Bion and many others. It is also similar to the mass political movement named in the common place as "the left".

There is no scarcity of members of the psychoanalytic movement displaying a tendency to be moved by "naïve idealism". Its main manifestation is a tendency to replace psychoanalysis proper by heterologous transplantations of other disciplines: in our days, mainly literature, myths, postmodernism's philosophy, or positivist-oriented approaches (Sandler, 2001, 2013b, 2015a,b,c). Is it a deep, if unwitting, attack against Freud's achievements?

> To turn to psycho-analysis; the erudite can see that a description is by Freud, or Melanie Klein, but remain blind to the thing described. Freud said infants were sexual; this was denied or reburied. This fate could have befallen the whole of psycho-analysis had there been no one to confer, as Horace said of Homer, immortality. If psycho-analytic intuition does not provide a stamping ground for wild asses, where is a zoo to be found to preserve the species? Conversely, if the environment is tolerant, what is to happen to the "great hunters" who lie unrevealed or reburied?
>
> (Bion, 1975, p. 5)

Or, in more theoretical terms:

> The individual analyst has two main contacts: his patients and society. In the first certainly, and in the second probably, he will have it brought home to him how little he knows and how poor

> his work is . . . when concentration is focused predominantly on psychotic mechanisms, the non-psychotic aspects of the work must be as present to the analyst's mind as his awareness of the non-psychotic aspects of the psychotic patients' personality are in the analysis he is conducting.
>
> (Bion, 1959, p. 24)

Are we analysts free from acting out their own psychotic personality through non-psychotic (under the view of society) actions, such as increasing in the quantity of analysts and patients – a highly prized political act that can be rationalized under a series of plausible reasons, for example, economical, of social class, etc. – at the expense of the quality of their work? This is not reserved to lay or non-lay analysts. Nevertheless, some members in the psychoanalytic movement, driven by the simplistic, wishful, rationalistic and positivist beliefs of causality and cure, who argue that psychoanalysis cures narcissistic or paranoid traits. As this is a pure logical conclusion based in belief, they are countered by other members of the psychoanalytic movement, who argue that they are wrong. Their counterargument is also driven by rationalistic logic – they belief that psychoanalysis is able to improve one's narcissism, because to them the cause of the illness is the lack of one's narcissism. Other people fantasize that a patient is glued to the paranoid-schizoid position and to get a cure, analysis make the patient to be glued to the depressive position. What was just an abstract, scientific model, our theory is now taken as if it was a concrete thing. Still, another people fantasize that a patient is cured when the analyst makes public confessions of countertransference in written works. The last one is just a complication of another idea, that one may use his countertransference, as if this phenomenon could be dealt with outside the analyst's personal analysis.

Along the whole history of the psychoanalytical movement, those facts emerged both with people who have the medical formation or not – the "lay analysts". As Freud tried to show, some "lay analysts", due to their experiences in life, could be much more "medical" than the "non-lay analysts". And some "medical analysts" could be much more informed in all the areas alien to the medical formation highlighted by Freud. Being himself, the prototype of them.

In brief: (1) are the "real lay analysts" or the people who despise, albeit unconsciously, real analysis those who espouse idealized ideas of cure rather than *practice* of a physician's methods of diagnosis and care, or treatment ("therapeutiké", or the mix of "iatriké" and "therapeutaz"), as observed Winnicott (1968); (2) are the "real lay analysts" those who display a *furor curandis* typical of young people who submit themselves to either the medical or to the psychological formation?; (3) are the "real lay analysts" those who replace psychoanalysis with erudition, those who replace psychoanalytic actions with "psycho-babble" duly disguised as theories, using terms that were created to describe facts but now are snobbishly uttered into plausible, palatable but unreal verbal constructs to delight audiences?

If one accepts the following minor addiction based on more than a half century of experience to Freud's text extracted from page 246 of The Question of Lay Analysis, one may conclude that:

> Analytic training, it is true, cuts across the field of medical education, but neither includes nor excludes the other. An analyst, privately or in any institutionalized training, must have an introduction to depth-psychology, or psycho-analysis; to theory of science, for psycho-analysis is the most pure practical theory of science; biology, mathematics, the science of sexual life, the symptomatology of psychiatry; must have a deep and real contact and dealing with people who meet death and life-threatening menaces; of obstetrics and palliative medicine; must be deeply informed in the history of civilization, mythology, psychology of religion, military and economics; and in the science of literature.

Would it be a timely advice – in a troubled epoch like ours – when people, either supporting or against psychoanalysis, issue statements, with no vestige of scientific doubt, that psychoanalysis is a false science? That it is just another form of literature? A time in which some "lay analysts" regard the words "psychiatry" and "physician" as dirty words? After all, in regards to quantity, "lay analysts" are today the vast majority in the psychoanalytical movement. It is possible to put forth the following hypothesis: one of the results of this is that anyone who dares to practice analysis four or five times a week will be fated to make it secretly. Are those analysts fated to follow the first Christians, who had to pray in the catacombs? To state this kind of practice publicly is an invitation to the opprobrium: to be labeled as "anachronic". Anyone in some places in the world who studies Freud's metapsychology or makes research into psychic reality is labeled as anachronic (Green, 2003). As it occurred in Freud's time, the same argument is bandied both by people who are self-styled as "pro-analysis" or "against psychoanalysis". "All colors agree in the dark," observed (Bacon, 1625, p. 61).

Notes

1 In a personal communication in 1981 by typewritten letter to one of the organizers of this book who wished to apply Wallerstein's ideas about this doctorate in the Faculdade de Saúde Publica da Universidade de São Paulo agreed with the hypothesis that there were evidences that Freud could not be too appreciative of such an enterprise.

2 Studies in large groups about the prevalence of mental and neurological diseases and birth order could not establish any kind of statistically significant correlation between those two facts. Three of those studies as well as a complete review can be seen in Sandler and Sandler (1978, 1981).

3 For example: an Italian who makes part of a Mafia syndicate; a Scottish, Arab, Jew, French or North American who makes part of any kind of money-making industry and is seen as if he or she is stingy; a foreigner who immerses himself in theaving, etc.

4 Rationalization and denial: the most basic modes to warrant the prevalence of the psychotic personality (Freud, 1911b, 1925; Bion, 1957).

5 Historically, since 1950, named chlorpromazine, imipramine, diazepine and others, which interfere in the functioning of a special kind of peptides, called by neurologists as the "neuromediators". It is just a very tiny known stage into an unknown range of electro-chemical transmission of impulses along the nervous system.

6 Who, among us psychoanalysts, take into account, in our written contributions to our field, the financial factors? It would be a digression to dwell about it now.

7 For example: dream work; research into the unconscious system (then unfavored, due to the more fashionable inception of ego-psychology); the need of training of analysis; attention to the here and now; the critical scrutiny of unwittingly ad hoc application of theories.

8 Who, outside the utterly tiny psychoanalytic movement, had heard about or given importance to the lawsuit in Austria against "the medical malpractice" made by a Prof. Theodor Reik?

9 Whose name was misspelled by Ernest Jones (op. cit, 1957, p. 315).

10 In Freud's usage of the German language, *Vorstellung*. Unfortunately, most translations to the English language (and other languages, too) mistake "presentation" with "representation", which would better correspond to *Die Vertretung*. We cannot dwell on the question of translation

now, for reasons of space and scope of the introduction to this book. It is widely acknowledged that those questions do exist, despite Strachey's strenuous effort to include detailed notes justifying or marking his options as a translator.

References

Adorno, I.W., Frenkel-Brunswlk, E., Levinson, D.J., and Sanford, R.N. (1950). *The Authoritarian Personality*. New York: Harper & Row.

Anderson, D.J. and Zalta, E. (2004). Frege, Boolos, and Logical Objects. *Journal of Philosophical Logic*, 13: 1–26.

Arendt, H. (1958). *The Human Condition*. Chicago: University of Chicago Press.

Arendt, H. (1979). *The Origins of Totalitarianism*. San Diego: Harvest Books, Harcourt & Brace.

Arendt, H. (2006 [1963]). *Eichmann in Jerusalem: A Report on the Banality of Evil*. London: Penguin.

Aristotle. (c. 360 B.C.). Physics, VI, chapters 1–8. English version by R.P. Hardie and R.K. Gaye. In: *The Great Books of Western Hemisphere*. Chicago: The Encyclopedia Britannica Inc.

Bacon, F. (1625). Of Vicissitudes of Things. In: J. Pitcher (Ed.), *The Essays*. London: Penguin, 1985.

Bell, E.T. (1937). *Men of Mathematics*. Touchstone Books, Kindle edition, Seattle: Amazon.com, 2014.

Bennett, C., Baird, A.A., Miller, M.B., and Wolford, G.L. (2009). Neural Correlates of Interspecies Perspective Talking in the Post-Mortem Atlantic Salmon: An Argument for Multiple Comparisons Correlation. *Journal of Serendipitous and Unexpected Results*, 1: 1–5. Extraído de www./prefrontal.org.

Berlin, I. (1974). *Against the Current: Essays in the History of Ideas*. Londres: Pimlico, 1997.

Bernays, E. (2004/1928). *Propaganda*. Seattle: Kindle edition, Amazon Digital Services.

Bion, W.R. (1957). The Differentiation of the Psychotic and Non-Psychotic Personalities. In: *Second Thoughts*: London: Heinemann Medical Books, 1967.

Bion, W.R. (1959). *Common Sense*. Ed. Francesca Bion. London: Karnac, 1992.

Bion, W.R. (1961). *Experiences in Groups*. London: Tavistock Publications.

Bion, W.R. (1962). *Learning from Experience*. London: Heinemann Medical Books.

Bion, W.R. (1963). *Elements of Psychoanalysis*. London: Heinemann Medical Books.

Bion, W.R. (1965). *Transformations*. London: Heinemann Medical Books.

Bion, W.R. (1967a). Notes on Memory and Desire. In: Francesca Bion (Ed.), *Cogitations*. London: Karnac, 1992.

Bion, W.R. (1967b). Commentary. In: *Second Thoughts*. London: Heinemann Medical Books.

Bracher, K. (1968). *The German Dictatorship*. New York: Penguin, 1991.

Bion, W.R. (1970). *Attention and Interpretation*. London: Tavistock Publications.

Bion, W.R. (1975). *A Memoir of the Future*. Volume I: The Dream. London: Karnac, 1991.

Bion, W.R. (1977). *A Memoir of the Future*. Volume II: The Past Presented. London: Karnac, 1991.

Blass, R.B., and Carmeli, Z. (2015). Further Evidence for the Case Against Neuropsychoanalysis: How Yovell, Solms and Fotopoulo Response to Our Critique Confirms the Irrelevance and Harmfulness to Psychoanalysis of the Contemporary Neuroscientific Trend. *International Journal of Psychoanalyis*, 96: 1555–1573.

Bullock, T.H., Bennett, M.V.L., Johnston, D., Robert Josephson, R., Marder, E., and Fields, R.D. (2005). The Neuron Doctrine, Redux/. *Science*, 5749, 310: 791–793, doi:10.1126/science.1114394.

Campos, R. (1994). *Lanterna de Popa: Memórias*. Rio de Janeiro: Topbooks Editora.

Cannetti, E. (1935). *Crowds and Poor*. English version, by Carol Stewart. New York: Viking Press, 1962.

Cassirer, E. (1906–20). *El Problema del Conocimiento en la Filosofia y en las Ciencias Modernas*. Spanish version by W. Roces. Mexico: Fondo de Cultura Economica, 1957.

Castiglioni, A. (1941). *História da Medicina*. Versão Brasileira, por R. Laclette. São Paulo: Companhia Editora Nacional, 1947.

Charlton, B.G. and Walston, F. (1988). Individual Case Studies in Clinical Research. *Journal of Evaluation in Clinical Practice*, 4: 147–155.

Coelho Filho, J.C., Takenami, I., and Arruda, S. (2013). Revisiting Rich's Formula: An Update About Granulomas in Human Tuberculosis. *Brazilian Journal of Infectious Diseases*, 17: 234–238.

Coelho, R.G.A. (1969). *Estrutura Social e Personalidade*. São Paulo: Livraria Pioneira Editora.

Comte, A. (1896). *The Positive Philosophy of Auguste Comte*. English version by H. Martineau. Londres; George Bell & Sons; reprinted electronically by Batoche Books, Ontario, 2000: http://socserv2.socsci.mcmaster.ca/econ/ugcm/3113/comte/Philosophy3.pdf.

D'Arcy, M.C. (1953). *St. Thomas Aquinas*. Dublin: Clonmore & Reynolds.

Darwin, C. (1871). Mental Powers of Man and the Lower Animals. In: *The Descent of Man. Origin of Species*. In: Mortimer Adler (Ed.), *The Great Books of the Western World*, Chicago: Encyclopedia Britannica Inc., 1994.

Dennis, W. (Ed.) (1948). *Readings in the History of Psychology*. East Norwalk: Appleton-Century-Crofts, pp. 206–213: Elements of Psychophysics, por G.T. Fechner; versão inglesa por H.S.Langfeld.

Einstein, A. (1916/1952). Relativity: The Special and General Theory; English version by Robert. H Lawson. In: *The Great Books of the Western World*. Chicago: Encyclopedia Britannica Inc.

Ellenberger, H. (1970). *The Discovery of the Unconscious*. English version, by New York: Basic Books.

Eysenck, H., and Eysenck, S. (1985). *The Decline and Fall of the Freudian Empire*. Londres: Penguin, 1988.

Fenichel, O. (1945). Neurotic Acting-Out. In: *The Collected Papers of Otto Fenichel*. New York: W. W. Norton and Company, 1954. This paper seems to those organizers as the best review of Freud's concept of acting-out hitherto published.

Fonagy, P. (2015). The Effectiveness of Psychodynamic Psychotherapies: An Update. *World Psychiatry: Official Journal of the World Psychiatric Association*. Retrieved in http:/www.researchgate.net/publication/277779884.

Franco da Rocha, F. (1919). *A Doutrina de Freud – resumo geral indispensável para a comrehensão da psicoanalise: segunda edição de pansexualismo*. São Paulo: Companhia Editora Nacional, 1930.

Frazer, J. (1890). The Golden Bough. www.templeofearth.com/books/goldenbough.pdf

Freud, F. (1925). Negation. *SE*, XIX.

Freud, S. (1891). *On Aphasia*. English version, by E. Stengel. New York: IUP.

Freud, S. (1900). The Interpretation of Dreams. *SE*, VI.

Freud, S. (1905). Three Essays on the Theory of Sexuality. *SE*, VII.

Freud, S. (1909). Five Lectures on Psycho-Analysis. *SE*, XI.

Freud, S. (1910). Wild Analysis. *SE*, X.

Freud, S. (1911a). Formulations on the Two Principles of Mental Functioning. *SE*, XII.

Freud, S. (1911b). Psycho-Analytic Notes on an Autobiographical Account of a Case of Paranoia. *SE*, XII.

Freud, S. (1912a). The Dynamics of Transference. *SE*, XII.

Freud, S. (1912b). Recommendations for Physicians on the Psycho-Analytic Method of Treatment. *SE*, XII. This paper was enlarged in 1924.

Freud, S. (1913a). The Claim of Psychoanalysis to Scientific Interest. *SE*, XII.

Freud, S. (1913b). Totem and Taboo. *SE*, XII.

Freud, S. (1915). On Narcissism. *SE*, XIV.

Freud, S. (1920). Beyond the Pleasure Principle. *SE*, XVIII.

Freud, S. (1922). Group Psychology and the Analysis of Ego. *SE*, XI.

Freud, S. (1926a). The Future of an Illusion. *SE*, XX.

Freud, S. (1927). The Question of Lay Analysis. *SE*, XX.

Freud, S. (1930). Civilization and Its Discontents. *SE*, XXII.

Freud, S. (1933–36). New Introductory Lectures in Psycho-analysis, XXXV: On the Question of a Weltanshauung. *SE*, XXII.

Freud, S. (1937a). Analysis Terminable and Interminable. *SE*, XXIII.

Freud, S. (1937b). Constructions in Analysis. *SE*, XXIII.

Freud, S. (1938a). Moses and Monotheism. *SE*, XXIV.

Freud, S. (1938b). An Outline of Psychoanalysis. *SE*, XXIII.

Freud, S. (1985). Project for a Scientific Psychology. *SE*, I.

Gay, P. (1998). *Freud – A Life for Our Time*. New York: W. W. Norton and Company.

Gilham, N.W. (2001). Sir Francis Galton and the Birth of Eugenics. *Annual Review of Genetics*, 35: 83–101.

Goleman, D. (1988). Health: Psychologists and Psychiatrists Clash over Hospital and Training Barriers. *The New York Times*, May 12.

Gray, P. (1993). The Assault of Freud. *Time*, November 29.

Green, A. (2003). *Quatro Questões para André Green/Quatre Quéstions pour André Green*. P.C. Sandler, Org. São Paulo: Departamento de Publicações da Sociedade Brasileira de São Paulo.

Grob, G.N. (2005). Public Policy and Mental Illness: Jimmy Carter's Presidential Commission on Mental Health. *Milbank Quarterly*, 83: 425–456.

Grunbaum, A. (1984). *The Foundations of Psychoanalysis: A Philosophical Critique*. Berkeley: The University of California Press. Seattle: Kindle Edition.

Hartmann, N. (1960). *A Filosofia do Idealismo Alemão*. Versão portuguesa, por J.G. Belo. Lisboa: Fundação Calouste Gulbekian, 1983.

Heath, T.L. (1956). *The Thirteen Books of Euclid's Elements*. Cambridge: Cambridge University Press.

Heisenberg, W. (1958). Physics and Philosophy. In: *The Great Books of the Western World*. Chicago: Encyclopedia Britannica Inc., 1994.

Hunink, M.M. (2004). Does Evidence Based Medicine Do More Good Than Harm? *British Medical Journal*, 329: 1051.

Jaques, E. (1960). Disturbances in the Capacity to Work. *International Journal of Psychoanalysis*, 41: 357.

Jaques, E. (1986). *A General Theory of Bureaucracy*. Londres: Heinemann.

Jaynes, J. (1976). *The Origin of Consciousness in the Breakdown of the Bicameral Mind*. Boston: Houghton, Mifflin Co., 1990.

Jones, E. (1957). *Sigmund Freud: Life and Work*. Volume III, *The Last Phase: 1919–1939*. London: The Hogarth Press.

Kant, I. (1781). Critique of Pure Reason. English version by M.T.Miklejohn. In *The Great Books of the Western World*. Chicago: Encyclopaedia Britannica Inc., 1994.

Kahnemann, D. (2011). *Thinking, Fast and Slow*. New York: Farrar, Strauss & Giroux.

Kandel, E. (2012). *The Age of Insight: The Quest to Understand the Unconscious in Art, Mind and Brain*. New York: Random House.

Karamanou, M., Liappas, I., Antoniou, Ch., Androutsos, G., and Lykouras, E. (2013). Julius Wagner-Jauregg (1857–1940): Introducing Fever Therapy in the Treatment of Neurosyphilis. *Psychiatriki.*, July–September, 24(3): 208–212.

Kernberg, O. (1984). Cambios En La Naturaleza De La Formación Psicoanalítica, En La Estructura y en las Normas de Formación. *API Monografias* # 4.

Klein, M. (1934). A Contribution to the Psychogenesis of Manic-Depressive States. *International Journal of Psychoanalyis*, 16: 145–174. Reprinted in *Contributions to Psycho-Analysis*. Londres: The Hogarth Press and the Institute of Psycho-Analysis, 1950.

Klein, M. (1946). Notes on Some Schizoid Mechanisms. In: M. Klein, P. Heimann, S. Isaacs, and J. Riviere (Eds.), *Developments in Psycho-Analysis*. Londres: The Hogarth Press and The Institute of Psycho-Analysis, 1952.

Klein, M. (1957). *Envy and Gratitude*. London: Tavistock Publications.

Klein, M., and Riviere, J. (1936). *Love, Hate and Reparation*. Londres: The Hogarth Press and the Institute of Psycho-Analysis, 1953.

Le Bon, G. (1895). *The Crowd*. English version. Michael Hart, editor. www.gutenberg.org/ebooks/445, 1996.

Lévy-Strauss, C. (1955). *Tristes Trópicos*. Brazilian version by W. Martins. São Paulo: Anhemby, 1957.

Mackay, C. (1841). *Extraordinary Popular Delusions and the Madness of Crowds*. Introduction by N. Stone. Hertfordshire: Wordsworth Editions, 1995. We owe our knowledge of this work as well as the possession of this book to Mrs. Francesca Bion.

McNall Burns, E. (1949). *História da Civilização Ocidental*. Brazilian version, by L.G. Machado, L.S. Machado e L. Vallandro. Porto Alegre: Editora Globo, 1981.

Malinowsky, B. (1929). *La vida sexual de los salvages*. Spanish version by R. Baeta. Madri: Ediciones Morata, 1975.

Marcondes, D. (1926). *O symbolismo esthetico na literatura. Ensaio de uma orientação para a crítica literária, baseada nos conhecimentos fornecidos pela psycho-analyse*. São Paulo: Secção de Obras D' O Estado de São Paulo.

Martins, C., and Sandler, P.C. (1980). Avaliação critica da psiquiatria comunitária. *Arquivos de Neuro-Psiquiatria*, 38: 65–75.

Marx, K. (1844). Manuscritos Economico Filosóficos. Versão brasileira, por J.C. Bruni. In: *Os Pensadores*. São Paulo: Abril Cultural, 1974.

Marx, K. (1852). *The Eighteenth Brumaire of Louis Bonaparte*. New York: Mondial, 2005.

Merton, R.W. (1948). The Self-Fulfilling Prophecy. *The Antioch Review*, 8(2): 193–210.

Natterson, J.M. (1966). Theodor Reik. In: F. Alexander, S. Eisenstein and M. Grotjahn (Eds.), *A História Da Psicanálise Através Dos Seus Pioneiros*. Rio De Janeiro: Imago, 1981.

Nietzsche, F. (1878–1880). *Humano, demasiadamente humano*. Brazilian version, by R.R. Torres Filho. In: *Os Pensadores*. São Paulo: Abril Cultural, 1978.

Nietsche, F. (1885–1885). *Para Além do Bem e do Mal*. Brazilian version by R.R. Torres Filho. In: *Os Pensadores*. São Paulo: Abril Cultural, 1978.

Onians, R.B. (1951). *The Origins of European Thought About the Body, the Mind, the Soul, the World, Time and Fate*. Cambridge: Cambridge University Press, 2000.

Pacheco e Silva, A.C. (1955). *Psiquiatria Clinica e Forense*, segunda edição. São Paulo: Livraria Vademecum.

Pascal, B. (1657). Pensées. English version by W.F. Trotter. In: *The Great Books of the Western World*. Chicago: Encyclopedia Britannica Inc., 1994.

Perron, R. (2002). Análise profana. In: A. Mijolla (Ed.), *Dicionário Internacional da psicanálise*. Rio de Janeiro: Imago, 2005.

Pichón-Rivière, E. (1980). *Teoria do Vínculo*. Brazilian version, by Eliane Toscano Zamikhouwsky. São Paulo: Martins Forntes Ed.

Pisani, R. (2000). *Elementi di Gruppoanalisi*. Rome: Edizioni Universitarie Romane.

Planck, M. (1949). Scientific Autobiography. In: *The Great Books of the Western World*. Chicago: Encyclopedia Britannica Inc., 1994.

Plato. (c. 380 BC a). Republic, VII, 514–517. In: *The Great Books of Western Hemisphere*. Chicago: The Encyclopedia Britannica Inc, 1994.

Pope, A. (1709). *An Essay on Criticism*. Originally published in 1744. www.poemhunter.com/poem/an-essay-on-criticism.

Pope, A. (1711). *An Essay on Criticism*. Originally published in 1744. www.poemhunter.com/poem/an-essay-on-criticism

Popper, K.R. (1963). *A Lógica da Pesquisa Científica*. Brazilian Version, by por A. Aiex. Cultrix, 1974.

Porter, R. (1999). *The Greatest Benefit to Mankind: A Medical History of Humanity*. Nova Iorque: W. W. Norton and Company.

Pray, L.A. (2008). Discovery of DNA Structure and Function: Watson and Crick. *Nature Education*, 1: 100.

Rabi, II, Millman, S., Kusch, P., and Zacharias, J.P. (1939). *Physical Review*, 55: 526.

Reik, T. (1940). *From Thirty Years with Freud*. New York: Farrer & Rinehart.

Reik, T. (1948). *Listening with the Third Ear*. New York: Grove Press.

Rickmann, J. (1950). The Factor of Number in Individual and Group Dynamics. In: W.C.M. Scott and S. Payne (Eds.), *Selected Contributions to Psycho-Analysis*. London: The Hogarth Press and The Institute of Psycho-Analysis.

Roudinesco, E., and Plon, M. (1997). *Dicionário De Psicanálise*. Rio De Janeiro: Zahar, 1998.

Russell, B. (1903). *Principles of Mathematics*. Cambridge. https://ia800303.us.archive.org/20/items/principlesofmath005807mbp/principlesofmath005807mbp.pdf

Sackett, D.L., Rosenberg, W.M., Gray, J.A., Haynes, R.B., and Richardson, W.S. (1996). Evidence Based Medicine: What It Is and What It Isn't. *British Medical Journal*, 312: 712.

Sandler, P.C. (1997). *A Apreensão da Realidade Psiquica*. Volume I. Rio de Janeiro: Imago editora.

Sandler, P.C. (1982). Modelos Teóricos em Psiquiatria Social. *Revista da Associação Brasileira de Psiquiatria*, 4: 8–14.

Sandler, P.C. (2000). *As Origens da Psicanálise na obra de Kant*. Rio de Janeiro: Imago Ed.

Sandler, P.C. (2001a). O Quarto Pressuposto. *Rev. Bras. Psican.*, 35: 907–934.

Sandler, P.C. (2001b). Le Projet Scientifique de Freud en Danger un Siécle Plus Tard? *Revue Française de psychanalyse*, Número hors-série, 181–202.

Sandler, P.C. (2005). *The Language of Bion*. London: Karnac.

Sandler, P.C. (2006). The origins of Bion's work. *International Journal of Psycho-Analysis*, 87: 180–201.

Sandler, P.C. (2012). Publicões, psicanálise e o movimento psicanalítico. In P. Montagna (Ed.), *Dimensões, Psican.lise. Brasil*. São Paulo: SBPSP.

Sandler, P.C. (2013a). The Sixth Basic Assumption. In: *A Clinical Application of Bion's Concepts*. Volume III: Verbal and Visual Approaches to Reality. London: Karnac.

Sandler, P.C. (2013b). Truth. In: *A Clinical Application of Bion's Concepts*. Volume III: Verbal and Visual Approaches to Reality. London: Karnac.

Sandler, P.C. (2015a). *An Introduction to 'A Memoir of the Future' by W.R. Bion*. Volume I: Authoritative, not Authoritarian Psychoanalysis. London: Karnac.

Sandler, P.C. (2015b). *An Introduction to 'A Memoir of the Future' by W.R. Bion*. Volume II: Facts of Matter or a Matter of Fact? London: Karnac.

Sandler, P.C. (2015c). Commentary on "Transformations in hallucinosis and the receptivity of the analyst" by Civitarese. *International Journal of Psychoanalyis*, 96: 1139–1157.

Sandler, P.C. (2016). Meritocracia Técnica e Politica: o curso de Psicoterapia Psicanalítica. In: R. Simon, K. Yamamoto, and G.K. Levinzon (Eds.), *Novos Avanços em Psicoterpaia Psicanalítica*. São Paulo: Zagadoni Editora.

Sandler, P.C. (2018). Wirkliche Psychoanalyse ist wirkliches Leben. *Jahrbuch der Psychoanalyse.*, 76: 181–220.

Sandler, P.C. and Sandler, E.H. (1978). Epilepsia e ordem de nascimento. *Arquivos de Neuro-Psiquiatria*, 33: 244–251.

Sandler, P.C and Sandler, E.H (1981). Esquizofrenia e ordem de nascimento. *Arquivos de Neuro-Psiquiatria*, 36: 46–66.

Shakespeare, W. (1601–1602). *Hamlet*. II. ii. Ed. Bernard Lott. Harlow: Longman, 1982.

Shakespeare, W. (1603–1606). *King Lear*. I. iv, 99W IV.115. Ed. Bernard Lott. Essex: Longman Group Ltd, 1974.

Shedler, J. (2015). Where Is the Evidence for "Evidence-Based" Therapy? *The Journal of Psychological Therapies and Primary Care*, 4: 47–59.

Smith, A. (1776). *Uma investigação sobre a Natureza e Causas da Riqueza das Nações*. Brazilian version by N.P.Lima. São Paulo: Hemus Editora, 1981.

Snyder, T. (2010). *Bloodlands: Europe between Hitler and Stalin*. New York: Basic Books.

Strachey, J. (1959). Editor's Note. In: Sigmund Freud (Ed.), *The Question of Lay Analysis*. *SE*, XX.

Sulloway, P. (1978). *Freud, Biologist of the Mind: Beyond the Psychoanalytic Legend*. New York: Harper Collins, 1980.

Taylor, L. (2011). About Higgs Boson. CERN, http://cms.web.cern.ch/news/about-higgs-boson

Thorner, H.A. (1973). Das Idol. *Psyche*, 34: 221.

Toynbee, A. (1934–1961). *A Study of History*. Oxford: Oxford University Press, 1972.

Trotter, W. (1919). *Instincts of the Herd in Peace and War*. Middletown: Simplicimus Book Farm, 2016.

Wallerstein, R.S. (1990). *The Doctorate in Mental Health*. Lanham, MD: University Press of America.

Warner, S.L. (1989). Freud and Money. *Journal of the American Academy of Psychoanalysis*, 17: 609–622.

Weber, M. (1905). *A Ética Protestante e o Espírito do Capitalismo*. Brazilian version by R.M.I. Szmrecsányi e T.J.M.K. Szmerecsányi. São Paulo: Livraria Pioneira Editora, 1967.

Winnicott, D.W. (1955). Metapsychological and Clinical Aspects of Regression within the Psycho-Analytical Set-Up. In: *D.W. Winnicott: Collected Papers*. London: Tavistock Publications, 1958.

Winnicott, D.W. (1968). *Home Is Where We Start From*. Eds. C. Winnicott, D. Goldberg, and S. Stephansky. New York: W. W. Norton and Company, 1986.

Wolfgang, M.E. (1961). Pioneers in Criminology: Cesare Lombroso (1835–1909). *The Journal of Criminal Law, Criminology, and Police Science*, 52: 361–391. Retrieved in www.jstor.org/stable/1141263?origin=crossref&seq=1#page_scan_tab_contents.

Yovell, M., Solms, M., and Fotopoulo, A. (2015). The Case for Neuro-psychoanalysis: Why a Dialogue with Neuroscience Is Necessary but Not Sufficient for Psychoanalysis. *International Journal of Psychoanalyis* 96: 1515–1563.

Young-Bruhel, E. (2008). *Anna Freud: A Biography*. Yale: Yale University Press.

INDEX

Aberastury, A. 170
Abraham, K. 74, 240, 248
academic training in psychoanalysis 137–138, 249–250
Agejas, E. 175
aggression 83, 112, 140–141, 145
Alexander, F. 278
alike applications of psychoanalysis 46–48; discussion and conclusion on 64–67; Freud's message about 48–51; how to read Freud's message about 52–56; inequality in 57–59;
ways of 60–64
American Balint Society 60
American Psychoanalytic Association 7, 17; exclusion of lay analysts by 8, 59; lawsuit against 52
"analysability" 17
Ancient Greek verbal formulations 273–274
annihilation anxiety 142
anticipation/expectation 106
anxiety disorder 225
Anzieu, D. 197
applied psychoanalysis 57
Aquinas, T. 273
Arendt, H. 262
Argentine Psychoanalytic Association 169–170, 173
Aristotle 145, 161, 257, 259, 273
Aslan, C. M. 184
attention, poised 75–76
Attention and Interpretation 205
Auden, W. H. 9
Australia 5, 21
Australian Psychoanalytic Society 5
authoritarianship 259–260
authority *vs.* nonconformity 16
"Autobiographical Study, An" 24
Avicenna 257

Bacon, F. 261
Badaracco, J. G. 172
Balint, M. 60
Balint Society, UK 60
Baranger, M. 170, 177
Baranger, W. 170
Barber's paradox 56

basic theoretical model in psychoanalysis 99–102
Beck, A. T. 258
Bell, D. 49, 57
Berger, H. 254
Bergmann, M. 16
Bergson, H. 233
Bergstein, A. 2, 215
Bernard, C. 257
Bernays, E. 262
Bernays, M. 20
Bernfeld, L. 196
beta-elements in thinking 223–224
Beyond the Pleasure Principle 269
Bicudo, V. L. 197–198, 211, 212, 265
biographies as source of data 241–245
Bion, W. R. 1, 3–4, 30, 41, 64, 93–94, 122, 200, 255, 262; on analysts abstaining from memory, desire, and understanding 201; on analysts as like a poet, artist, person of science, or theologian 209; on analysts two main contacts 278–279; on analyst training 208–209; on institutionalizing reaction 216; integration of work of Freud, Klein, and others by 268–269; on learning from one's own experience 204; on model of medicine 205–206; on non-truths 42, 193–194; on pain 33; on primal fantasy 100–102; on psychic factors 105, 106; on psychoanalysis parallels with medicine 215, 216–217; on psychoanalysts' analysis of both the conscious and unconscious 204–205; on psychotic state of mind 229–231; on spectrum of senses and perceptions 226–229; on theory of transformations and invariants 275; on the unconscious mental state 220–224; on vision in darkness 219; on working from inside out 202
bisexuality and bilaterality 126
Bleger, J. 170
Bollas, C. 41, 197
Bolognini, S. 31–32, 34, 187
Book of Genesis, The 251
Botella, C. 219
Botella, S. 219
Brazilian Congress of Psychoanalysis 41
Breuer, J. 130
British Psychoanalytical Society 196, 243
Britton, R. 141
Browne, T. 261
Brücke, E. 232

Camden, V. J. 49
Cannetti, E. 262
Cáramo, C. 170
Carneiro, C. A. 2, 192
Carter, J. 249–250
cathected memory-trace 104–106
causal thinking 222
Cavafy, C. P. 122
Charlton, B. G. 259
Chasseguet-Smirgel, J. 197
cognitive science 127
Cohen, P. 63
compulsion to confess 81–83
"Compulsion to Confess and the Need for Punishment, The" 81
Comte, A. 252
conjecture 79–80
consciousness *see* unconscious, the
constellation 101
Cooper, A. M. 138, 146, 150
Costa, G. P. 1, 237
counter-transference 60, 71, 95; *see also* transference
Cratylus 143
creative-persecutory power 42
'Current' Psychoanalysis at the Interface of the 'New' Sciences, The 200

Darwin, C. 275
da Vinci, L. 241–242

death instinct theory 139–142
Dennis 259
depth-psychology 20
Descartes, R. 138, 145, 150, 273
Die Presse 239
Dirac, P. 275
discovery of ignorance 203
dissidences 278
dreams 125, 126–127, 257
Dufresne, T. 50
Dutch Psychoanalytic Institute 75

education, application of psychoanalysis to 60–64
ego, the: mental apparatus and 183–185; psychic disorders and 107–112
Ego and the Id, The 183–184, 224–225
Einstein, A. 148, 155, 275
Eissler, K. R. 142
Eitington, M. 240, 242
Eitington Model 12, 176
empiricism 145, 151
endless analysis 201
Envy and Gratitude 269
Esman, A. H. 48, 57
Essay on Criticism 262
European rationalism 145
evidence-based medicine 258, 259
evil 260–263
extenders 16

Fainstein, A. 2, 168
false medicine 252–255
fantasy, primal 100–102, 111–113
Fechner, G. 272
feminism 19
Fenichel, O. 141
Ferro, A. 71
Fiorini, L. G. 177
Fliess, W. 125, 126
Fonagy, P. 10
Forel, A. 257
forgotten memories 78
Formulations on the Two Principles of Mental Functioning 268–269
Fragment of Great Confession 75
Franco da Rocha, F. 264, 265
Frazer, J. G. 258, 261
free association 223, 257
freedom of thought 15
French, R. 66
frequency of psychoanalysis 43–44
Freud, A. 8, 17, 239, 242
"Freud in the Antipodes" 21
From Thirty Years with Freud 244
Future of an Illusion, The 49–50, 131–132
"Future of an Illusion, The" 136

Galen 251, 254, 257
Galton, F. 253
Garma, A. 169, 170, 173
Garma, B. 170
Gawande, A. 233
Gay, P. 52
Gerber, I. 203, 212
gestalt 102
Goethe, J. W. von 74, 99, 242, 252
Goldberg, A. 149, 150–152, 162–163
Goldenberg, M. 172
Goldstein, M. 174
Golgi, C. 257
Golland, J. H. 61
Göring, M. 264
great man 133
Green, A. 219
Greenson, R. R. 55
"Group Psychology and the Analysis of the Ego" 116
Grunberger, B. 243
guilt 81
Guyomard, P. 182

hallucinations 99–100, 230
hallucinosis 261
Hanly, C. 2
Harari, Y. N. 203–204
Hardoy, G. F. 170
Hartmann, H. 142
Harvey, W. 257
Hawking, S. 275

Heisenberg, W. 275
heretics 16
Highs, P. 275
Hippocrates 251, 254
historical truth 132
Horovitz, M. 2, 122
hostile transference 39
Hume, D. 146
hypnosis 252

id versus superego 15
ignorance, acceptance of 203–204
Impartial Person 5–6, 10–11, 22, 98–99, 113–114, 115, 169, 202, 239–241, 264
independence of mental life 126–127
Inhibitions, Symptoms and Anxiety 125
Inquisition, the 273
instinct, human 109–111
"Instincts and Their Vicissitudes" 146
institutionalizing reaction 216, 226
Instituto Latinoamericano de Psicoanálisis (ILAP) 176
"intellectual cramps" 135
International Balint Association 60
International Psychoanalytic Association (IPA) 2, 4, 5, 41; authorised institutes of 19, 169, 170–171; equality law and lawyerization affecting 264–266; exclusion of lay analysts from training by 23; Fonagy's study published by 10; non-medical analyst members of 7–8, 196; on psychoanalysis of the analyst 178–182; psychoanalytic movement and 237–239; as responsible for training analysts 31, 174–176, 208
Interpretation of Dreams, The 125, 126, 130
interpsychic level 100
intersubjectivity 151
intrapsychic level 100
Introductory Lectures 55
intuition 147–148
irreducible subjectivity 154–156
Issacs, S. 196

Jones, E. 66, 97, 242, 247, 248–249
Joseph, B. 196
Journal of Applied Psychoanalytic Studies 61, 62
Judaism 127
Jung, C. G. 71

Kandel, E. 272
Kant, I. 100, 105, 146–149, 233, 267, 277
Karr, J. A. 258
Katrin Kemper, A. 264
Kernberg, O. 176, 178, 179, 265
Kirsner, D. 176
Klein, M. 30, 140, 142–144, 196, 220–221, 243, 268–269, 278
Koch, R. 257
Kohut, H. 138–139, 153
Kölliker, A. von 257
Kristeva, J. 197
Kusché, C. A. 62–63

Lacan, J. 129, 276
laissez faire policy 16
Langer, M. 170
Laplanche, J. 116
Laurents, A. 93
Lay Analysis-Life Inside the Experience 8
lay analysts 1–5, 117–118, 168–171; analysis of 178–182; candidates' desire to become 11–16; comparison of past and present 6–23; counter-transference in 60, 71, 95; depending on non-sensuous experience 204–207; early attitudes toward 66–67; emerging from the opening to the unconscious 211–213; essential characteristics of 30, 37–45; Freud's posture about existence of 246–249; Impartial Person 5–6, 10–11, 22, 98–99, 169, 202, 239–241, 264; influence of 40–41,

186–187; lay knowledge of the unconscious and 198–204; mental apparatus and its structure and 182–187; motives of 53–54; new kind of knowledge from 194–195; Nissen on need for 96–118; partnership between patient and 29; patient preference for 54–55; personal analysis by 24–35, 40; physicians as 16–20; prominent 196–197; psychoanalytic movement and psychoanalysis proper and 237–239, 276–281; quack 52–53; quantity and quality of presentation and 266–275; relationship to medicine 124–133; self-analysis in 71, 72–73, 94, 135–137; social questions surrounding 275–277; as tradition in psychoanalysis 195–198; training analysis in 56; training of 40, 171–172, 207–209; working tools of 258–260; *see also* psychoanalysis
lay knowledge of the unconscious 198–204
layman, definition of 19, 192–193
Le Bon, G. 261
Liberman, D. 170
libido theory 38, 115, 142
"Lies and the Thinker" 42
line of division 124
Lipps, T. 126, 127–128
listening and silence in psychoanalysis 76–78, 246
Listening with the Third Ear: The Inner Experience of a Psychoanalyst 75, 78, 246
little learning 278–281
Locke, J. 138, 145, 157, 259
Lombroso, C. 253
low frequency psychoanalysis 43–44

Maimonides 257
Malignant Deceiver 150
Malva, F. R. 212
Mannoni, M. 197
Mannoni, O. 197
Marucco, N. 187
Marxism 3, 132
masochism 83–84, 140, 143
Masochism in Modern Man 74, 82, 83–85
material reality 218–220, 267
Matter of a Lay Analysis: Dialogues With an Impartial Person (Die Frage der Laienanalyse: Unterredungen mit einem Unparteiischen), The 239
medicine: ancient 251, 254, 257, 259; authoritarianship in 259–260; evidence-based 258, 259; as manifestation of "scientific nucleus" of humans 268; mesmerism and 252; parallels between psychoanalysis and 13–14, 215, 216–217; Positivist Religion and false 252–255; relationship of lay analysis to 124–133; social empowerment of 256–258; *see also* physicians
Meltzer, D. 220
mental apparatus 182–187
mental life, uncharted 220–224
Mephistopheles 27–28
Merleau-Ponty, M. 145
Merton, R. 262
mesmerism 252
Miller, J. A. 173
Mitchell, S. 141
modifiers 16
Moise, C. 174
Money-Kyrle, R. 25, 196
moral courage 80
Moses and Monotheism 125, 127, 131–133
Murphy, N. 245
myelinization 143–144

"naïve idealism" 278
narcissism 94, 142
National Psychoanalytic Association for Psychoanalysis 75

Natterson, J. M. 240, 244, 245
negative transference 39
Neue Freie Presse 196
neuroscience 126–127, 143–144, 257, 258, 272
New Freie Presse 239
new kind of knowledge 194–195
New York Psychoanalytic Society 75
Nietzsche, F. 262
Nissen, B. 2, 96
Nissl, F. 257
non-events 219
non-truths 42, 193–194
"Normal Counter-Transference and Some of Its Deviations" 25
Notes on Some Schizoid Mechanisms 269
noumenal world of things 148

objectivity 151–152, 154
Oedipus complex 62, 82, 83–85, 136–137, 145; contrary Freudian and self-psychological theories of 138–139, 149–150; *see also* sexuality role in psychoanalysis
Ogden, T. 71
"On Dreams" 126, 131
oneness 101
On Narcissism: An Introduction 183
On Negation 269
"Open Door Review of Outcome Studies in Psychoanalysis, An" 10

Pacheco e Silva, Dr. 265
pain in psychoanalysis 33, 225–226
Panajian, A. 2, 70
Panteleeva, I. 2, 46
Parens, H. 141
Pasteur, L. 257
Patient, the Therapist and the State, The 210
patients: favoring of lay over professional analysts by 54–55; harsh treatment of 26–27; inequality of distribution of 59; influenced by lay analysts' personal situations 40–41; interview with Theodor Reik's former 85–93; lost case 25–26; partnership between lay analyst and 29; transference in 25, 39, 47–48, 55–56, 81, 137, 256; unconscious mental state in 220–224
pedagogic child analysis 59
perceptual identity 103
personal influence of analysts 40–41, 186–187
Petrucci, J. L. F. 2, 37
Pfister, O. 50, 124, 125, 131, 234
Philips, F. 197
philosophy 138, 143–145
phrenology 252
physicians: ancient 251, 254, 257, 259; declining interest in analytic training in 32–33; differences between tasks of psychoanalysts and 205–206; medical school training of 26–28, 35n1–6, 37–38, 216; trained as analysts 16–20; in university hospitals 26–27; working as analysts 28–29, 52–53, 171–172; *see also* medicine; psychiatry
Pigman, G. 65–66
Planck, M. 275
Plato 143–144, 147, 157, 261, 269, 274
pleasure principle 39, 261
Plon, M. 243–244
pluralism, psychoanalytic: death instinct theory and 139–142; defined 138; distinction between appearance and reality in 157–158; Goldberg on 149, 150–152; intersubjectivity and 151; irreducible subjectivity in 154–156; Kant's transcendental deduction of space and 147–149; objectivity and 151–152, 154; Oedipus complex and 138–139,

145, 149–150; philosophy and 138, 143–145; Schafer on 151–154, 156–157; scientific realism in 146; subjectivity of experience and 154–162
Poetics 145, 161
poised attention 75–76
political correctness 38–39
politics of psychoanalysis 123–124
Pontalis, J.-B. 116, 122, 197
Pope, A. 254, 262
Positivist Religion 252–255
Postscript to The Question of Lay Analysis 232
power and psychoanalysis 41, 42–43, 44–45
"Preface to Aichhonr's Verw Ahrloste Jugend" 25
preschool classroom, therapeutic 62–63
primal fantasy 100–102, 111–113
Proclus 269
Project 125, 129
Protagoras 147, 151, 157
psyche and physis, splitting between 274–275
psychiatry 26, 32, 126–127; clashes with psychoanalysis 211; medical school curriculum in 34–35; public perceptions of 32; social empowerment of 256–258; *see also* physicians
psychical apparatus 126, 127, 130–131
psychic disorders 107–112
psychic intensity 272
psychic reality 218–220, 267
psychoanalysis: academic training and 137–138, 249–250; alike applications of 46–67; of the analyst 178–182; applied to education 60–64; attempts to shorten 40; in Australia 21; basic theoretical model of 99–102; biographies as data source in 241–245; as both art and science 79; clashes with psychiatry 211; clinical, as "pure gold" 57–58; clinical model of 102–106; clinical vignette of 112–113; compulsion to confess and need for punishment in 81–83; conjecture in 79–80; defined in "tri-partite" manner 9; difference between speaking about and practicing 204; efficacy and relevance of 9–10; flourishing of 9; frequency of 43–44; Freud's clarity in communicating ideas of 29; and gap between theories presented in books and everyday life 27; important literature on 29–30; institutionalizing reaction in 216; integration into medical school curriculum 34–35; international spread of 196–197; intervention of law enforcement in 181–182; as lay in its essence 192–213; lay knowledge of the unconscious and 198–204; lay tradition in 195–198; listening in 76–78, 246; medical school training in 26–28, 35n1–6, 37–38; mental apparatus and its structure in 182–187; as murky career path 25; need for laypersons in 96–118; non-events in 219; Oedipus complex in 62, 82, 83–85, 136–137, 138–139; organizations for training in 31; outcome studies on 10; pain in 33, 225–226; parallels and differences between medicine and 13–14, 215, 216–217; physicians and 16–18; political correctness and 38–39; politics of 123–124; power and 41, 42–43, 44–45; practice by non-medical analysts 171–172; problem of pluralism in 138–164; psychoanalytic movement and 237–239, 276–281; quantity and quality of presentation in 266–275; role of sexuality in 114–116; scientific view of 122; self-analysis

in 71, 72–73, 94, 135–137; short clinical vignette on 106–107; social empowerment through 250–255; specificity of 122–123; spectrum of senses and perceptions in 226–229; state regulation as a thorn in the flesh of 209–211; suffering of training analysis in 40; surprise in 72; technology in 257, 258; training in 31, 34–35, 40, 137–138, 171–178; treatment effects of 113–114; truth and 42; working tools of 258–260; *see also* lay analysts
Psychoanalytic Institute Eastern Europe (PIEE) 176
psychoanalytic methods 17
psychoanalytic movement 237–239, 276–277; little learning in 278–281
psychology, social empowerment of 256–258
psychotic personality 256
psychotic state of mind 229–231
psychotic transference 38
"Puberty Ritual of the Primitives, The" 74
public hypnosis 252
punishment, need for 81–83
"pure forms of intuition" 147–148
Putnam, H. 147, 150–151

quackery 15–16, 16–17, 47, 52, 74, 247, 252; false medicine and 254–255
Question of Lay Analysis, The 2

Rabi, I. 275
Ramón y Cajal, S. 257
Rangell, L. 153
Rank, O. 196
Rascovsky, A. 170
reality: versus appearance 157–158; psychic versus material 218–220, 267
"Reflections on the History of Psychoanalysis" 16
Reik, A. 74–75
Reik, C. T. 73
Reik, E. 74–75
Reik, Marija 75
Reik, Max 73
Reik, Miriam 75
Reik, Theodor 2, 4, 22, 37, 52, 168, 170, 195–196, 239, 244; accused of quackery 74, 211, 247, 263; on analytic process as "work shop" 81; on the compulsion to confess and the need for punishment 81–83; discussion and conclusion on 93–95; early years of 73–75; on Freud as entirely visual 76–77; as a Freudian 70–71; Freud's relationship with 239–240, 244–246; on importance of self-analysis 72–73; interview with former patient of 85–93; on listening and silence 76–78; on listening with the third ear 75, 78–81; on masochism 74, 82, 83–85; on the Oedipus complex 82, 83–85; on poised attention 75–76; on self-analysis 94; significance of work of 70, 94–95; view of analytic process of 71–72
Reik, Theodora 75
religion: historical truth of 132, 133; as illusion 50; positivist 252–255
Renik, O. 154–156, 161, 162–163, 187
resistance 39, 42
Rezende, A. M. de 200, 203, 212
Riviere, E. P. 170, 172
Rivière, J. 196, 271
Roudinesco, E. 197, 210, 243–244
Rustin, M. 58, 65

Sachs, H. 196
sacral function of medicine 129
Sandler, A. 62, 155
Sandler, E. H. 2, 24
Sandler, J. 62
Sandler, P. C. 1, 219–220, 237
Santayana, G. 3

Sapiens-A Brief History of Humankind 203
Saragnano, G. 2
Sartre, J.-P. 145
Schafer, R. 151–154, 156–157, 161, 163
Schneider, M. 197
Schneier, M. 242
Schnitzler, A. 74
Schreber, D. P. 241–242
Schrödinger, E. 275
Schröter, M. 59
science, limitations of 31
scientific analysis 124
scientific empiricism 148
scientific function of medicine 129
scientific medicine 129–130
scientific realism 146
Searles, H. F. 55, 94
Secret Self, The 75
Segal, H. 140, 232
self-analysis 71, 72–73, 94, 135–137
self-assault 270
self-object differentiation 142
self-preservation 141, 142–143
self-psychology and the Oedipus complex 138–139, 149–150
self-punishment 81
sensuous reality 218–220
sexuality role in psychoanalysis 114–116; bisexuality and bilaterality and 126; *see also* Oedipus complex
Shakespeare, W. 99, 242
Simonelli, T. 66
social empowerment 250–252; of medicine 256–258; Positivist Religion and false medicine in 252–255
Solms, M. 184, 272
specificity of psychoanalysis 122–123
spectrum of senses and perceptions 226–229
Spielman, R. 2, 5, 6
Spinoza, B. 145, 261, 273
state of mind, psychotic 229–231
state regulation of psychoanalysts 209–211
statu nascendi 103
Stone, L. 17
Strachey, J. 96, 169, 241
"Studies on Hysteria" 102–103, 130
subjectivity of experience 154–162
Sulloway, P. 243
surprise in analytic work 72, 79
Szasz, T. 51

technology in psychoanalysis 257, 258
theory of seduction 125
thing presentation 104–105
Thomä, H. 62
Thompson, C. 182
thought identity 103
"Thoughts for the Times on War and Death" 131
training, psychoanalytic 31, 34–35, 40, 137–138, 171–178, 207–209
training analysis 12
transcendental deduction of space 147–148
transference 25, 39, 47–48, 55–56, 81, 137, 256; *See also* counter-transference
Trotter, W. 261
truth 193–194; historical 132; non- 42, 77; religion and 132, 133; verbal analogies for 274
Turilazzi Manfredi, S. 30
Tustin, F. 220
"two-body" psychology 249
Two Encyclopedia Articles 51
two forms of existence 276

Ulloa, F. 178
uncharted mental life 220–224
unconscious, the 81, 101; analysts emerging from the opening to 211–213; Enlightenment philosophy of 145; lay knowledge of 198–204; as psychical reality 128; uncharted mental life and

220–224; unrepressed state of 224–226
Unconscious, The 224
unrepressed unconscious, the 224–226

verbal formulations 259, 272–274
Vieira, C. de A. 212
Vienna Psychoanalytic Society 74, 81, 196
V International Psychoanalytic Congress 209
Virshow, G. 257
Voltaire 203
von Helmholtz, H. 272

Wagner-Jauregg, J. 253
Waldeyer, H. G. 257
Wallerstein, R. 7, 23, 48, 59, 249–250, 265
Walston, F. 259
Weber, M. 262
Weltanschauung 66
"What Do Teachers Want (From Psychoanalysts)?" 61
"What Works for Whom? A Critical Review of Psychotherapy Research" 10
Widlocher, D. 173
"wild analysis" 260
Wilson, W. 241–242
Winnicott, D. W. 30, 219, 280
Wittgenstein, L. 135
word-representation 271
Wundt, W. 259

Young-Bruhel, E. 242

For Product Safety Concerns and Information please contact our EU representative GPSR@taylorandfrancis.com
Taylor & Francis Verlag GmbH, Kaufingerstraße 24, 80331 München, Germany

www.ingramcontent.com/pod-product-compliance
Ingram Content Group UK Ltd.
Pitfield, Milton Keynes, MK11 3LW, UK
UKHW022218190926
475702UK00003B/421
* 9 7 8 0 3 6 7 0 7 5 0 8 8 *